STRATEGIC MANAGEMENT OF THE
HEALTH CARE SUPPLY CHAIN

STRATEGIC MANAGEMENT OF THE HEALTH CARE SUPPLY CHAIN

Eugene S. Schneller
Larry R. Smeltzer

Foreword by Lawton Robert Burns

JOSSEY-BASS
A Wiley Imprint
www.josseybass.com

Published by Jossey-Bass
A Wiley Imprint
989 Market Street, San Francisco, CA 94103-1741   www.josseybass.com

Jossey-Bass books and products are available through most bookstores. To contact Jossey-Bass directly call our Customer Care Department within the U.S. at 800-956-7739, outside the U.S. at 317-572-3986, or fax 317-572-4002.

Jossey-Bass also publishes its books in a variety of electronic formats. Some content that appears in print may not be available in electronic books.

Library of Congress Cataloging-in-Publication Data

Schneller, Eugene Stewart.
  Strategic management of the health care supply chain / by Eugene S. Schneller and Larry R. Smeltzer.
    p. ; cm.
  Includes bibliographical references and index.

  ISBN 978-1-118-19342-6

  1. Medical care—Administration. 2. Medical facilities—Business management. 3. Strategic planning. 4. Business logistics.
    [DNLM: 1. Materials Management, Hospital—organization & administration—United States.
  2. Efficiency, Organizational—United States. 3. Purchasing, Hospital—organization & administration—United States. WX 147 S359s 2006] I. Smeltzer, Larry R. II. Title.
    RA395.A3S3665 2006
    362.1'068—dc22   2005021213

FIRST EDITION
HB Printing 10 9 8 7 6 5 4 3 2 1

CONTENTS

FOREWORD

We academics who teach in graduate health administration programs often talk about adopting a "system view" or taking a "systemic approach." For example, we take a system view of quality improvement (Don Berwick's work) and health care reform (the Institute of Medicine's recent publications). We also surely spend a lot of time studying hospital systems and organizational issues within hospitals. But do we really study hospitals systemically?

If you look at the voluminous research that has been done on hospitals over the past forty years or so, you will find little research that examines hospitals externally as part of wider systems of economic activity or internally as chains of value that use raw inputs to produce a given product. Apart from looking at the demographic and regulatory communities in which hospitals operate, researchers have paid much too little attention to the economic trading partners with which hospitals interact. And apart from looking at the personnel inputs such as medical and nursing staff, researchers have paid much too little attention to the raw materials with which these personnel have to work.

This book by Eugene Schneller and Larry Smeltzer addresses this critical shortcoming in the health administration literature. One basic thesis of their book is that materials matter. Raw materials such as medical devices, pharmaceutical, and medical-surgical supplies comprise a large share of the total costs of any hospital; so do the activities involved in the sourcing, procurement, and distribution of these materials. Moreover, the percentage of national health care spending being devoted to raw materials is also growing. Within twenty years, the percentage of national expenditures devoted to drugs and devices will approach what we as a nation spend on hospital care now. And yet this is a largely unexplored frontier in health care cost containment. Why is this so?

My belief is that hospital executives have spent the past fifteen years focused on the downward portion of their value chain: their bargaining and negotiations with private sector payers and their lobbying against dwindling reimbursement from the Medicare-Medicaid system. By contrast, they have not focused on their negotiations with upstream firms that supply their raw materials, but instead have delegated these issues, as well as the management of raw materials, to their vice presidents for materials management.

If we are ever to manage health care costs, we must tackle the thorny issue of managing the supplies that medical professionals (such as physicians and nurses) order and use in treating patients. To do so, researchers and practitioners need a systemic view on how hospitals transact with the producers and purchasers of these raw materials outside their walls. The producers are the various product manufacturers; the purchasers are the group purchasing organizations. They will also need to know how hospitals can work with the real buyers of products inside their walls: the physicians and nurses (particularly those in the operating room).

This book provides the first systematic treatment of these managerial issues, covering both external and internal management of the hospital's supply chain. Appropriately, the book focuses on the managerial processes that need to be managed: sourcing, purchasing, distribution, value analysis, and standardization. The book not only provides a rich conceptual framework for managing these processes, but also supplements the authors' conceptual work with rich studies of hospitals and health systems that have implemented process improvements in these areas.

The book is essential reading for students of health administration, as well as practitioners already out in the hospital field, who wish to make a dent in the growing problem of rising supply costs. This problem is "where the puck is going to be" in the future. We need systemic approaches to solving it. Programs in health administration and hospital executives today must engage this problem more deeply than they have in the past.

I commend the authors for their achievement here. I am also grateful to have had the opportunity to know and consult with Smeltzer during the time he and Schneller prepared the original manuscript. And, finally, I am thankful that the Center for Health Management Research has continued to express its support for research like this.

December 2005   Lawton Robert Burns
                                                   Wharton School
                                                   Philadelphia, Pennsylvania

PREFACE

This book is based on three years of supply chain–focused research in hospitals and hospital systems by faculty at the W. P. Carey School of Business at Arizona State University. The goal of the research was to provide the knowledge base, rationalization, and strategies necessary for influencing hospitals and systems to position the supply chain function for improved performance and savings. It is our hope that management at both the senior and operations levels will recognize that effective supply chain management has the potential to make a difference in achieving both a positive bottom line and goals associated with clinical safety, outcomes, and client satisfaction.

The research did not aspire to identify the full range of best practices associated with supply chain management Rather, our goal was to chronicle the ways that progressive organizations differentiate themselves in the supply chain marketplace and understand the variability in progressive practices in what many consider leading hospitals and systems.

The Team

The research team, consisting of Eugene Schneller and Larry Smeltzer, brought the perspectives of both health sector management and supply chain management to address the issues pertaining to progressive health sector supply chain practices.

Schneller, a faculty member in the School of Health Management and Policy, has spent his career scrutinizing hospital structure, health system managerial competencies, and management strategy in the health sector. His work also has a strong focus on the role of physician and nonphysician managers in leadership and organizational change.

Smeltzer, who passed away prior to the completion of the manuscript for this book, was a faculty member in the Department of Supply Chain Management at the W. P. Carey School of Business. As both an educator and consultant, he worked to improve the supply chain for a wide range of business types, including hospitals. Over the course of his academic career, he carried out research and executive education that was focused principally outside the health sector. With a history of studying such diverse companies as Motorola and John Deere, he brought to this project an in-depth understanding of how the nonhealth sector had used supply chains to achieve success.

Smeltzer's fascination with the hospital supply chain was grounded in his observation that hospitals and hospital systems are organizational entities that have difficulty understanding materials as assets. He would argue that perhaps this is because materials in the health sector are fairly inflexible in their range of use and it is difficult to dispose of them in ways that may differ from their designed function. A company such as Dell, he pointed out, consistently saw inventory as an asset. The important question is how to cart products that can be quickly marketed to a demanding pool of customers. Such opportunities are infrequent in the health sector, where patient demand is driven by episodic illness and only infrequently by pressures to engage in preventive behavior. He constantly challenged supply leaders in health to articulate a vision for the field more clearly. This book is about how that vision is developing in progressive hospital and hospital systems.

The Problem

Much of the impetus for this book was grounded in observations of the enormous variability in supply chain performance in hospitals and hospital systems across the United States. This is reflected in performance metrics from a group of fifteen similar hospitals within close proximity on the East Coast in the United States. These organizations all had a somewhat similar mix of services, and none were academic health centers. Among this group, hospital supplies ranged between 12 and 25 percent of operating revenues and between 13 and 25 percent of operating expenses. The supply cost per hospital day (adjusted for case mix) ranged between $150 and $333. Within the same group, supply cost per adjusted discharge ranged between $244 and $1,640. Large percentage differences between very similar organizations in supply performance need to be understood as a precursor to improvement.

For the hospitals in this group and similar hospitals, the potential for savings by merely bringing the underperformers to the level of average performers could be the difference between loss and profitability in their previous year of operations. Thus, there is good reason to understand the strategies that the better performers employ. This book reports on the successful strategies that progressive hospitals and hospital systems throughout the United States use.

The Audience

This book was designed with several audiences in mind. Top-level hospital and system executives can read it to understand the advantages that can be achieved by moving supply chain management to a more strategic position in the managerial structure. Vice presidents, directors, and managers of the supply chain will learn how progressive supply chain organizations work and will find strategies they can use and reshape for their own organization to transform the supply chain function by improving quality, constraining cost, and improving overall organizational performance.

This book will also be a useful tool for managers in purchasing partner organizations, who can use the book to better comprehend their own customers: hospitals, hospital systems, and, perhaps of greatest importance, the new generation of hospital supply chain executives who are committed to increasing the value they receive as products travel from the manufacturer to the patient. Hospital supply chain executives who hope to manage effective and strategic supplier and purchasing partner organizations can use this book to better manage a wide range of supplier and purchasing partner relationships, especially as they pertain to distributors and group purchasing organizations.

Students of health services management will find that the materials presented in this book sensitize them to the challenges they will encounter in managing the spiraling increases in the costs of materials in hospitals and hospital systems. The book fills a distinct need for these students: although supply chain management has occupied a pivotal position for change in other sectors, leading to a proliferation of interest in this topic in graduate management education in the United States, supply chain management strategy occupies an almost nonexistent role in graduate health services management education.

There is scant mention of the hospital in major supply chain management textbooks. While faculty in departments of supply chain management frequently report that the differences between the health sector and other sectors are not so dramatic as to require separate attention, those who do research in the sector find that health care supply chain managers face a combination of challenges that are unique to the sector and that there is a fairly steep learning curve associated with the production, distribution, financing, and consumption of products.

Students in the field may already know that the most basic challenge to supply chain managers is to ensure that on a day-to-day basis, their organizations are prepared to provide patients and customers with the best products, at the best price, for the best outcome. This book will show them that they must also address and understand the desires of a clinical staff who have little focus on resource use and that, most important, the supply function must move beyond what many have seen as a narrow purchasing or procurement function. Progressive practices will assist managers in meeting the challenges posed in designing, managing, and monitoring an effective supply strategy; understanding purchasing partners; hiring competent supply managers; and ensuring accountability. Students will also recognize that failed distribution systems can lead to lost revenues as well as the inability of hospitals and systems to provide necessary services. There are risks to be avoided by developing an effective supply chain.

Graduate students who are not enrolled in health sector management programs frequently find employment in companies that have hospital and health sector clients. This book will show them how to improve sales and services to hospitals and hospital systems by gaining a thorough understanding of health care clients. They will understand that the centrality of professionals (especially physicians and nurses) requires product development and marketing strategies that meet special requirements of design acceptability, clinical efficacy, safety to professional and patient, and improved patient outcomes. Converting business opportunities into reality requires mastery of the culture, structure, and regulatory environment of the hospital and the materials and services it consumes.

ACKNOWLEDGMENTS

In 1999, as a result of a referral by Howard Zuckerman and Lawton (Rob) Burns to a funding sponsor, I was fortunate to work on a project that scrutinized the ways integrated delivery networks used group purchasing organizations in their materials-contracting efforts. The in-house publication associated with that research, *The Value of Group Purchasing*, which is reprinted in this book as Study 1, quickly became a standard reference for understanding a number of challenges associated with the health care supply chain. My colleague at Arizona State University's W. P. Carey School of Business, Department of Supply Chain Management, Larry Smeltzer, took a special interest in the publication, suggesting that many factors beyond group purchasing contributed to the unique nature of supply chain practice in the health sector. Thus, in 2000, when funding became available to carry out a more systematic study of the health care supply chain, Larry urged me to join him in what would be an incredible journey for the two of us into an area where we were both "half-novices."

Larry knew a great deal about supply chain and a little about the health sector, and I know a good deal about aspects of health care organizations and very little about the whole area of supply chain management. What began as a curiosity became an all-encompassing project for the two of us. Over a two-year period, we traveled across the nation holding focus groups, visiting hospitals and systems, and carrying out executive education. Larry was a wonderful collaborator and friend. He continually asked penetrating questions, built confidence in research subjects, and ensured that as investigators, we left organizations with some measure of value. Without him, this research would not have been conceived, and many of the chapters would not appear as they are found in this book. Larry died suddenly in January 2004. His death came one day after we had completed, drawing on many of our observations from this study, a three-day program in executive education at HCA. In those sessions, we recognized that armed with our observations, there was much that the findings of our research could contribute to the improvement of the performance of supply chain practice in hospitals and systems across the United States.

Students who participated in our sessions at HCA and elsewhere will tell you that Larry made them, for the first time, self-reflective about both their work and their place in the workforce. Larry, of course, did this wherever he went, and he is dearly missed by many people. Much of what I have written comes from what I learned from and with him. And for this I am very grateful. If there are faults in the final book, they are, of course, my own. But he put me onto this journey with a great grounding. Many people contributed to the shaping of this research and the successful implementation of the research plan. First and foremost, the corporate members of the Center for Health Management Research are credited with asking penetrating questions about the importance and performance of the health care supply chain. Those not familiar with the center are referred to its Web site (http://depts.washington.edu/chmr/research/). Douglas Conrad (University of Washington) and Thomas Rundell (University of California, Berkeley) skillfully guided the request for proposals associated with the funding of this work and provided important commentary on the research in progress. Howard Zuckerman, who was the founder of the center and a consultant to the center, provided valuable input at the early stages.

As the researchers, we benefited significantly from discussions and consultation with Lawton Burns from the Wharton School at the University of Pennsylvania. He continually challenged the investigators to turn their focus "upstream" from the perspective of the end users themselves. His early work, presented in his book, *The Health Care Value Chain* (2000), systematically characterized the various organizations (including distributors and group purchasing organizations) involved in the purchasing and supply function in the U.S. health care system. Our goal was to find out how, in the presence of the purchasing partners that Rob had so carefully documented, supply chain strategy was put into practice. It is worth noting that there has been relatively little systematic attention given by health services researchers to the health sector supply chain. Burns's *The Health Care Value Chain* continues to provide the only real access for students and practitioners who want to "quick start" their understanding of the field.[1] This book, as a companion piece to Burns's book, provides insight into the world of supply chain through the eyes of hospitals and systems themselves. On numerous occasions, Rob and I have discussed the fact that fellow health services researchers have frequently thought that we have cut off a rather unremarkable aspect of the field for inquiry. At least one critic has suggested that the supply chain focus takes us far away from issues associated with health services management. I hope that this book contributes to the small but growing research-based literature that will lead to a recognition that materials and their management matter.

In the early stages of the research, an advisory panel provided valuable input through telephone interviews and at a focus group held in Chicago. It was their insistence that supply chain issues would constitute a continuing area of strategic importance that helped us to focus on issues that transcend a transactional view of supply chain management.

They believed that the then newly released Institute of Medicine study on medical error provided a "burning platform" for bringing supply and value management issues to the forefront as a set of practices by which general hospital and system management could help to shape the improved performance of their organizations.[2] As detailed throughout this book, the repositioning of this function is in general very slow.

A number of graduate research assistants at the W. P. Carey School were involved in the research at various stages, including Vidya Ramagathan, Anuj Girdhar, James Chaney, and Amber Coan. Anuj and James provided great insight into the initial drafting of the concluding chapter. James's and Amber's continuous commitment to the project helped to ensure a manuscript that would meet the needs of both students and the field of practice. Amber methodically reviewed each chapter, asked penetrating questions, and, through the eyes of a graduate student with no experience in the field of practice, had the courage to continually ask, "What do you mean?" To their credit, they quickly lost any reserve frequently associated with the teacher-student relationship, insisting that the final product had a level of consistency and focus to help drive supply management decisions. Dave Patton, my colleague in the development of the Health Sector Supply Chain Initiatives at Arizona State University provided editorial input on the early chapters. Having served as a chief executive officer in several health care systems, he asked the kinds of questions that only someone who had a firsthand interface with the hospital supply chain function could raise.

In fall 2003, I was fortunate to visit England to carry out a series of interviews on the supply chain management strategy being employed for the National Health Service (NHS). I visited a number of leading systems in London, Oxford, and Plymouth, as well as the NHS Purchasing and Supply Agency. While there are important differences between the delivery of health services in the United States and England, my visit to Plymouth led to my meeting Ian B. Shepherd, procurement and logistics manager of Plymouth Hospitals NHS Trust, who had developed an important case study, "Clinician, Supplier and Buyer Working as One to Improve Patient Outcomes." The case, with Shepherd's permission, appears as Study 2 in this book. The case demonstrates many of the key issues that characterize the supply chain in both nations and illuminates the possibilities for supply managers to work with clinicians to improve system performance and increase clinician satisfaction.

I am grateful to the following individuals for their assistance in an advisory capacity in the early stages of the project (asterisks in the following list denote members of the Center for Health Management Research at the time of the launch of the University/Center for Health Management Research Study project):

James Bruss, Advocate Health System

John Cashmore, Rush Presbyterian St. Luke's Medical Center

David Dearman, Tenet Healthcare

Patricia Fitzpatrick, Strong Memorial Hospital, University of Rochester

James Francis, Mayo Clinic

Cathie Furman, Virginia Mason Medical Center*

Jim Gleich, JBC Healthcare

Milt Hamerly, Catholic Health Initiatives

Van Johnson, Sutter Health*

Patrice Lange, Summa Health*

Ian Leverton, Sharp Healthcare*

Neil Marks, Washington Healthcare*

Rosalind Parkinson, Ohio State University Health Center

Sister Theresa Peck, Catholic Health Partners

Ken Peterson, Aurora Health Care

Robert Petzel, UpperMidwest Healthcare Network, Department of Veterans Affairs*

Nancy Pratt, Sharp Healthcare*

Jeffrey Selberg, Exempla

Michael Valentio, Department of Veterans Affairs

Bruce L. Van Cleve, Trinity Healthcare (Michigan)*

David Zimba, West Penn/Allegheney

This project required many days of travel to collect data and writing time that frequently can detract from important aspects of family life. A day never went by when we were on the road when Larry failed to talk about Toni and the family he had gained in their marriage. Perhaps there is a symmetry as lives go on both independently and separately. Toni Smeltzer, Larry's wonderful companion and wife, told me that Larry's newly developed focus on the health care supply chain had invigorated his interest in his work and challenged him to apply what he had learned in manufacturing and other sectors to improve the performance of the health care delivery system. As those who know Larry would expect, he fully engulfed himself in the project, and in doing so he was able to share his satisfaction, excitement, and happiness with his family.

I know that Ellen, my wife and best friend, wondered how a sociologist who had so little exposure to the supply chain could become so engulfed in topics such as distribution, supply risk, and inventory. And when I started to talk to her about topics such as supply chain clockspeed, not part of the vocabulary of one who considers himself a very traditionally trained sociologist, she wondered just how far one might go to reinvent oneself and refocus a career. But throughout my immersion in the area of supply chain management and in my undertaking this research, she was patient, understanding, and always ready to listen. I am very grateful for her understanding, consistent support, and encouragement.

Finally, I am grateful to Arizona State University, W. P. Carey School of Business, and its School of Health Management and Policy for granting me a sabbatical to work on this book. Jeffrey Wilson, director of the school, bought into my argument that our commitment to training the next generation of leaders for strategic health sector supply chain management was dependent on an accessible knowledge infrastructure by which students could better understand the field. It is my hope that this book is a contribution to that aspiration and will allow students to emerge as evidence-based managers.

December 2005   Eugene S. Schneller

THE AUTHORS

Larry R. Smeltzer was professor of supply chain management at the W. P. Carey School of Business, Arizona State University. His primary research focus was supply strategies, and his work was published in such journals as *Supply Chain Management Review, European Journal of Purchasing and Supply Management, IEEE Transactions on Engineering Management,* and *Sloan Management Review.* He also published descriptions of best practices through the Center of Advanced Purchasing Studies. Smeltzer received his Ph.D. in business from Northern Illinois University in 1980 and a master's degree in organizational science from the University of Nebraska in 1971.

Eugene S. Schneller is professor of health management and policy at the W. P. Carey School of Business, Arizona State University. He is director of the Health Sector Supply Chain Initiatives and codirector of the Health Sector Supply Chain Research Consortium. Schneller is a frequent speaker on issues pertaining to group purchasing organizations and strategic management of the health care value chain. His publications appear in a variety of health management journals, including *Hospital and Health Services Administration, Health Care Management Review, American Journal of Public Health, Social Science and Medicine,* and *Frontiers of Health Services Management.* He received his Ph.D. from New York University in 1973 and an honorary P.A. degree from Duke University Medical Center in 2004.

STRATEGIC MANAGEMENT OF THE HEALTH CARE SUPPLY CHAIN

A BURNING PLATFORM FOR CHANGE

As health care costs escalate and hospital operating margins decrease, there is a growing consensus that the next generation of leaders in the health care system will require a new set of competencies to position their organizations for success in a competitive marketplace. With supplies and purchased services accounting for the second largest cost component for a hospital (Figure I.1), it is increasingly recognized that supply chain management is one of the principal areas for improvement in organizational performance.

A focus on the supply chain comes at a time when hospitals and systems are questioning the value obtained from hospital system redesign and merger strategies that have not always achieved anticipated net income. These organizations are also reevaluating cost reduction efforts associated with improved management of care.[1] Looking toward supply chain management in an environment where the cost of materials is escalating and other industries are heralding savings associated with such strategy is emerging as an attractive new focus.

Supply-related savings can come from many different supply chain management strategies. Industry analysts believe a hospital can reduce its overall expenses by at least 2 percent through the deployment of better inventory and distribution processes.[2] This represents a percentage of total expenses, not just the amount providers spend on supplies and pharmaceuticals.[3] Nationally increasing process efficiencies could result in a savings of approximately

FIGURE I.1.   HOSPITAL OPERATING EXPENSES.

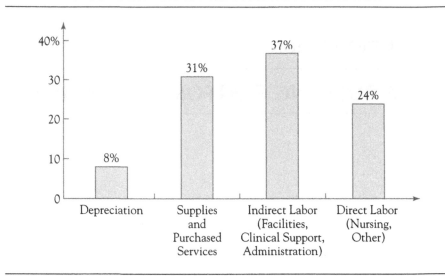

$16.5 billion.[4] This figure targets process costs alone and does not even consider the ever increasing purchase prices of goods and services.[5] In addition, there needs to be dramatic improvement in the ways materials are purchased and used from the point of manufacturer to the point of decision at the bedside. The potential benefits are significant and constitute the grounds for change in managerial focus.

Further supply chain management benefits beyond cost are associated with improved safety and outcomes as a result of purchasing standardization. Cost, safety, and improved outcomes, considered together, constitute a "burning platform" for elevating the contribution of efficient and effective supply chain management. As reimbursement formulas reward pay for performance, where rates are calculated on the basis of improved outcomes and adherence to standardization in patient care, additional savings from effective supply chain management may be on the horizon. The field of supply chain management and strategy, however, continues to be characterized by an absence of useful knowledge and documented best practice.[6]

To achieve performance improvement, it is important to build an inventory of successful and cutting-edge health sector supply chain management to enable decisions on the basis of evidence. This book identifies and scrutinizes progressive practices and strategies associated with managing a hospital or hospital system supply chain.

The Sponsors and Their Questions

The research for this book was supported by the National Science Foundation–sponsored Center for Health Management Research (CHMR). CHMR, an Industry University Cooperative Research Center, is supported and governed by health systems from across the United States, including John Muir/Mt. Diablo Health System (California), Sharp HealthCare (California), Spectrum Health (Michigan), Sutter Health (California), Swedish Medical Center (Seattle), Virginia Mason Medical Center (Seattle), and the VA Midwest Health Care Network-VISN23 (North Dakota).

These organizations recognize the growing costs of supply chain management and the lack of systematic information available for guiding themselves and informing the field in the area of supply chain management. At least one of the sponsor executives indicated that this is an arena where they have "assumed competency" and transferred both oversight and responsibility to others within their organizations. As a senior leader explained, "There has been no real interest in managing the supply chain." Others, while not taking such a strong backseat perspective, did not see supply chain management as an area for strategic emphasis. In other instances, the CHMR members pointed out that with their strong purchasing partners, especially group purchasing organizations, they did not have to worry about managing the supply chain. At the same time, they wondered if their purchasing partners were the best possible purchasing partners. Several even questioned the need of having such partners. Only one of the CHMR members, Swedish Medical Center (Seattle), had no group purchasing affiliation and believed that it had achieved substantial savings by managing its own sourcing and contracting with suppliers.

The CHMR members also expressed concern that their ability to manage costs was becoming increasingly difficult. They were being told by consultants that there were hospitals and hospital systems that take the supply function very seriously and were reporting substantial savings as a result of better management of the supply chain. These executives also expressed a sense of frustration and futility associated with their efforts to work with physicians and other customers to achieve their goals in savings and improving supply chain performance. At least one of the CHMR member systems pointed out that they were not able to influence clinician behavior around issues pertaining to supplies and had basically withdrawn any attempts to shape performance by managing materials. It is with these challenges in mind that the CHMR commissioned us to scrutinize the best performers and report on their findings.

The Arizona State University research proposal to the CHMR addressed four principal research questions:

1. What are the characteristics of the more progressive hospital and hospital systems in managing the supply chains?

   How do the business strategy, organizational structure, personnel capabilities, and environmental and competitive forces of the organizations with more progressive supply chain practices differ from the organizations with less progressive supply chain practices?

   What is the role of leadership by clinicians and nonclinicians in organizations characterized by progressive supply chains?

2. What conditions predisposed these organizations to have leading-edge supply chain structures and practices?
3. What are the enablers and barriers to progressive supply chain management practices in hospitals and hospital systems?

   What guidelines will lead to progressive supply chain practices?

4. What progressive supply chain practices can hospital and system managers best use from leading practices in manufacturing and retail supply chains?

These questions were addressed from focus groups with panels of experts, site visits to systems that were identified as progressive, and scrutiny of systems that appeared to pay little attention to managing the supply chain. Early in the research process, the team held a focus group in Chicago with leaders from a number of major systems, including Aurora Health Care, Catholic Health Initiatives, Mayo Clinic, Ohio State University Medical Center, Tenet Healthcare Corporation, and the Veterans Administration.

To provide guidance to the field of practice, the research team's work scrutinizes the value brought to end users (hospitals and systems) by progressive supply management strategy. Discussions with executives in leading group purchasing organizations (GPO) and with distributor organizations provided insight (from the perspective of purchasing partners) to the investigators on the factors associated with effective supply chain management. However, the goal for the research was not to understand progressive organizations from the GPO or distributor perspective but from the perspective of the hospital or the system. Throughout the book, the research team's observations are referenced as findings from the Arizona State University/Center for Health Management Research Study (ASU/CHMR) study. The chapter appendix provides an account of the research methodology employed.

The Unique Health Sector Supply Chain

The analysis in this book draws on the fields of strategic management and supply chain management in order to better understand managing the hospital and hospital system supply chain. Supply chain management tasks, such as sourcing of materials, forecasting demand, selecting and employing distribution models, and assessing risks associated with supply inefficiency, all apply to the health sector. Knowledge of these tasks serves as a building block for supply management excellence.

For instance, although the supply function in hospitals has traditionally been seen as having a limited scope under the term "materials management," progressive hospitals have adopted the idea of a supply chain, which presents a more robust or expansive view of the world of materials. Chopra and Meindl define supply chain management as the sum total of "parties involved, directly or indirectly, in fulfilling a customer request."[7] This is a very broad customer-centric definition that considers new product identification and development, marketing, operations, distribution, finance, and customer service as part of supply chain management.

Applied to hospitals and health systems, such a definition can be interpreted to include the flow of products and associated services to meet the needs of the hospital and those who serve patients.[8] In fact, the health care supply chain is in many ways more complex and working on many different dimensions from the supply chain in other sectors. Thus, the perspective in this book is quite different from the perspective one would take to scrutinize a manufacturing firm such as General Motors, a high-technology firm such as Dell, or a continuous processing industry such as Exxon. When considering the unique challenges that a hospital or hospital system supply leader faces, it is necessary to consider four macro processes associated with the hospital and hospital system supply chain. The first three processes are related to what Chopra and Meindl have identified as customer relationship management (CRM), internal supply management (ISM), and supplier relationship management (SRM).[9] Given the unique nature of the health care sector, the hospital supply chain manager frequently sees himself or herself as having relationships with a wide variety of organizations that bridge the gap between suppliers and the hospital. These relationships extend to distributors, information intermediaries, and GPOs. These purchasing partners must also be carefully managed in a fourth macro process, identified and detailed in this book as purchasing partner management (PPM). Purchasing partners are frequently distinct from suppliers and characterized by strong relationships both upstream (with manufacturers) and downstream (with the hospitals they serve).

This unique supply chain requires that the successful manager adopt a shifting perspective: keeping focus on the ISM aspects related to end user preference for products while also looking upstream from the hospital, considering how suppliers, distributors, GPOs, and other purchasing partners affect the marketplace for products. This shifting perspective between an internal and external supply chain focus challenges the manager to think in multiple dimensions while juggling a number of factors.

Mix of External and Internal Clients

Physicians, nurses, and others who are end users of products are discussed in this book as part of the supply chain CRM function. In other words, they are internal clients, as they are often employees of the organization and daily participants in the selection, supply management, and use of products. Many of these categories of workers reside only temporarily within the hospital or system. As attending physicians or registry nurses, they may practice in several different organizations and find themselves with minimal involvement in the supply chain management function. At the same time, they have expectations that the supply chain will provide them with the services necessary to accomplish their work. When supplies are not available or are unacceptable, the organization faces increased risk that it cannot perform a function or that a function will be performed improperly. Nonperformance leads to loss of revenue, and improper performance may lead to risk of even greater loss of assets.

The patient, of course, is the ultimate client or beneficiary of an effective supply chain. For many procedures, good materials contribute to great outcomes. The supply chain also ensures the availability and quality of many of the necessities for high levels of satisfaction, including food and room amenities. Materials also ensure that the purchaser of services, government, private insurance companies, managed care organizations, and self-paying patients receive value for their money. The unique combination of internal and external clients complicates the work of hospital and hospital system supply leadership.

The Centrality of the Physician

In most business sectors, decisions of what product to buy are not left to the discretion of thousands of different employees serving thousands of different clients whose needs change daily. Once product decisions are made, standardization prevails, and the supply chain is managed by sourcing professionals.

In contrast, hospitals have thousands of physicians who are serving the needs of many more thousands of patients. Clinicians, principally physicians, diagnose illness and decide, within the context of acceptable parameters, how to approach the care of their patients. Physician assessment of how much demand or stress a patient will place on a product (such as a hip implant) results in significant variability in materials choice, even for patients with similar demand characteristics. Such lack of standardization in choice also contributes to variability in the need for hospitals to stock many different kinds of basic products such as sutures. While nonclinicians are increasingly involved in setting standards for best practices, the decisions of physicians also influence patients' length of stay in the hospital and other factors that affect the consumption of hospital materials and resources.

Furthermore, patients come in many different sizes and shapes. Disease in any one individual is frequently characterized by its "emergence," or change, rather than a steady state. Health care requires that many different products be available to meet these changing needs. The anticipated need for a product for a patient on a given day may be quite different from what was believed to be needed the previous day. Again, uncertainty, in a field characterized by customized applications of technologies, prevails.

Clinicians also have long-standing relationships with suppliers and preferences for certain products. Physicians have frequently trained in organizations that have favored one supplier over another and participated in supplier-supported product development. They also become dependent on suppliers for continuing education and technical support in their use of products. Clinicians are often loyal to certain products and resistant to changing products and processes, even in the face of new developments. Yet medicine, more than other sectors, is characterized by an enormous research and development environment in both the public and private sectors. For the supply chain manager, this is a complex environment, where the preferences of the clinician must be weighed against the organization's need for improvement and change.

The Changing Clockspeeds of the Hospital

Charles H. Fine has advanced the concept of clockspeed to understand the rates of evolution and change in products, processes, and organization in different industries.[10] He refers to the extraordinary rapid clockspeed of the entertainment industry, the somewhat slower clockspeed of the semiconductor industry, and the even slower clockspeed of the aircraft industry. Taking a patient's ailment as the focal point for a health care product, Fine sees the clockspeed of the health care industry (except for emergency care) as dispersed, modular, and slow in both time and space.[11]

Although Fine's view of the health care industry is true in some cases, perhaps what is most remarkable about the hospital is the various clockspeeds associated with different departments, their products, and the relationship between products and stakeholders. In departments where there is little introduction of new technologies, such as internal medicine and psychiatry, the clockspeed may be very slow. This is very different than the fast clockspeed in cardiac surgery, where new products, processes, and expectations continually challenge both the organization and the individual players. Similarly, the supply organization for food catering for patients, employees, and visitors has a very different clockspeed from the hospital's computer information technology department, which supports decisions on an organizationwide, or enterprise, basis.

In many instances, the clockspeed within a department itself changes with the introduction of new technologies. A desktop specimen analyzer, for example, may mean that a physician can move ahead with treatment at the same visit as diagnosis. The ripple of such an innovation can be felt throughout the organization. What was once very modular and requiring several visits to many different specialists is now tight and integral, requiring products expertise and a highly coordinated organizational structure and effort. Furthermore, this new technology may lead not only to the dissolution of the relationship between the hospital and an outside laboratory that formerly provided the test but also necessitate an on-demand inventory of the product.

Outside Authority

While many daily decisions are left in the hands of physicians and other clinicians, a vast regulatory environment is associated with health care and influences product selection and use. New products and reprocessed products must go through rigorous testing, and aspects of the reuse of a product are subject to extraordinary scrutiny.[12] Thus, although there may be several approaches to solving problems, those that are acceptable generally meet the criteria developed by outside authorities such as the Food and Drug Administration.

In the environment of medicine, product specification to suppliers is not usually developed on a hospital-by-hospital basis. Rather, there is a high level of standardization that is required even before a product comes into the marketplace. In this environment, the hospital supply chain executive must monitor the marketplace and work closely with internal clients to better understand the shifting environment. This executive, charged with securing approved products, runs the risk of buying a product that is later deemed unacceptable or of procuring too much of a product as new ones emerge.

A good example of the quickly changing and complex environment that materials managers face was the introduction of new and improved stents. Stents are cagelike products used to support the coronary artery following angioplasty (see Case I.1). They have been used for a number of years in their original "bare metal" form but are undergoing a revolution in both design and function. In April 2003, the drug-eluting stent was introduced into the marketplace as an improvement over uncoated metal stents that failed to prevent restenosis, or the reblocking of the artery. Many factors, as discussed in Case I.1, "Stent Wars," resulted in a high level of competition between manufacturers and tension in the marketplace, including uncertainty over which supplier's stents would be introduced and approved for clinical applications, whether drug-eluting stents would be used exclusively for a patient or if there would be a mix of drug-eluting and traditional stents in a single surgery, the differences in performance between the emerging products, the costs associated with the stents, and the chances for improved reimbursement. The FDA is continually assessing changes associated with this new technology.

◆ ◆ ◆

Case I.1 Stent Wars

The status and availability of drug-eluting stents are the subject of many legal disputes and other factors, which some time ago we labeled "Stent Wars." Since marketing analysts predict that drug-eluting stents are so successful clinically that they will double the current world market for stents to $5 billion annually, it is easy to understand the flurry of activity among and between all of the competing device manufacturers.

Currently two drug-eluting stents, the Cordis Cypher sirolimus-eluting stent and the Boston Scientific Taxus paclitaxel-eluting stent system, have received FDA approval for sale in the United States (the Cypher stent in April 2003; the Taxus stent was just approved in March 2004) as well as the CE Mark for sale in Europe. In addition, the Cook V-Flex Plus is available in Europe. Medtronic and Guidant both have drug-eluting stent programs in the early stages of clinical trials and are looking to 2005 or 2006 for possible approval. Both the Taxus and Cypher stents have shown significant reduction of restenosis in clinical trials and in the field as well. In October 2003, the FDA issued a warning regarding cases of sub-acute thrombosis (blood clotting) with the Cypher stent that resulted in some deaths. Upon further study, it seemed that the incidence of thrombosis is no greater than that with bare metal stents. . . . The TAXUS stent uses a different drug coating—while more data is being collected, it seems from the preliminary results that the TAXUS stent may have properties that are beneficial to treating diabetic patients as well. . . . Developments in the "Stent Wars" can be fast and furious in the race to market.

Source: http://www.ptca.org/articles/des1.html.

◆ ◆ ◆

Although the drug-eluting stent has been on the market for only a short period of time, observations of patient-benefit have quickly led to changes in material use. Recognition that certain categories of patients benefit more from open heart surgery than from angioplasty places new demands on hospital facilities and demands a different mix of products. With the introduction of a second drug-eluting stent supplier, supply strategy has shifted to benefits that are accrued by standardization through one supplier and the different clinical appropriateness of each product. This is a difficult environment in which to manage. However, what was initially a clinical preference item was quickly becoming commoditized. As the exclusive use of multiple drug-eluting stents during a single surgery has increased, the substantial differences in costs between the more conventional stents and the drug-eluting stents have increased. The costs associated with such use are of great importance to hospitals, especially when they are paid on a capitated or diagnosis-related-group basis. Government, employers, and the commercial insurance industry are of course concerned with the substantial differences in costs associated with this new stent technology, especially as stents become used for a wider range of procedures. In March 2004 the Office of the Inspector General, in the face of increased use of drug-eluting stents, challenged "inpatient and outpatient claims involving arterial stent implantation to determine whether Medicare payments for these services were appropriate."[13] As the use of these devices continues to change, supply chain managers will want to understand not only the issues determining current use, but how use is likely to change in the future and how such changes will affect sourcing, contracting, and the demand for this challenging technology.

Many Procedures and Many Points of Use

Hospitals bring together advanced technology to solve the problems of people in need of care. There are over five thousand hospital units in the United States, some linked by affiliation, working to ensure that tens of thousands of products are available to meet the demand of clinicians and their patients.

The number of different disease categories, which in other industries might be thought of as discrete products, attests to the difficulty that analysts encounter as they try to understand the hospital. The International Classification of Diseases (Ninth Revision) lists twelve thousand diagnosis codes and thirty-five hundred procedure codes. While these diagnoses are frequently bundled or aggregated into a smaller number of aggregate procedures for purposes of payment, such as diagnosis-related groups, these reimbursement groups "mask clinically important details about procedures that were performed."[14] As suggested in the earlier discussion of stents, the differences in resource use for any one admission may vary substantially. Hospitalization for the various types of septicemia range from $24,878 (mean) for staphylococcal septicemia compared with mean charges of $16,149 for other types of septicemia.[15] Within and between categories, resource use differences are also substantial. One is challenged to think of another industry that has such a large number of units, operating at such an intense level, on a daily basis.

Despite the complexity of the hospital, there are few reports of stock-outs that lead to postponement of procedures or the turning away of patients. Perhaps one of the most notable examples of a stock-out that affected an entire population was the lack of flu vaccine in the fall of 2004. But one is hard pressed to think of other examples where the health sector could not meet demand because of supply-related issues. Finally, the outpatient environment is increasingly managed by hospitals and hospital systems themselves. Giving attention to both the inpatient and outpatient environment is a further complexity for the supply chain.

Separation of R&D, Purchasing, and Practice

Relatively few hospitals across the nation other than major medical centers can boast mature research and development programs. Often new products or approaches to treating disease arise as a result of clinicians' bringing new technologies and techniques into the hospital after exposure to them at conferences or through direct marketing by vendors. For these kinds of items, supply chain managers find themselves attending to the management of new technologies after client preferences have been developed and commitments between suppliers and clinicians have been cemented. Given this separation of research and development, purchasing, and practice, the materials management role has been seen as a set of tasks to provide clients with efficient access to materials, not a strategic role with the materials manager affecting a supply chain or enhancing value through assistance in product selection, sourcing, and delivery to the point of service.

With the separation of research and development from purchasing and practice, internal supply management has been the focus of the hospital and health system materials managers. Ensuring that customer-demanded goods are available to support the day-to-day hospital and system operations is a focal point for serving a wide variety of clinical and nonclinical customers. This activity alone demands sophisticated collaboration or coordination across the hospital or system. As discussed in great detail throughout the book, those involved in materials management are frequently marginalized from suppliers through unique health sector purchasing arrangements that include group purchasing. In addition, the very high status of the clinician end user and the strong relationships between clinicians and suppliers marginalize the materials manager even more. In only the most progressive systems has materials management in the health sector been involved in the full range of strategic supply management.

Toward Effective Health Care Supply Chain Management

Repositioning the supply function to improve hospital and hospital system performance is not an easy task. Even in many of the most progressive systems, the supply function remains a level below the executive suite. While it is fairly easy to point to the differences that can be made by reducing supply costs, developing a vision for a more central and strategic role of the supply function is more difficult. Hospitals and hospital systems characterized by progressive supply chain practices show not only reduced costs but stronger internal relationships and trust with clinical staff. They are also characterized by improved efficiencies and savings associated with the processes of care.

In the following chapters readers are challenged to think about:

- Developing a set of tools to analyze, or "frame," supply chain[16] for hospitals and systems
- Strategies for bringing customer value (through supply) to hospitals and systems
- Managing supply chain stakeholders
- Assessing the strategic fit between supply chain management practices and hospitals and hospital system characteristics

Skillfully employed, the marriage between building block skills and competencies and an understanding of the strategic factors associated with excellence in hospital and hospital system performance will benefit those who seek to improve their organizations.

Each of the chapters identifies supply chain management and supply strategy practices that characterize progressive organizations. Management and supply strategy practices were labeled "progressive" on the basis of improving some aspect of supply practice and contributing to the ongoing maturation of the health sector supply chain. This second criterion, maturation of the supply chain, requires special mention. An obvious requirement for hospital and hospital system performance is the presence of materials necessary to carry out clinical and non-clinical processes. Stock-outs (which are infrequent) prevent hospitals from carrying out procedures and lead to reduced revenues. They also lead to reduced customer satisfaction and the loss of both clinicians and patients. Thus, it should come as no surprise that hospitals and systems that are characterized at the most basic level define their own supply function as principally transactional; that is, materials are sourced, procured, distributed, and consumed as a result of end user demand and without a methodical, disciplined, and prudent approach to the comparative value of the product against competing products. It is from this baseline of success in carrying out everyday functions that progressive practices are identified and analyzed throughout this book. In order to help readers assess the value of each of the identified practices, we use the idea of developmental stages or levels of supply chain maturation to detail how these practices work to distinguish progressive hospitals and systems. The progressive practices that were identified relate to each of the macro processes: internal, customer, and supplier relationship management. In many instances, the customer of the health care supply chain is internal to the organization itself (for example, a physician or nurse). The hospital and system supply chain executives will need a strong set of skills to manage the diverse stakeholders across the supply chain.

It would be a mistake for supply chain managers to take a rigid approach in judging the appropriateness of their hospital's developmental stage. Not all systems will progress from one stage to the next in a systematic fashion. A dramatic change in leadership, for example, may move a system rapidly from one stage to another. Some do not progress at all or are characterized by regression to a previous stage. Similarly, a judgment of hospital and hospital system maturity level requires careful scrutiny. Some hospitals and systems find that an achieved stage of supply chain function truly fits its culture and positioning in the marketplace. Thus, it should not be concluded that an organization's level of achieved supply management maturity is a signal of a need for change or a marker of success or failure. Rather, knowing the maturity level of one's supply chain function allows an assessment of the advisability of engaging in self-development and potential opportunities.

It is important for readers to understand that the goals of management must not always be to try to move every organization in which they work to fit a specific mold. Different organizations achieve success through different strategies. Different organizational structures and positioning allow different levels of maturity. Only the most sophisticated and well-positioned organizations will achieve integration of the supply chain processes and their overall management strategies to qualify for an advanced stage of maturity.

Finally, the ideas in the following chapters were reviewed by the advisory board of the CHMR and reported in a morning-long educational session at the meetings of NCI (a large supply chain health networking and education organization) and at retreats and meetings sponsored by the two largest GPOs (Novation and Premier).

Organization of the Book

This book is organized to reflect the three hospital and health system supply chain macro processes that Chopra and Meindl identified as customer relationship management, internal supply management, and supplier relationship

FIGURE I.2.   ORGANIZATION OF THE BOOK.

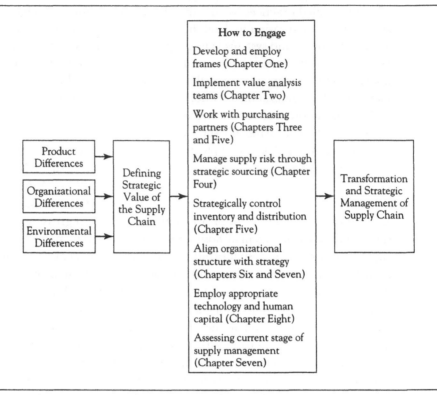

management, as well as key issues pertaining to purchasing partner management.[17] (See Figure I.2.)

Chapter One considers the current state of supply chain management in hospitals and systems. It differentiates between "merely" managing the supply chain
and developing "frames" for engaging supply strategy management and strategic
fit between the hospital or system and its supply chain management behaviors. An
important feature of Chapter One is the identification of the barriers associated
with repositioning supply chain management as a strategic function. Readers will
come away with the theoretical grounding for understanding strategic supply management in an environment as it relates to the broad field.

Chapter Two considers the types of costs that hospitals and hospital systems
experience in the purchasing process and the strategy, price, demand, and implementation risks associated with hospital purchasing. The chapter also provides
a detailed assessment of the strategic sourcing process that successful supply chain
managers follow, including their activities with suppliers and negotiations. Readers

of the chapter will be better prepared to understand and manage hospital and the hospital system risk, needs, and product complexity.

Chapter Three considers the issues related to product standardization for managing costs and improving clinical performance. Product standardization, a key to supply chain success in other industries, is difficult in hospitals where clinicians have strong preferences for the materials used in the course of their practice. Internal customer supply management is also challenging due to physician relationships with suppliers. The chapter details the hospital value analysis process and value analysis teams. It also provides a mechanism for assessing the mix of the medical staff in relationship to their participation in hospital supply chain management effectiveness. Read in concert with Studies 2 and 3, the chapter prepares readers to assess and manage the purchasing process with professionals.

Read in concert with Study 1, Chapter Four details the ways that hospitals and hospital systems engage GPOs as an outsourcing strategy to secure materials. With 96 to 98 percent of all hospitals in the United States using a GPO to carry out their contracting of goods and much of their strategic sourcing, this chapter is key to understanding the strategic alternatives that hospitals and systems have as they engage the marketplace. The principal focus of the chapter is on purchasing partner selection and management. A specific focus is on how the GPOs support hospital and system purchasing rather than on the structure and functioning of GPOs themselves to the extent that GPOs have many of the features of quasi organizations that act as agents to suppliers for the hospitals and systems.[18] The chapter also considers the extent to which GPOs represent a comprehensive strategy for securing goods in a changing health care marketplace and the ways they are changing in order to meet the needs of their hospital and hospital system customers. This necessitates that the focus of the chapter also be on the strategic fit between GPOs and their hospital members and clients. The chapter also considers, in the face of increased criticisms that group purchasing may restrict competition in the marketplace, a variety of ethical concerns relating to GPO and hospital system purchasing. GPOs must be seen as suppliers of services, including sourcing, contracting, and procurement financing management.[19]

Chapter Five provides a discussion of supply strategy decisions. While standardization and more effective purchasing are considered opportunities for savings, it is estimated that significant savings can be achieved by strategically managing the flow of goods from the supplier shipping dock to the point of use. The choices associated with insourcing and outsourcing the inventory and distribution functions are in many ways similar to the choices identified in the discussion of GPOs in Chapter Four.

As in other chapters, we draw on observations from the progressive practices in the ASU/CHMR study hospitals to assess the strategic questions that should be used to consider strategic fit between inventory, distribution, and performance. Readers will be able to assess the effectiveness of inventory and distribution strategy and understand how the design of this function can lead a hospital or system to manage its supply chain better as a series of assets.

Read in concert with Study 3, Chapter Six examines the options and opportunities for structuring the supply chain to effectively meet the needs of hospitals and hospital systems. It considers the important debate concerning the centralized or decentralized supply function within the context of the book's overall concern for achieving strategic fit and effectiveness of supply chain management. This question is important, but it must be considered within a multifaceted strategic framework of an organization with very different customer demands and clockspeeds. Chapter Six presents a series of strategic questions that will help the reader determine if a unitary or a hybrid—a combination of centralized and decentralized characteristics—approach is more appropriate for a hospital or system's supply function.

Chapter Seven details and refines the criteria that enable executives to determine their stage of transformation across several characteristics, including physician relationships, supply chain relationships, strategic cost management, and technological development. The chapter contains an extensive discussion of where a hospital or system falls on a continuum of organizational maturation and how well its positioning at that level is consistent with the organization's opportunities. The idea of stages of development is also closely aligned with the fulfillment of important managerial tasks, including strategic sourcing, contracting strategy, managing with the GPO, and inventory and distribution.

Chapter Eight examines a variety of technologies and human resources to accomplish the goals set out in this book. While the purpose of the ASU/CHMR research was not to scrutinize these technologies and human resource challenges, it became clear that it is impossible to move effectively along the strategic continuum without introducing new informatics and developing a workforce that can embrace the strategic frame to the supply mission. This chapter details the human resource skills that will be necessary for managing the internal and external networks associated with a health care system's supply chain. This skill set is dramatically different from the skill set that is required for managing in a supply environment where transaction and order fulfillment is the principal task.

The chapter also considers the enormous contribution that information management technology has brought to the health care supply chain environment and the ways these systems can assist in internal customer management, purchasing partner management, and internal supply management.

Finally, the chapter considers the future of supply chain management for hospitals and hospital systems and how it will be shaped by many factors. These factors include new products and technologies that will influence patient care, such as drug-eluting stents, which, as demonstrated in Case I.2, have dramatically influenced the arena of interventional cardiology and hospital practice. The factors also include new supply chain technologies and the elevation and repositioning of the supply chain function. Advancements in evidence-based medicine and pressures on clinicians to improve quality, safety, and outcomes have the potential to reposition the supply chain as a key player in the advancement of supply chain management in the hospital and hospital system.

◆ ◆ ◆

Case I.2 FDA Approves Drug-Eluting Stent for Clogged Heart Arteries

The Food and Drug Administration today [April 24, 2003] approved the first drug-eluting stent for angioplasty procedures to open clogged coronary arteries. In most cases, a stent is left permanently in the artery to keep the vessel open after angioplasty. The new stent slowly releases a drug, and has been shown in clinical studies to significantly reduce the rate of re-blockage that occurs with existing stents.

Drug-eluting stents may have a substantial impact on the occurrence of re-blockages for patients with heart disease. Each year 800,000 angioplasty procedures are performed in the United States to open clogged coronary arteries. In approximately 15%-30% of patients, the artery becomes clogged again (a condition called restenosis) within a year, and it must be treated again with a procedure such as angioplasty or bypass surgery.

"Today's approval represents a significant step forward in the treatment of heart disease," said HHS Secretary Tommy Thompson. "Patients who receive this device will need fewer repeat operations to unclog arteries, which can make a real difference in the quality of their lives."

The product is the Cypher Sirolimus-Eluting Coronary Stent (Cypher stent), made by Cordis Corporation, of Miami Lakes, Fla. It is a tiny metal mesh tube that is covered with the drug sirolimus. The company has a license from Wyeth Pharmaceuticals for the use of sirolimus.

The Cypher stent provides a mechanical scaffold to keep the vessel open while the drug is slowly released from the stent to prevent the build-up of new tissue that re-clogs the artery. In studies conducted by the firm, the stent reduced the rate of restenosis by about two-thirds.

"Drug-eluting stents combine drugs with medical devices to provide more effective care for many patients with heart disease," said FDA Commissioner Mark McClellan, M.D., Ph.D. "FDA is working to make sure its regulatory procedures encourage the quick and efficient approval of such safe and effective combination products."

FDA approved the stent based on a review of laboratory and animal tests and two clinical studies of safety and effectiveness conducted by Cordis, as well as review of manufacturing procedures for this new combination product.

In the U.S. study (called the SIRIUS study), 1058 patients received either the Cypher stent or an uncoated stainless steel stent made by Cordis. The patients in the SIRIUS study had blockages of 15mm to 30mm long in arteries that were 2.5 mm to 3.5 mm wide.

Results were similar for both types of stents in the weeks immediately following the procedure, but after nine months the patients who received the drug-eluting stent had a significantly lower rate of repeat procedures than patients who received the uncoated stent (4.2% versus 16.8%). In addition, patients treated with the drug-eluting stent had a restenosis rate of 8.9%, compared to 36.3% of patients with the uncoated stent. The combined occurrence of repeat angioplasty, bypass surgery, heart attacks and death was 8.8% for drug-eluting stent patients and 21% for the uncoated stent patients.

A smaller study of 238 patients conducted outside of the U.S. (the RAVEL study) was similar to the SIRIUS study, but it evaluated patients with shorter blockage of the coronary artery. That study also showed significant reductions in repeat procedures and restenosis.

This smaller study was the basis for the product's approval in Europe, and supported the product's approval in the United States. While the RAVEL study suggested that the Cypher stent showed promise, it was not large enough to assess the patients most likely to benefit from the device.

The U.S. study evaluated the product's safety and effectiveness in a much broader population. The additional evidence obtained from the U.S. study required by FDA should allow doctors to use the drug-eluting stent with more confidence about the benefits of the product in more patients.

The safety and effectiveness of the Cypher stent in smaller diameter arteries or for longer blockage that required more than two stents was not studied in either trial. Also, the safety and effectiveness have not been studied in patients who are having a heart attack, patients who had previous intravascular radiation treatment, or patients who had their blockage in a bypass graft.

The types of adverse events seen with the drug-eluting stent were similar to those that occurred with the uncoated stent.

Patients who are allergic to sirolimus or to stainless steel should not receive a Cypher stent. Caution is also recommended for people who have had recent cardiac surgery and for women who may be pregnant or who are nursing. Patients who receive the drug-eluting stent will likely need to take certain kinds of anti-platelet drugs for at least several months.

FDA is requiring Cordis to conduct a 2000-patient post-approval study and continue to evaluate patients from ongoing clinical trials to assess the long-term safety and effectiveness of the Cypher stent and to look for rare adverse events that may result from the use of this product.

Source: Food and Drug News, Apr. 24, 2003.
http://www.fda.gov/bbs/topics/NEWS/2003/NEW00896.html.

◆ ◆ ◆

This book contains four in-depth studies, which appear at the end of the book, that will help readers gain a stronger understanding of the advantages of strategic health supply management.

Study 1, "The Value of Group Purchasing in the Health Care Supply Chain," reports on an in-depth analysis of the group purchasing organization (GPO) utilization by ten major health care systems around the nation. The study demonstrates the high level of variability associated with GPO service use and reveals the expectations that supply chain managers have for their GPO partners. It also reveals the savings potentials associated with GPO utilization. As discussed in Chapter Three, the study also reveals the difficulties that some hospitals and systems encounter in working effectively with their supply partners and, as discussed in Chapter Two, managing risk.

Study 2, "Clinician, Supplier, and Buyer Working as One to Improve Patient Outcomes," was written by Ian Shepherd at the Peninsula Trust in Plymouth, England. The study provides an account of how a major system was able to work collaboratively with its medical staff as well as suppliers in high-cost cardiology products to achieve considerable savings and access to a wide variety of products. The case suggests that problems associated with managing strategic choice are similar across very different national health care delivery systems and that management of the supply chain truly can lead to efficiencies and opportunities. The case, read in concert with the book's extensive discussion of value analysis teams, supplier relations, and standardization, gives the reader the opportunity to view theory put into practice.

Study 3, "Metropolitan Hospital System—A Study of a Hybrid Organizational Design," provides insight into the restructuring of the supply chain function in a multihospital health care system. The case, which demonstrates the transition of the system toward a centralized supply chain function and the sustained role of supply management and leadership at the hospital level is an important supplement to the Chapter Seven discussion of organizational design.

Study 4 provides the full text of Office of Inspector General Advisory Opinion No 05–06. Case analysis by both students and practitioners will lead to a better understanding of the variety of constraints that affect the effective management of the supply chain and provide the opportunity to assess the extent to which gain sharing can be an effective incentive to reduce cost while sustaining high-quality patient care. The study is an important companion to Chapter Three, which addresses a role that value analysis teams (VATs) play in assessing products the attempt to achieve standardization to reduce costs and improve outcomes.

Appendix: Methodological Considerations for the ASU/CHMR Supply Chain Progressive Practice Study

The driving purpose of the ASU/CHMR Supply Chain Progressive Practice Study was to identify and systematically report empirically verified supply chain management strategies and tactics that would lead to greater efficiency and effectiveness in the health care supply chain. A limited amount of research had been conducted on the health care supply chain prior to this project. Therefore, it was not possible to use the extant literature to develop a tightly controlled research hypothesis for this project. To achieve the goal of the project by carrying out systematic case studies of progressive practices, the following kinds of materials were scrutinized:[20]

- System annual reports
- Overview statements of the supply chain function including:
    An organization chart of the system to show how the materials management or supply chain process relates to the other units within the system
    An organization chart of the materials management or supply chain group (to provide an understanding of the roles and responsibilities of the managers)
    A mission statement or list of objectives for the materials and supply function

- Descriptions of initiatives that the group was pursuing. This included anything from a simple set of PowerPoint slides used within the department to an elaborate business case designed for an executive review.

    During the site visits, information was gathered pertaining to:

- The overall supply chain philosophy and the history of the process that has evolved to its current status
- The internal flow of products, including warehousing and distribution technologies
- The current status and initiatives of any information technology activities that affect supply management
- The involvement of physicians in the standardization process and value analysis teams
- Technology and new product assessment
- Interrelationships with members of prominent supply chains such as the group purchasing organization (GPO) or distributors
- Expectations of the materials or supply process

The focus for the research methodology was to develop useful knowledge based on methodical scrutiny of a number of key issues and key cases.[21] The first step in this research was to develop a general idea of what is meant by the health care supply chain in order to have a focus for the study. Following Burns, the strategy was to gather information that encompasses the information, supplies, and finances involved with the acquisition and movement of goods and services from the supplier to the end user that enhance clinical outcomes while controlling costs.[22] The decision was made not to directly include the manufacturer's inbound supply chain; however, it was understood that the supplier's inbound supply chain may influence the other downstream components of the supply chain.

The second step of the project was to conduct an extensive review of the supply chain literature that directly related to the health care supply chain. Although a fair number of antecdotal articles were available, few empirical studies had been conducted within the health sector supply chain. Too few articles were available to develop a comprehensive analysis.

The third step was to review the general business and supply chain literature outside the health care sector. The purpose was to determine the extent to which studies could be generalized from other industry sectors to the health sector. The result of this review was a comprehensive paper that formed the basis for the qualitative analysis in the research reported here.[23]

Qualitative Research Methodology

Because it was not possible to establish quantitative research protocols based on previous studies, a preliminary qualitative case study approach was used. The research method to collect the information was the nondirective case field study and telephone interviews.[24] With this approach, the researcher provides a series of nondirective questions but uses extensive probes and summary questions to develop trends and themes from the interviews. An objective of the methodology is to aggregate themes across the interviews with as little researcher bias as possible.[25] The researchers had systematically studied qualitative methods and had conducted several studies using this technique. Their extensive experience and previous publications using this methodology add credibility to the assessments.

Some of the preliminary interviews were conducted individually so that each researcher could develop a general perspective for the research questions. Several subsequent cases were conducted with both researchers in order to ensure that the richness of the information was fully captured.[26] In other situations, critical incidents such as value analysis teams were directly observed and the primary participants subsequently interviewed. Finally, focus groups were conducted to obtain in-depth information on specific, direct questions.

The intensity and duration of case study activity depended on the value the researchers found in sustained data gathering at any one location. Some of the visits lasted two days, while others were a matter of only a few hours depending on the questions being addressed. An integral part of the case studies was document review. Whenever possible, we reviewed individual policies, procedures, meeting notes, memos, and any other related information. Regardless of the method, we shared and compared our observations in each case. This ensured that an objective conclusion was developed.

Research Sample

Hospitals and hospital systems that use progressive supply chain management practices constitute the primary sample for this research. Duplication of the "progressive" systems by respondents was used to develop the research sample.[27] This was achieved, first, by developing a list of systems or hospitals we knew in conjunction with other academics to use progressive practices. The resulting sample was based largely on the hospital or hospital system reputation among both informant practitioners and academics.

The second step was to solicit the viewpoint of consultants within the discipline. Their opinion allowed us to capture a broad range of progressive practice organizations. We believed that they would be able to identify the organizations that they considered the most progressive as a result of their business activities. We took care in the sample not to simply choose those that had been a firm's clients. The final step was to review practitioner magazines to identify the organizations most frequently identified as innovative and review conference speaker rosters to determine who were most frequently asked to speak.

Finally, an effort was made to include a variety of organizational structures (for example, centralized versus decentralized), affiliation (for example, religious order relationship versus secular), and missions (for example, investor owned versus nonprofit). A large freestanding hospital was included, as well as an extremely large integrated network. In addition, several academic teaching and research hospitals were included as well as community hospitals. Hospitals ranged in size from a fifty-bed rural hospital to a six-hundred-bed urban health center.

The emphasis was on hospitals and hospital systems that were considered to use progressive supply chain practices. However, not all systems visited or in which interviews were conducted and data were gathered were progressive on every aspect of their supply chain management. Thus, hospitals and systems have not been identified by name. For instance, one rather large system was included that had not initiated any strategic supply initiatives during the past several years. One freestanding hospital was included in which the director of materials had been in the same position for over ten years and was very comfortable with information systems that had not been altered for almost a decade. Another system indicated that its arrangement with its GPOs was strictly reactive, and no cost models were used. Understanding how such systems carried out the management of their supply function provides important perspective.

Choosing Respondents

Selection was guided by interviews with executives across the United States to determine progressive systems. An advisory board provided valuable information on leading organizations and strategies for thinking about how to select participating systems most effectively.

Within each system, the director of materials management was the principal respondent. In most systems, however, we spent time with other supply chain employees, department staff, and, in many instances, the individuals to whom the director of supply chain reported. This last person was most frequently the chief financial officer. Meetings with CEOs were rare, and most of the information gathered from CEOs was from interviews carried out in separate visits to systems and in the course of focus group participation. Although the overwhelming majority of hospitals or systems were willing to cooperate, several were not willing to participate in the study. The most common reason for noninvolvement appeared to be the amount of time required. However, in two situations, the primary contact was fearful that the information would be used incorrectly. Since a number of organizations asked that their input remain confidential, we have chosen not to identify, save in special cases, organizations we studied.

Four Primary Areas of Investigation

For each site we visited, we scrutinized a wide range of supply chain strategic factors:

1. Information flow

    Integration of cost, clinical, and charge systems

    What type of information systems do and do not work

    Internal communication of goals and missions

    Integration of distributors' information with internal systems

    Point-of-use information and data integration

2. Organizational dynamics

> Culture
>
> Leadership
>
> Organizational structure
>
> Physician relationships
>
> Change management

3. Metrics

> How goal achievement is measured
>
> How to determine cost reduction
>
> The relationship of supply chain goals to the larger enterprise goals
>
> The use of reward incentives

4. Supply chain relationship management

> How to manage cost, information, and improved efficiencies with manufacturers, GPOs, and distributors
>
> The relationship among units within a system or network

CHAPTER ONE

FRAMING AND REPOSITIONING MANAGEMENT OF THE HEALTH CARE SUPPLY CHAIN

With purchased goods and services accounting for the second-largest dollar expenditure in American hospitals (see Figure I.1),[1] the supply chain is a major component of the health care delivery system and accounts for a burdensome toll of expense. Supply-related savings could come from many different supply chain management strategies. Industry analysts believe a hospital can reduce its overall expenses by at least 2 percent through the deployment of better inventory and distribution processes.[2] This represents a percentage of total expenses, not just the amount providers spend on supplies and pharmaceuticals.[3] Nationally, increasing process efficiencies could result in an annual savings of approximately $16.5 billion.[4] This figure targets process costs alone and does not even consider the ever increasing purchase prices of goods and services. Given that materials reflect such a wide spread, those at the high end of the cost continuum have much to gain through effective management of the supply chain.

Those who wish to contribute to the development of an effective supply chain must possess the capability to clearly observe the supply chain in action, analyze the dynamics of supply chain processes, and craft solutions that will be acceptable to both internal and external stakeholders. This chapter provides a series of frames, or lenses, for understanding the current environment that characterizes the health sector supply chain and achieving managerial success.

The Current State of Supply Chain Management in Health

The world of health sector management is continually being challenged and undergoing change. At the end of the twentieth century, there was a growing consensus that the strategies associated with managed care were no longer bringing continued savings and cost reduction to the delivery of health services. The growing cost of care and pharmaceuticals, increased hospital acuity, and new technological developments led to unacceptable annual increases in health care costs. This was also a period when some leaders in the field, associated with the National Center for Health Leadership, were questioning the extent to which senior management in the United States was truly prepared to assume responsibility for the complexities of health care delivery.[5] Major professional associations, such as the American College of Healthcare Executives, were rethinking the competencies that would ground leadership for the future. While this questioning led to debates about where new leadership might find appropriate training and how to structure the management of education and practice, many progressive systems are leading change by demanding improved performance and strategic thinking from their managers. In these systems, there is a recognition that the management of the supply chain is one of the candidates for change.

External Influence

What is leading change of managing supply in hospitals and systems? As candidates from other sectors of the economy are recruited into the management of the materials function in hospitals, there is an increased presence of managers who have experienced environments in sectors of the economy where supply chain management occupies a central position in an organization's strategy for competitive advantage. Their exposure to supply chain is grounded in industry research and organizational experience in which materials and inventory are seen as a strategic asset. In industries outside health care, the assets have the potential to be manipulated in ways that increase organizational performance. In most instances, the factors associated with the management of the internal nonhealth sector supply chain are dramatically different than they are in hospitals where purchasing is influenced by clinicians.

Furthermore, scrutiny of the hospital balance sheet encourages consultants and other influential leaders to begin to give the health care supply chain some of the attention it has received in the manufacturing and retail industries. Information system companies such as Dell, manufacturing companies such as Toyota, and retail providers such as Wal-Mart proclaim that much of their success is attributable to strategically managing their suppliers, distribution, and inventory. While it is generally concluded that the health care supply chain is immature compared to other industries,[6] consulting firms, health information technology providers, and a new cadre of executives in the health sector are coming to believe that new strategies for improved supply chain management will bring lower costs and greater efficiencies to their organizations. In addition, supply chain managers believe that they can contribute to the demand for greater safety in hospitals as well as improved outcomes. For the first time, there is a growing belief that materials matter.

Barriers to Change

There are still many obstacles and barriers to change in the industry of supply chain. Health care is described by almost every commentator as highly fragmented and relatively inefficient. There is little evidence of a clear strategy or structure for managing the health care supply chain. Transaction costs continue to be relatively high, and variation in prices across the system is substantial. While those who finance health care services (both private insurance and government) have taken an interest in a more disciplined purchasing of services, they have expressed little interest in developing incentives to eliminate the supply-related inefficiencies that inflate health sector costs.

Although outside influences have brought a positive new focus on the supply chain, low executive expectations still exist on what can be accomplished, perhaps due to the failure of other faddish business principles once introduced into the health sector. In fact, looking outside the health sector is not new for hospital and hospital system executives. Urged to rethink their approaches to the provision of health care, they have, in the past, frequently looked toward the nonhealth sector for guidance. Some observers have even joked that hospital management can best be thought of as the implementation of the latest managerial strategy, frequently at a time when other sectors have already applied the new principle and moved on to other management strategies. Observers often reprimand health sector executives for desperately jumping "from one of these 'savior' recipes, with its attendant gurus, to another, and then yet another."[7] Many managerial fads and fashions, even when successful in other sectors, have led to disappointing results when applied in the hospital. A recent analysis of strategic management applied in health care points out that over the past decade,

> healthcare providers consistently and universally adopted "faddish" structures and programs, most of which produced unrealistic expectations that ultimately were not often fulfilled. These included the legitimization of the so-called

integrated systems' acceptance of the strategic rationale for hospitals and/or physician management companies purchasing physician practices and the ready adoption of "hot" management techniques (e.g., total quality management, reengineering, and corporate restructuring).[8]

Techniques developed in other sectors, such as Total Quality Management (TQM) were touted to be applicable to the health sector. Yet "the few studies that emerged after TQM diffused widely either suggest that it did not realize the promises made on its behalf, or focus only on hospitals that claimed successful adoption."[9] Perhaps this is because the techniques were not customized to the unique needs and diversity of health care organizations. The research reported here confirms that the supply chain is in need of careful examination and consideration of alternatives for transformation. Managerial strategies from other sectors are not likely to be quick-fix strategy for successful health sector performance improvement.

Except in the most progressive hospitals, executives' expectations of the impact of supply chain management are low. Perhaps inattention to this function accounts for the fact that the supply chain function is somewhat less vulnerable than other areas to managerial intervention and may account for low levels of hospital and system investment in performance improvement. The ASU/CHMR study's interviews with leaders in the hospital industry indicate that they frequently define the supply management function as transaction focused and substantially outsourced through group purchasing organizations (GPOs) and distributors. Few understand that a significant portion of purchasing functions, even if outsourced through membership in GPOs or distributors, are functions requiring careful management.[10] Study 1, "The Value of Group Purchasing in the Health Care Supply Chain," reports on an extensive set of interviews regarding GPO utilization and services to members by ten major hospital systems across the United States. The findings reveal that GPOs have been seen as organizations that are parallel to the hospital's own purchasing function and not as trusted purchasing partners, and that there is a great deal of variability in utilization of GPO contracts and duplication of GPO functions.[11] When the interviewers asked hospital and system supply managers about their use of group purchasing and costs associated with the purchasing process, the managers experienced difficulty in developing even a list of expenditure areas and expenditures amounts. One can interpret this as the failure to recognize the area as substantially under their control with or without a GPO relationship. The absence of information also raises the issue of their inability to routinely benchmark their own performance against other hospitals and systems.

What Is Strategic Management of the Supply Chain?

As managers assess how to best work with purchasing partners or to engage internal clients such as physicians, it is critical to clarify the role of supply chain management and to develop a tool box of frames, or lenses, to view the system. Supply chain management in the health sector has traditionally been viewed as a transactional activity, with supply chain managers understanding their work as a set of encounters, both internal and external, to source, purchase, and deliver goods to the point of service. The transactional frame, although operationally important, is insufficient by itself for taking advantage of the ways supply chain can bring value to a hospital or system. Managers must ask themselves, "What is meant by managing the supply chain?" and more important, "What does 'supply chain management strategy' mean?"

The Health Care Perspective on Supply Chain Management

In the Introduction, we defined *supply chain* as the "parties involved, directly or indirectly, in fulfilling a customer request."[12] When considering the role of hospital supply chain management and specific managerial mandates, this customer-centric perspective extends the limited view of a purchasing department as restricted to developing better and more responsive suppliers.[13] Jonathan Byrnes points out:

> Hospital managers are making significant progress toward mastering the buying portion of procurement, but this is just the tip of the iceberg. They need to master extended supply chain management, downstream to the complex networks that are being created, and upstream to the major distributors who are providing their products and manufacturers who are producing their products. The huge potential gains that will flow from supply chain rationalization can provide desperately needed resources to offset major cost pressures coming from obligations such as indigent care.[14]

How one views a supply chain depends on where one sits in the process. From the supplier's perspective, hospital and health system supply chains are predominantly downstream from their own operations. The downstream supply chain incorporates the distributor and proceeds through the provider institutions, which include clinics, hospitals, hospital systems, integrated delivery networks (IDNs), and the final customer.[15] Sometimes the final customer in the health care supply chain is the patient, such as when a patient orders a medical device over the Internet. However, with patients having a relatively minor voice regarding what products they consume during a hospital stay, the true customer is frequently the nurse, physician, or other hospital worker.[16]

When viewed from the perspective of the hospital supply chain manager, the supply chain's focus is most fundamentally on managing the processes associated with securing products. From this viewpoint, the supply chain must consistently be seen as a series of sourcing, procurement, and distribution services that satisfy a very specific set of customer needs, especially clinicians who work at the point of service. It is the "service-centric" aspect of the supply chain emphasized throughout this book that distinguishes the health sector as more complex than supply chains in other fields.[17]

Supply management, or "materials management," is frequently seen as the function in which a single manager is "responsible for planning, organizing, motivating, and controlling all of those activities principally concerned with the flow of materials into an organization." The key functions for such a manager are:

- Anticipating material requirements
- Sourcing and obtaining materials
- Introducing materials into the organization
- Monitoring the status of materials as a current asset[18]

The application of these four basic functions includes those tasks identified in Figure 1.1. This model fails, however, to reveal the enterprisewide complexities that exist in the supply chain.

Supply Management Versus Supply Strategy

Health sector supply chain refers to the information, supplies, and finances involved with the acquisition and movement of goods and services from the supplier to the end user in order to enhance clinical outcomes while controlling costs.[19] The term *supply chain management* refers to the traditional materials management function of product selection, procurement, and distribution. Operationally, the supply chain management functions combine "related functions such as purchasing, inventory, control, and stores under the authority of one individual," who is charged to "solve materials problems from a total system viewpoint rather than the viewpoint of individual functions or activities."[20] It includes the upstream aspects of purchasing that require planning, "forecasting, and scheduling material flows from suppliers" and downstream aspects that include internal "distribution channels, processes, and functions that product passes through on its way to the end customer."[21]

FIGURE 1.1. SUPPLY CHAIN MANAGEMENT FUNCTIONS AND RELATED PROCESSES.

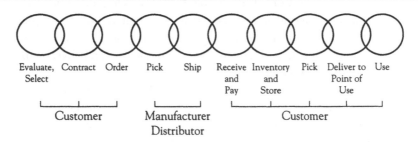

1. Identify product need and equivalencies (via value analysis teams and other sourcing schemes).
2. Assess volume and anticipated contract compliance (assessing physician use patterns, commitment to contract compliance, and the extent to which substitute products are anticipated in the market).
3. Assess risk.
4. Match product and anticipated volume to product pricing, strategic sourcing, and contracting strategy.
5. Make commitment to resources to carry out strategic sourcing and contracting strategy (for example, GPO, self-contracting, fact-based negotiation).
6. Determine transportation, distribution, and storage and warehousing strategy on the basis of product type and considerations such as consignment inventory (for example, commodity versus physician preference).
7. Consider options for receiving, picking, and distribution of goods.
8. Track utilization.
9. Determine product effectiveness and assess replenishment strategy.

Note: Nine processes associated with completing interlocking functions as identified by Schneller, E., and Smeltzer, L. Unpublished study in collaboration with HCA, 2002.

Source: Ten interlocking functions identified by Kowalski-Dickow Associates, Inc. (1994). *Managing Hospital Materials Management.* Milwaukee: American Hospital Publishing.

Supply chain management also includes internal functions associated with transforming the inputs from suppliers into units that could be applied at the point of service.[22] Senior management rarely recognizes this as a complex role requiring an individual who has extraordinary human relations, operations management and research, informatics, and financial skills. As the hospital becomes more complex, it also requires an individual who can shift perspectives. Effective managers will understand their role in facilitating transactions concomitantly and understand the more strategic aspects of supply chain management. Therefore, it is important to differentiate between tasks associated with supply chain management and more critical cognitive or thinking aspects of strategic supply chain direction. This more strategic role includes giving attention to the variety of internal and external actors who come together in a modern hospital or health care system to gain advantages through "cost reduction, technology development, quality improvement, cycle time reduction, and improved delivery capabilities to meet customer requirements."[23]

Supply management strategy is a term used to reflect the decisions and actions that supply management professionals take in the course of their work to improve organizational performance. This focus reflects the fact that "managers have been pressured into constantly seeking new methods of adding value, either through improved performance of their product or through the development of the 'service package' and service delivery system that surround it."[24] Successful implementation of supply strategy requires a new overarching and differentiating logic. For the sophisticated supply chain executive, the vision must be very broad to facilitate "the integration of supply activities within firms in dyadic relationships, in chains of firms and in inter-organisational networks."[25] Finally, supply management strategy is a perspective that allows managers to capture change and understand the importance of repositioning the supply function to meet the organization's mission.[26]

Luke, Walston, and Plummer's review of writings about management strategy suggests that strategy consists of the "key concepts and ideas that organizations use (or have used) to achieve and sustain competitive advantage over their rivals."[27] Hospitals and hospital systems, in seeking to achieve and sustain competitive advantage through supply management, develop strategies that extend to their current and potential purchasing partners. These partners include suppliers, distributors, GPOs, and information management and technology vendors.

Burns suggests that purchasing partners represent a complex set of stakeholders, each having impact on the organizations they are intending to serve.[28] Just as hospitals have gone through mergers and acquisitions and changed many of their services in the face of new technology and reimbursement schemes, hospital and hospital system trading partners have become more strategic in their thinking and more diversified in their offerings. There is a growing need for supply chain executives to be linked to both the business aspects of supply strategy (such as e-commerce and improved distribution models) and the quickly changing clinical terrain (such as the introduction of new products, for example, drug-eluting stents). Success for progressive systems appears to rest on a new set of managerial competencies that are highly strategic and applied in an environment that in the past has been characterized as "transactional" (Table 1.1).[29] While progressive systems are working vigorously to develop strategies to improve the knowledge and performance base of the supply chain

TABLE 1.1.   SUPPLY CHAIN MANAGEMENT ORIENTATION.

Supply Management Orientation, 1999	Supply Management Orientation, 2009
Product, commodity oriented	Process focused
Price focused	Total cost oriented
Operational expense	Outcome and revenue focused
A silo perspective that sees departments and units as the principal focus	Information based
Material manager	Supply strategy management
Inefficient process	Efficient processes
Many points of contact	Paperless
Decentralized	Centralized

Source: Schneller, E., and Smeltzer, L. Unpublished study in collaboration with HCA, 2002.

workforce, the absence of a clear vision for supply chain management continues to serve as a barrier.

Repositioning Strategic Supply Management Leadership

The reporting level for purchasing managers reveals a great deal about the importance of purchasing.[30] Few purchasing managers occupy a seat at the vice-presidential level. The majority of purchasing managers in centralized purchasing departments report "directly to the executive officer responsible for profitable operation—president, executive vice president or general manager."[31] In the majority of health organizations, purchasing, even if reporting to a vice-presidential level, is removed from operations. Supply management has not yet reached the point where it is part of the executive management team. From ASU/CHMR focus groups with senior system managers, it is apparent that only a minority of chief executive officers or chief operating officers attribute importance to this area when they articulate their hospital or system's values, vision, or mission.[32] Research reveals significant differences in perceptions by senior executives and supply chain managers regarding problems, achievements, and opportunities in the supply arena. This suggests a disconnect between how management views supply chain and how supply chain managers see their work (Table 1.2). Yet there is somewhat greater convergence (Table 1.3) regarding how they assess the future.

What accounts for this positioning of purchasing at a lower level? Interviews carried out for the ASU/CHMR study reveal that many CEOs and CFOs value their materials management departments as providing a series of necessary but rather routine and uncomplicated procurement transactions. Supply chain

TABLE 1.2.   VIEWS BY HOSPITAL EXECUTIVES AND SUPPLY CHAIN MANAGERS ON RECENT SUCCESS.

Rank of Recent Success Area	Executives	Supply Chain Managers
Involving clinicians in standardization	1	5
Reducing operating room costs through standardization	2	2
Investing in information technology	5	3
Reducing labor due to automation	6	3
Improving demand forecasting for the operating room	7	7
Lowering cost due to GPO contracts	3	1
Lowering the operating room cost through improved processes	4	6

Source: McKesson and Healthcare Financial Management Association. "Resource Management: The Healthcare Supply Chain 2002 Survey Results." Chicago: Healthcare Financial Management Association, 2002. http://www.hfma.org/resource/focus_areas/scsurvey.pdf.

TABLE 1.3.   VIEWS BY HOSPITAL EXECUTIVES AND SUPPLY CHAIN MANAGERS ON FUTURE OPPORTUNITIES.

Future Opportunities	Rank of Opportunity Area by Executives	Rank of Opportunity Area by Supply Chain Managers
Involving clinicians in standardization	1	1
Reducing operating room costs through standardization	2	2
Investing in information technology	3	4
Reducing labor due to automation	4	7
Improving demand forecasting for the operating room	5	3
Lowering cost due to GPO contracts	6	7
Lowering the operating room cost through improved processes	7	6

Source: McKesson and Healthcare Financial Management Association. "Resource Management: The Healthcare Supply Chain 2002 Survey Results." Chicago: Healthcare Financial Management Association, 2002. http://www.hfma.org/resource/focus_areas/scsurvey.pdf.

managers express the view that their overarching goal and expectation from purchasing partners has been to simply obtain demanded materials at the lowest price possible.[33] Advancing the role of supply chain in the managerial hierarchy requires recognition that the area can contribute to the bottom line and improve clinical performance in ways that are directly related to the organization's quest for competitive advantage.

Framing the Health Care Supply Chain

Achieving savings through supply management in hospitals and systems is dependent on the rethinking of the field to a point that deemphasizes the transactions between suppliers and hospitals and redirects management focus to a comprehensive view of asset use and deployment. To move in this direction, a unitary framework for understanding the supply chain is probably not a reasonable aspiration. Rather, there must be the development of a set of frames for understanding supply chains and recognition of the value they can provide, individually and in concert, for system improvement.

A *managerial frame* is a lens or set of lenses employed by individuals to better understand the world of how to view the supply chain and serves as a basis for managerial action.[34] A manager who tends to look at problems through a political frame will operationalize problems differently from a manager who sees the issues through a frame grounded in an organization's culture or human relations. The ability to see problems through multiple frames provides managers with the ability to become more analytical in designing solutions.

Smeltzer and Manship document the extent to which manufacturing industries see the supply chain as the function that represents their most important competitive weapon.[35] Since hospitals and hospital systems are highly heterogeneous, analytical frames from other industries should be cautiously applied in the health sector. Without a perspective or frame, one can manage only toward the problems of a given moment, in a highly reactive manner. The challenge of finding the right way to frame the health care supply system has always been difficult, but the need to do so has become overwhelming in the turbulent and complicated world of the twenty-first century. Forms of management and organization that proved effective only a few years back are now obsolete.[36]

The ASU/CHMR research reveals that supply chain managers draw on a number of rather specialized frames for assessing their environment and world of work:

• *Supply chain as transaction.* The transactional frame judges activities, actions, and actors (individuals) on the basis of their ability to facilitate the movement of goods and services from manufacturer to the point of service. This frame lends itself to quantitative analysis and benchmarking that tracks products over time and workers on the basis of completed contracts, goods received, and procedures completed. Ease of access and price, rather than contribution to the larger enterprise, is key to transaction analysis. As a frame, transaction pushes the supply chain manager to think strongly in terms of tactics and the need to complete the job at hand.

• *Supply chain as service*. The service frame, which is dependent on the transactional frame, aligns the supply function with ensuring satisfaction for internal customers (for example, clinicians) across the hospital and the system. Materials in this scenario are satisfiers for highly valued processes, which could not be undertaken without materials. They also provide satisfaction to specific workers by meeting their preferences and ensuring few inconveniences to workforce participants. In this frame, supply chain is generally reactive, although it can become part of a larger system's goals, such as improving patient satisfaction through purchasing better raw materials to increase service quality.

• *Supply chain as orchestration*. The supply chain function in the modern hospital and hospital systems represents the intersection of many customer demands and broader system requirements for knowledge. Success requires orchestration: working to bring together, through sourcing decisions, contracting, and logistics, combinations of products that enhance performance. This orchestration frame is operational when supply chain executives can channel their decisions to support organizational goals that transcend a single procurement order. A focus on safety, for example, might lead supply chain managers to prefer "sharps" products that work well together to avoid needle sticks or, when used together, promote reduced length of stay (which is associated with reduced patient injuries).

Materials executives now have at their disposal a variety of metrics, such as total supply expenses percentage of patient revenue, GPO total spend, total supply expense per adjusted patient day, and surgical supply expense per adjusted discharge. Such information allows them to take a broad view of how different products come together, in different hospital settings, to contribute to the care of patients. When data on individual hospitals and systems are available, materials executives are also able to benchmark their own organization's performance within their system and against other systems. Using such information, the orchestration lens provides a broad view of the supply function in the organization. It leads to understanding that while materials must be present (transactions must have transpired), there is much more to understanding the organization than the sum of transactions. As demonstrated in our discussion of value analysis teams and standardization, supply chain as orchestration is much more complex than the service orientation.

• *Supply chain as transformation*. The transformational frame has a strong dependency on the transactional frame; it tends to judge products on the basis of their contribution to some organizational or clinical goal (such as improved safety) and individuals on the basis of their ability to advance the goals of the organization. The transformational frame thinks of materials as one input into improving organizational performance. It assists managers in seeing resources as assets and not just pass-through or potential liabilities. In this frame, materials are synergistic. They allow procedures and processes to be completed more effectively. Materials in the transformational model are selected because they lead to better services, outcomes, and new ways of working. Materials processes are selected on the basis of their sustaining the hospital's agility and adaptability in a quickly changing environment. The transformational lens is sensitive to both the changes in the health care delivery environment and the ongoing changes in the supply chain environment. Within this idea of supply chain as transformation, there are a number of subthemes, including supply chain as value and supply chain as quality. These are the principal ingredients of transformation.

Managing with Frames

No one frame is sufficient for effective health care supply or strategy management. Progressive supply chain leadership should be judged by the extent to which its activities are continually adding value. In the broadest sense, value is multidimensional: reducing supply cost, improving clinical outcomes and safety, improving service quality, and increasing customer satisfaction. Those who employ such frames in managing the supply chain must be simultaneously coordinators, advisers, information brokers, relationship brokers, and knowledge and information managers.[37] They must manage the organization's risks, collaborate with professionals, engage in collaborative relationships with trading partners such as GPOs, and adjust the organization's supply design as new challenges arise.[38]

Orchestration requires working closely with physicians, nurses, technicians, and a wide range of nonhealth professionals to manage the products and the technological innovations that characterize modern hospital practice. As in other industries, the management of such an environment requires skills associated with motivating and leading with technical professionals, managing innovation, providing leadership in the innovation process, managing knowledge as it relates to work, and designing organizational processes for innovation.

Many organizations find it difficult to use frame analysis and change their view on a set of issues that has long been defined as a service area. The health sector supply chain has been "viewed largely in supplier-centric terms, with a focus on distribution, logistics and purchasing products into the user base."[39] The inadequacy of such a definition rests in the fact that while everyone knows that health care providers cannot work without materials, the transaction frame does not let managers transcend questions regarding price of goods. If one begins to see health sector supply chain as a "provider-centric model," it is possible to view the supply chain as a pipeline to products and services.[40]

The customer-centric view of supply chain management in hospitals and systems demands "a holistic approach to managing operations within collaborative inter-organizational networks allowing the formation and implementation of rational strategies for creating, stimulating, capturing and satisfying end customer demand through innovation of products, services, supply network structures and infrastructures in a global, dynamic environment."[41] This suggests a robust set of ideas to approach the area of supply and materials for producing excellence in health care. The idea of supply within a set of interorganizational and intraorganizational networks makes it possible to see the supply function through frames for analysis. It also becomes much easier to see the supply chain through a frame that considers the value of supplies or materials as potential assets within the organization. The task of management is to search for a mix that brings value to organizations.

In recognition of the potential for the supply chain to contribute to the organization's success and of the complexity related to managing supply strategy, a few bright trends are emerging that indicate the environment for supply chain management is changing. In the hospitals and systems that are recognized by the ASU/CHMR, the supply chain management position is elevated to a strategic role. In addition, there is an active effort to recruit more highly qualified professionals for these positions. The importance of managing this issue is receiving attention in the executive suite as more technology expenditures are being allocated to the supply function, and a few hospital executives are beginning to define the outcomes of the supply process in terms of assets rather than only expenditures. As a result, search firms are challenged to identify candidates who have both highly developed supply chain management skills and the ability to deploy strategic frames.

Contingency theory is based on the notion that there are no universal prescriptions in management.[42] Contingency theory posits that the correct management principle or technique to be applied should be related to the existing set of circumstances or situation. The theory envisions good management as the ability to perceive the significant or limiting factors in a situation. Table 1.1 identifies a number of the contingent issues that organizations must grapple with as they attempt to improve organizational performance.

Successful managers, recognizing the contours of given circumstances, apply multiple management frames and develop consequent strategies for obtaining value from the supply chain.[43] The idea of multiple frames for envisioning the supply chain is consistent with the contingency theory precept that there is no one best way to manage, but as circumstances demand, there may be best approaches to problem solving. Thus, a supply chain manager interested in understanding more fully how to satisfy physician demands might employ the service frame in seeking a solution. When interested in working with physicians on standardization, to improve outcomes and safety, as well as to reduce costs, the transformational frame might be a more powerful perspective.

The Complexity of Value

The overarching purpose of the ASU/CHMR project, as identified in the Introduction, is to identify progressive practices that add value through effective management of the supply environment within hospitals and systems. But what is value? Is it reduced cost? Or is it assurance that the correct supplies are available when needed? Some would say that value is defined as the correct supplies at the right place at the right time at the best possible price. This perspective on value is extremely general. An even more general definition is what value is worth to the organization in its attempt to meet organizational objectives. Does this mean that the hospital system should decrease the amount spent on a particular type of supply? Or that supply chain management should increase safety, improve customer service, or improve value in providing leading-edge health care?

These questions are not easy to answer because value varies depending on the organization and the product or service involved. If the product is a highly technical and unique medical device such as a specialized pacemaker, the supply process is much different than if it is an order of bed linens or even standard pharmaceuticals. Whereas the supply chain manager may have a level of comfort exercising judgment in the purchase of linen, the purchase of the clinical preference item will require close attention to medical staff preferences, new developments in the technology marketplace, and technical and service requirements. Also, a facility maintenance service such as housekeeping differs vastly from temporary nursing services, where there must be great vigilance in the selection of individuals who will assist to produce the expected levels of clinical outcomes. The risk of poor housekeeping is low customer satisfaction. The risk of poor nursing can be disastrous to the well-being of a patient. Similarly a capital expenditure such as MRI equipment, given its special requirements for shielding, electricity, and acceptability to clinical staff, cannot be considered the same as a capital expenditure for desktop computing.

New technologies, such as desktop analyzers for tests, have the potential to significantly affect the nature and flow of supplies away from laboratories to the point of service. Accompanying this kind of change may be the ability to change the entire protocol for patient care from multiple visits to a single visit for an episode of care. Different supplies derive a different value for the hospital.

To add to the complexity pertaining to value, the significance of a product is not evaluated the same from organization to organization. Hospitals differ in many ways, such as their mission, size, and geographical configurations. Table 1.4 suggests that value may be affected by both product and hospital differences. Large systems or specialty hospitals, for example, may be able to purchase products in a large volume at a reduced price. This may lead to a system seeing the product as an asset, that is, contributing to revenues for certain kinds of surgical procedures.

**TABLE 1.4.   VALUE DIFFERENCES DERIVED FROM PRODUCT
AND HOSPITAL DIFFERENCES.**

Hospital or System Differences	Product or Service Differences
Mission: specialties, research, academic	Commodities
Size	Medical surgical devices
Geographical concentration or dispersion	Physician preferences
Stakeholders	Capital equipment
Physician relationship	Support services
Managerial capability	Technology
Ownership	

An academic health center with well-trained surgical teams may have the expertise to use a complex surgical product. A surgeon performing the same kind of surgery in a community hospital may value a product for its ease in application.

Not only do different organizations and people value different products in different ways, hospitals and systems have developed diverse strategies in solving their supply chain challenges. Some have decided to manage the entire process internally. Others outsource as many functions as possible. Many systems involve physicians and other clinicians intensely in their purchasing deliberations, while others keep clinical staff at an arm's length. Among organizations that are considered progressive (effectively managing and sourcing information and relationships), many different combinations are observed. Contingency management is necessary to respond to this complex environment.

Strategic Fit and Misfit

It would be naive to think that all managerial lenses produce equally desirable outcomes for organizations. A physician-led organization may, for example, differ from a nonphysician-led organization across a wide number of dimensions that reflect aspects of culture, power, and human resources. Mayo Clinic, one of the systems studied in the course of the ASU/CHMR research, employs the vast majority of its medical staff and relies on physician-led committees to drive decisions across the Mayo system. Implementation of decisions reached in such a way is not nearly as significant a problem as it is in other systems. At the same time, Mayo's strong clinical culture and commitment to physician autonomy may mean that it, like other systems, experiences difficulty achieving consensus on product selection. Discussion of cosmopolitan and local physician orientations in Chapter Three provides important insights into the ways medical staff are oriented to collaboration. Managerial decisions must meet the demands of the organizations in which they

FIGURE 1.2.   THE DYNAMICS OF ACHIEVING STRATEGIC FIT.

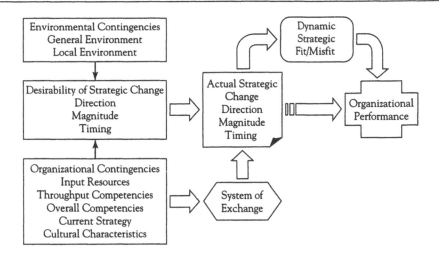

Source: Adapted from Zajac, E. J., Kraatz, M. S., and Bressler, R.K.F. "Modeling the Dynamics of Strategic Fit: A Normative Approach to Strategic Change." *Strategic Management Journal,* 2000, *21*(4) 429–455.

are employed. The idea of strategic fit can be drawn on to explain how different solutions may represent progressive practices in different organizations.[44]

The positioning of strategic fit considerations in determination of decisions regarding supply performance improvement is detailed in Figure 1.2. Outsourcing and insourcing decisions regarding an area such as distribution provide a succinct example for understanding the idea of strategic fit. The University of Nebraska Medical Center, a nationally recognized leader in academic practice, has made the decision to outsource its entire inventory and distribution process to a single distributor. While this appears to be a successful strategy for a single-site academic health center that can establish a successful and trusting relationship with a distributor, such a decision may be unworkable for a multisite, multicity system where it would be difficult for the distributor to meet, equally, the demands of all of the different entities within the system. The same system also made the decision to outsource a great deal of its purchasing through its group purchasing organization, Novation, which provides the opportunity to participate in an exchange system for the purchasing of many of their goods. For the University of Nebraska, these decisions are seen as consistent with the centrality of its educational goals. Throughout the book, a great deal will be said about the systems of exchange in which hospitals and systems participate. Chapter Seven revisits the "system of exchange" idea to reveal that there are options for hospitals and systems as they engage the marketplace for materials, supplies, and services.

Strategic fit and misfit reflects the alignment with the vision and values of a hospital or hospital system and its culture. Whether set by the CEO of a large investor-owned or integrated delivery system or by the government, vision and values provide the orientation, which is a calculus for judging the advisability of opportunities as well as frames for understanding threats. To better understand the issue of strategic fit, the ASU/CHMR study assessed the relationship between vision and value in the English National Health Service. "Value for money" is one overarching theme guiding the National Health Service. This theme is linked to a vision of a series of expectations for the system to which supplies, in addition to price, can be judged by:

- Contribution to successful clinical outcomes in the eyes of patients
- Contributions to successful clinical outcomes in the eyes of providers
- The extent to which the product results in increased use (for example, as a result of emergency room turnover)
- Improved access as a result of savings
- Improved safety to the patient
- Improved employee safety
- Reduced total expenditures per admission

Study 2, "Clinician, Supplier and Buyer Working as One to Improve Patient Outcome" (all studies are placed at the end of the book) explains how a large hospital in Plymouth, England, has been able to capitalize on vision, extraordinarily strong management, and physician collaboration to effectively manage one of the more expensive supply areas associated with cardiology.

In the United States, no common set of values drives health policy and, consequently, delivery. Many of the items listed above resonate with how progressive supply chain leaders in the United States view their roles. In an ASU/CHMR focus group, over ten U.S. health systems indicated that the Institute of Medicine study on patient and hospital safety, *To Err Is Human*, is a "burning platform" for the supply chain manager in his or her attempts to shape the materials environment.[45] In addition, as the introduction of new technologies into the practice arena accelerates and stresses even further the ability of the hospital to achieve a positive bottom line, attention will be paid to the issue of materials.

Summary and Conclusion

Effective and efficient supply chain management represents an opportunity to add value and decrease costs in the U.S. health care system. To accomplish this end, it is necessary for top-level executives and supply chain managers to reframe and transform their approach to the supply chain. Each hospital or system must determine what value can be achieved through the supply chain and structure itself to meet its goals. This will vary depending on product, organization, and environment. Study 3, "Metropolitan Hospital System: A Hybrid Organizational Design," outlines how one large U.S. hospital has organized itself successfully to meet its supply challenges.

The objective of supply chain management is to maximize the overall value of the product or service while reducing costs. Supply chains are dynamic systems[46] that must be designed to fit the product or service involved if they are to reduce costs.[47] To ensure that the supply chain design fits the product, the processes integral to the industry must be considered. "The ultimate competency," Fine argues, "is the ability to choose capabilities well.[48] For managers to achieve competitive advantages, they need to adapt and incorporate elements responsible for supply chain success in their industry.[49] Industries that do this well understand their own "clockspeed."[50] This idea proposes that there are various rates of change and demand posed by different industry-related products, processes, and organizational design. Information management companies where technology is changing quickly are characterized by a faster clockspeed than automobile manufacturers. The health sector overall is characterized by a fairly slow clockspeed. However, different departments and specialties are characterized by distinctive rates of change. Rapid innovation in cardiology implants and medical imaging, for example, require an agile supply chain due to their fast clockspeed. In contrast, mental health services change at a much slower pace.

How well hospitals and systems are able to judge their clockspeeds and adjust accordingly requires careful scrutiny. Smeltzer and Ramanathan have questioned the extent to which the health care sector can learn from other industries, especially manufacturers, as they seek the right advantage.[51] Their work suggests seven key areas for comparison between hospital and other industry supply chains including differences associated with: (1) customer, (2) task, complexity, specialization, and professionalism, (3) organizational structure, (4) organization-employee relationship, (5) product, (6) markets, and (7) information management. The following chapters are attentive to these comparison areas, with the hope that those now managing and making contributions to supply management strategy will find success.

CHAPTER TWO

MANAGING SUPPLY RISK
AND COST REDUCTION

As supplies become an increasingly large proportion of hospital costs and levels of patient acuity rise, the probabilities and consequences of risk associated with purchasing increase. Few hospital and system managers, however, identify risk management as a focal point of their job. Rather, they consistently identify cost reduction as their major challenge—and the metrics associated with cost as constituting the ways their performance is most likely to be evaluated. The ASU/CHMR case studies reveal that progressive systems are engaged in risk reduction. Most systems have a special focus on risk as it applies to cost reduction, and the most progressive systems engage in cost management. The avenue for this activity is most frequently strategic sourcing. This chapter scrutinizes the ways that progressive systems manage risk associated with purchasing and cost reduction.

Drawing on the work of major supply chain theorists, Young defines risk "as the potential to be deprived of use either by reason of long lead time, non-delivery or unacceptable quality."[1] Risk also relates to the chance of purchasing goods that will not satisfy end users or customers. Risk management reduces the chance that the cost of goods will be harmful to the production of a certain product or service and ultimately to the success of the organization. The following discussion reviews the types of costs that can be reduced and managed through strategic sourcing. This is important because not all costs can be treated the same. Next, the meanings, types, and costs of supply risk are reviewed. Finally, a strategic sourcing process that has been derived from the numerous ASU/CHMR case studies will be presented and discussed in the context of cost and risk.

Types of Cost

Three kinds of costs are associated with hospital and hospital system purchasing: purchase (or price), transaction, and administrative costs.

Purchase Cost

Purchase cost represents the price of the good or the service being acquired. By far, this is the most frequent type of cost mentioned by hospital supply managers. In fact, it is common for managers to refer to cost when considering only purchase price. The other types of costs are only sidebar conversations by many managers in discussions of their roles in pricing strategies. However, the more progressive supply chain managers differentiate among the types of costs when making supply chain decisions.

Transaction Costs

Transaction cost[2] is incurred with the exchange of goods between the buyer and seller.[3] Transaction costs range from high-cost efforts by staff to hand-prepare and fax an order to a supplier that is using low-cost computer-assisted ordering. Transaction costs also include the costs associated with purchasing partner fees and commissions, paying for assurances of safety for product delivery, and the monitoring of order fulfillment. Because transaction cost is much more difficult to measure than purchase price, it is less frequently mentioned or included in annual supply management goals. Also it is infrequently monitored nor reported as part of the cost of ownership. Much of what occupies the attention of supply managers is actually cost related and how to avoid transaction cost risks.

Firms that work together over long periods of time develop trust and frequently are able to reduce transaction costs by developing interorganizational mechanisms for reducing conflict and adapting to each other's cultures.[4] The selection of purchasing partners, as discussed throughout the book, represents an important strategy in reducing not just the price paid for goods, but also the potential costs associated with ownership of goods over time. An overwhelmingly high proportion of respondents to the ASU/CHMR research and "The Value of Group Purchasing in the Health Care Supply Chain" (Study 1) report that much of their behavior stems from the belief by supply managers that they receive lower purchase prices in the marketplace than through GPO contracts. These managers charge their staff to use time to research price opportunities beyond their current market pricing. While there may be lower-cost purchasing opportunities, a solid cost-benefit methodology to understand the costs and value associated with such search and purchase efforts is infrequently implemented. Given this narrow focus, the investment of a hospital or system by engaging in activities that might well be carried out more efficiently by others (that is, outsourced) is rarely calculated as part of transaction costs. Study 1, "The Value of Group Purchasing in the Health Care Supply Chain," however, reveals that not all transaction costs are avoided by outsourcing the contracting and sourcing by hospitals and systems.

Administrative Costs

Administrative cost is the internal cost incurred by the buyer for such items as accounts payable and receivables and the typical errors that occur in these processes. Many administrative costs are affected by the direct transactions that the hospital or system chooses. This is also a difficult type of cost to measure so it is often not included in annual cost reduction goals.

Study 1 identifies the wide range of costs (which are certainly price items) associated with hospital sourcing, negotiating, and contracting. The ten systems scrutinized for that study, however, were not able to produce regularly reported data associated with such costs and did not routinely track those costs. The absence turns the focus of the supply manager, charged with the goal of cost reduction, to a focus on purchase price. It is noteworthy that relatively few health care organizations point out that they approach most cost items, other than major capital items, with a view of total cost of ownership. Total ownership costs include aspects of inadequate product management tools, disruptive scalability, poor health product reliability and performance, and compromised product efficiency.[5] Total cost of ownership analysis allows the firm to better select supply sources and distribution channels, improve supplier and distributor performance, define performance expectations, increase supply chain partner accountability and control, select preferred supply partners, and introduce measurement.[6] Such cost analysis can make the purchase price of a good appear trivial. In discussing basic office equipment, Steele Case, an office furniture company, includes the following cost metrics as important in measuring the total cost of ownership:[7]

- Planning and design
- Selection process and purchasing activities
- Delivery and installation
- Orientation and training
- Movement of management and reconfiguration
- Refurbishing maintenance
- Disposal

Case 2.1, developed by Steelcase, one of the nation's largest manufacturers of office equipment, depicts a methodical and disciplined view of total cost of ownership that can be applied by supply chain managers to a variety of products that characterize the health care delivery environment.

◆ ◆ ◆

Case 2.1 Total Cost of Ownership

. . . It's possible that in identifying total cost of ownership a company may discover that a low-cost product may carry significant management costs. In this scenario, a company's most significant savings might be in streamlining management of the product in the workplace rather than trying to simply procure the product at a lower price. Or another strategy may involve selecting a different product that carries lower management costs. In this last option, a product whose purchase price is higher might actually offer a lower total cost of ownership.

A comprehensive understanding of the total cost of ownership is critical for leveraging the return on your company's investment in workplace furniture and furnishings.

"Digital Equipment's Swedish operation in Stockholm redesigned their office for maximum flexibility. The redesign has produced a 50% reduction in space use, a 50% decline in energy consumption, a 60% decline in cleaning costs, and more highly motivated employees" (Personnel Management, Aug. 1993).

The illustration [below] attempts to depict the allocation of cost of ownership elements based on overall industry experiences.

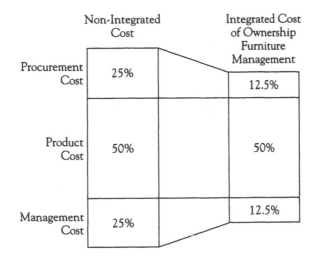

What It Might Look Like

The illustration [shown on the previous page] provides a glimpse of how a new approach to cost of ownership might be structured. This is an illustration of how new views of life-cycle costs may affect the business impact of the workplace.

How It's All Connected

A focus on cost of ownership and its impact on the furniture configurations and the workplace does not exist in isolation. No company can be successful by focusing only on costing and the impact of this factor on the work environment.

As companies get a clearer picture of true costs of ownership, businesses will also be focusing on issues, such as:

- Financing alternatives: the new strategies being developed to more effectively leverage company investments in facilities and furnishings, creating an even more integrated approach to linking the workplace to business success
- Organizational shape: the new structures, management styles, team patterns, and work culture and their collective impact in creating a new set of needs for the workplace
- Health and safety: the collection of issues that affect the safety, health, and comfort of the workplace, and the impact of those issues on workplace design

A holistic integration of these and any other relevant workplace factors will ensure that a new approach to designing and furnishing the workplace will create a more effective place for people to work and companies to succeed.

Source: "Cost of Ownership: New Ways to Calculate Costs." http://www.steelcase.com/na/knowledgedesign.aspx?f=10255&c=10903.

◆ ◆ ◆

The Nature of Supply Risk

Risk exists when (1) outcomes are uncertain, (2) goals are difficult to achieve, and (3) there is potential for extreme consequences.[8] Another way to look at risk is the potential inability to succeed in meeting project, process, or system objectives. These two definitions specify the relationship between risk and cost reduction. While a goal for health care is cost reduction, risk can prevent the ability to meet this goal. The level of risk is generally estimated using two components: (1) the probability that the risk event will occur and (2) the consequences of the risk.[9]

Risk, an essential element of the overall supply management task, is not easy to see and quantify.[10] Table 2.1 provides a summary of the types of supply risk in hospitals and systems, along with their causes and results.

TABLE 2.1. TYPES OF RISK.

Type of Risk	Cause of Risk	Result of Risk
Strategy risk: Inappropriate strategy for good or service	Inappropriate match between product and supply strategy Poor knowledge of supply strategies	Product not delivered at the right place at the right time at the best price
Market risk: Inappropriate strategy for market conditions	Lack of knowledge about cost trends within the market	Purchase incorrect goods or service Pay too much for good or service Use technology-inferior goods
Demand risk: Buying too much or too little of the good or service	Volatility of customer demand Over- or underspecifying requirements	Incorrect inventory levels Overpay for unnecessary product specifications Use of inappropriate materials Poor customer relationship
Implementation risk: Supply strategy is appropriate but not implemented correctly	Poor information and communication within the hospital	Inventory costs too high Materials unavailable Unnecessary administrative costs

Source: Adapted from Clouse, M., and Busch, J. "How to Identify and Manage Supply Risk." Oct. 2003. http://www.supplychainplanet.com/e_article000195015.cfm.

Risk can be divided into four major categories: strategy risk, market risk, demand risk, and implementation risk.[11] Each type of risk has very different characteristics and can be attributable to a variety of different causal factors.

Strategy Risk

Inappropriate strategy for hospital goods or services is frequently related to the lack of knowledge by supply chain managers about the availability of a product in the marketplace. This kind of risk occurs as a result of supplier manufacturing difficulties, breakdown in distribution channels, and the internal handling of products. Issues regarding shelf life are critical for many health-related products such as pharmaceuticals and infusion products. For such products, strategy risk must revolve around the ability for timely and frequent movement of fresh supplies to the proper location and monitoring product availability at the point of use.

Strategy risk can also be related to the supply chain manager's not properly understanding how a product will be used in the hospital and whether there are preferences for specific brands by clinicians.

Monitoring strategy risk for products that are quickly changing in marketplace demand and use (such as bare wire stents) is extremely important. Progressive systems hedge against this risk by achieving a balance for commitment based on volume or loyalty. This is done by developing a contracting system that has well-developed escape clauses specifying the conditions under which contract conditions can be altered or cancelled.

The level of strategy risk is attributable to the competencies and abilities of the supply chain manager and staff to understand the materials marketplace and develop action plans to mediate risk. Substantial costs are associated with poor performance in this area, especially purchase price and transaction costs. Hospitals can afford few stock-outs. When goods are not available for a surgical procedure or for carrying out a diagnostic test, the hospital or system is forced to take immediate action or suffer a loss of revenue to another facility.

The ASU/CHMR study found that high levels of activity associated with next-day delivery are defined by some supply executives as a supply strategy; others, however, recognize it as costly and a signal of a lack of strategy. Supporters of next-day delivery point out that the large number of deliveries represents the hospital's deliberate strategy to secure a rarely used item and avoid inventory. Those who question the costs of such deliveries report that the volume of just-in-time deliveries through the loading dock represents a breakdown in the ability of the supply chain management staff to anticipate the demand for certain products. Few supply chain mangers carefully monitor or manage such shipments or understand the true cost of managing risk in this manner. Virginia Mason, a hospital system in Seattle, recently reported that its central service and sterile processing distribution department, serving a 336-bed hospital and related outpatient and physician clinics, received thirty thousand UPS and Federal Express packages in 2004. Although that was three thousand fewer deliveries than in the previous years, it represents a significant proportion of the supply acquisition costs in the preparation of materials for 15,500 surgical cases.[12] Virginia Mason, working with supply specialists, was able to cut more than $755,000 in savings in its central services area. The costs of such transactions continue to be of great concern to suppliers, who see the transaction costs associated with such delivery modes as contributing to increased costs.

Market Risk

Unavoidable health sector market risk is related to the lack of price transparency in much of health sector purchasing. Progressive systems increasingly benchmark their prices with information obtained from consulting firms and intelligence gained through networking discussions. As discussed in greater detail in Chapter Four, there is a great reliance on purchasing partners, such as GPOs, to assist in understanding cost trends. GPOs provide cost data comparisons on a national basis as well as benchmark their own members, nationally and regionally, on metrics associated with price, cost, and other key outcome variables. While purchasing at an inappropriate price may not lead to purchasing inferior technology or goods, it can clearly result in reduced operating margins, thus resulting in the inability to provide high-quality services.

Market risk is associated with upstream supply availability and how such availability affects the willingness of suppliers to offer flexibility in their pricing. The inability to manage market risk, if it does result in purchasing inferior products, may lead to increased dissatisfaction from medical staff. One of the ASU/CHMR research sites encountered problems with a recently acquired hospital that had done an inadequate job of managing market risk. Physicians were accustomed to demanding goods regardless of price and ease of availability. In this instance, failure to manage market risk led to both higher purchasing prices and inordinately high transaction costs.

Demand Risk

Demand risk is related to (1) uncertainty associated with disease patterns in a hospital or a system's population, (2) the supply manager's lack of understanding of disease trends, (3) failure to understand and manage clinician preferences, and (4) ability to carry out value analysis effectively. Demand risk is especially costly when applied to hospital physician preference items and the failure to manage the medical staff. The inability to manage demand risk also affects the customer relationship efforts carried out by supply chain managers.

Implementation Risk

Hospitals and systems face significant problems implementing their supply chain strategies. Hospitals are highly departmentalized organizations. They frequently lack general, fundamental protocols to facilitate communication regarding materials that are used in an integrated fashion to produce outstanding clinical outcomes. In progressive systems, organizational redesign and increased centralization counter the risk that units will not collaborate. Knowledge management in the health sector is, however, in its infancy.[13] If the health sector is to capitalize on its information base adequately, increased investment in knowledge management systems will be necessary.

Research demonstrates a wide range of variability throughout hospitals and hospital systems in their participation in contracts in conformance to centralization efforts.[14] BJC HealthCare in St. Louis, among the most progressive systems, has put into place strategies to reduce implementation risk. BJC HealthCare–affiliated hospitals are closely aligned to centralization strategies, and methods are in place to ensure that manufacturer representatives, even when working closely with clinicians, do not counter the BJC HealthCare effort to enforce the contracts it has in place. Similar programs at Sharp HealthCare in San Diego have led to a realignment of relationships between suppliers and the Sharp hospitals.

Strategic Sourcing

Strategic sourcing is a supply chain process for managing risk and reducing cost in the acquisition of goods and services. When this process is executed properly, it works to ensure that the organization is able to achieve its supply chain mission and strategy.

Large-scale empirical research on strategic sourcing indicates that this process can have a major impact on a hospital or system's goals.[15] The health systems scrutinized, however, do not carry out all of the activities as they relate to cost reduction and risk management in a sequential manner. In fact, only a few systems or hospitals that may be considered progressive actually used all steps. There are seven principal activities of strategic sourcing:[16]

1. Category and spend analysis
2. Market analysis
3. Strategy development
4. Supplier relationship strategy
5. Supplier analysis
6. Cost and price analysis
7. Fact-based negotiation

Category and Spend Analysis

This strategy must be adapted to fit the nature of the supply strategy, which in the hospital industry varies dramatically. The different types of products may be conceptualized as a triangle seen in Figure 2.1.[17] The figure is shaped like a triangle because a continuum exists between each of the product categories. Some products are pure commodities (bed linens) or capital items (gamma camera), while others may be halfway between a commodity and a physician preference item (basic heart pacemaker).[18]

FIGURE 2.1. SUPPLY CATEGORIES.

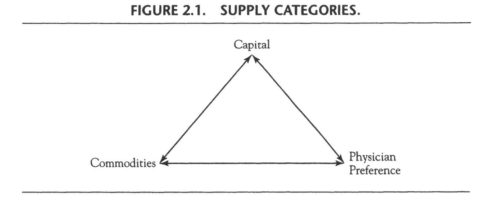

An important aspect of category analysis, as developed by the Aberdeen Group, is the determination of the purchase size, or "spend analysis," for each category. Three levels of spend analysis have been identified: [19]

> *Level 1: Spend summary.* This summary information of the dollar and quantity spend on specific items at individual sites influences buyers to develop sourcing strategies on perception rather than on comprehensive fact-based summaries.
>
> *Level 2: Category data.* Categorical data typically classify supplies into families of spending that offer the greatest leverage. Data on entire categories, such as paper and cotton goods, constitute categorical data. This level, while providing strategic direction, can also be deficient. The trouble is that a single supplier can provide multiple and different categories of goods. The consequence is that opportunities for leverage across the product groups of a supplier may be lost. With the emergence of products that span pharmaceuticals and materials categories, such as drug-eluting stents, classification becomes even more difficult.
>
> *Level 3: Consolidated spend data.* This is the aggregation of 100 percent of the data into a single consolidated view of the spend. This detail enables a precise view of spending with each supplier for each commodity in the system, hospital as well as the buyer level. This allows for comprehensive sourcing strategies.

Following the Aberdeen Group criteria, only one system in the ASU/CHMR study approaches level 3; most are at level 1. The main reason is that most systems lack the information systems to aggregate the data. This makes it extremely difficult to assess a variety of purchasing partner strategies such as a GPOs and distributors. It also makes it difficult to assess the effectiveness of purchasing partners. However, even when spend analysis is at level 1 or 2, it is still possible to use the subsequent strategic sourcing steps on certain items. For instance, one system has a clear spend analysis of all hip replacements across the four hospitals within the system. This makes it possible to use strategic sourcing and drive value on this one item even though many other items have poor spend visibility. Spend analysis and aggregation of data may well be the foundation for supply chain improvements. The databases provided by companies such as Global Health Exchange and Neoforma increasingly provide their clients with advanced spend and opportunity information. Yet not all systems take advantage of such information.

Category analysis requires the classification of goods or services on the dimensions of risk, cost, or value that different kinds of goods bring to the organization.[20] Figure 2.2 depicts how the categories may be placed in a quadrant with risk on one axis and value on the other. Risk may have an impact on internal operations as well as customer service. If a customer (physician or patient) demands a certain good or service and it is not available, poor customer service may result. Poor supply function can affect patient satisfaction in other ways, including decreased comfort due to the unavailability of appropriate materials. Price does not necessarily affect the potential risk of poor customer satisfaction.[21]

The products or services placed in each of the quadrants in Figure 2.2 require a different sourcing strategy. A low-risk, low-cost item is much different from a high-cost, high-preference item. Also, the strategy will vary depending if the product is a commodity,[22] capital good, or physician preference item. Broadlane, a GPO, distinguishes among health products as follows: (1) low-volume commodities such as soaps and slippers, (2) high-volume commodities such as intravenous solutions and custom surgical trays, and (3) clinical preference items such as spinal implants.[23] Most physician preference items would likely fit into the upper-right-hand

FIGURE 2.2.   CATEGORY OF PRODUCTS.

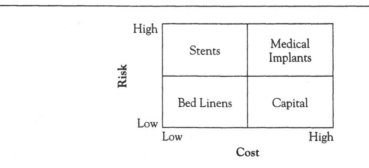

quadrant, and the subsequent strategy would be entirely different from items in the lower-left-hand quadrant. The strategy would also differ on the success of standardization efforts by the hospital to gain physician consensus. It is important to keep in mind that such analysis permits the supply manager to engage in leveraging as "a straightforward strategy that follows directly from an organization's commodity strategy development process."[24]

The range of engagement in outsourcing and insourcing is a further confirmation of the contention that the best management strategies are highly contingent on a wide variety of organizational strategic fit factors. Intuition may tell many managers that low-cost, low-risk items do not justify their time and attention. However, a consideration of the total cost of ownership of such items may lead managers to engage the market to reduce costs for the system. Insourcing and outsourcing advantages have been closely scrutinized by supply chain analysts with a focus on the level of control that one desires to have over inputs, flexibility, economies of scale, investment risk, cash flow, and labor.[25]

Technology, such as reverse auctions,[26] where prequalified bidders are awarded contracts on the basis of their offering the lowest bid, has been used to facilitate the hospital commodity purchasing process.[27] Sourcing and purchasing strategies require careful analysis to determine if the transaction costs associated with the auction (including qualifying suppliers dealing with logistics and returns, and engaging in supplier relationships with the firms under contract) are worth the price savings achieved. Careful analysis is especially important for items in the low-cost, high-risk quadrant, where it is difficult to easily determine if a GPO or internal strategic sourcing will produce the best prices for the least costs. It may depend on the nature of the risk, the dollars involved, the personnel capabilities available, and the relationship with the GPO.

Disciplined supply chain management requires careful consideration of insourcing and outsourcing options for important supply functions. Outsourcing the identification of products and contracting through GPOs (Chapter Four) and aspects of logistics and distribution (Chapter Five) is an option continuously assessed by progressive systems. While a number of progressive systems report that they routinely manage their own sourcing and contracting for high-dollar physician preference items, a number of progressive systems have used GPOs to engage the marketplace collaboratively to drive the market.

Market Analysis

Market analysis establishes the supply market structure, forces, and trends in order to determine how to best purchase items. It is important to know the basic market structure—perfect competition, imperfect competition, oligopoly, or monopoly—in order to determine how much power and influence the hospital or system has on pricing. For instance, in a near monopoly, as might be the case with a highly specialized dual-head gamma camera, the buyer has little power to influence pricing. In fact, the buyer may be on a waiting list to receive the capital item. However, in a perfect or imperfect market structure, many suppliers may exist, so it may be possible to have a greater influence on the market price, as is the case with items such as bedding, gauze, and gloves. An oligopoly may exist with pharmaceuticals that have lost their patent protection. Although only a few competitors may exist, intense competition may prevail through the introduction of generic drugs that drive prices down. Thus, markets may be classified in terms of the complexity in the number of suppliers in a given market structure, unique versus standardized or commoditized products, and new versus changing versus established technologies. The buyer usually has little power in markets that are characterized by few suppliers, unstandardized products, and new technology. Simple markets are much easier to buy from as they have many suppliers, stable products, and mature technologies.

From the perspective of management, the most popular approach to market analysis is to use the Five Force model developed by Porter, which is presented in Figure 2.3.[28] The use of this model allows the market analyst to determine (1) the

FIGURE 2.3.   THE FIVE FORCES.

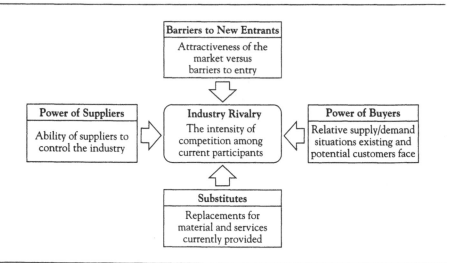

presence of substitutes for a product, (2) barriers pertaining to the entrance of new competitors into the market, (3) the power of the suppliers, (4) the power of buyers, and (5) industry rivals or the overall market competitiveness. With the result of this analysis, it is possible to determine the current power of the buying system and how to obtain additional influence through appropriate supply strategies.

Only one of the progressive systems in the ASU/CHMR study reports using the Five Forces analysis to develop a sourcing strategy. In this instance, it is used to assist in the purchase of heart defibrillators. The system has one hospital with a highly regarded and busy cardiac center. Given this unique market positioning, the system uses its unusually high demand for heart defibrillators to help secure very low prices. Demand was not the only factor working in this hospital's favor. It determined that the market, although an oligopoly, was extremely competitive, and the hospital could develop purchasing power by leveraging its volume. An additional source of power was its strong reputation in cardiology. The manufacturers therefore wanted the business in order to use the hospital's reputation in future promotional efforts. Furthermore, through a disciplined product analysis, the supply team, in consultation with cardiovascular surgeons, determined that several of the brands of defibrillators had nearly identical product characteristics. This created substitution power. The supply management team made a compelling argument to the cardiac physicians demonstrating how the system could dramatically reduce prices. In addition, the selected manufacturer was willing to present a research grant to the hospital. When the physicians agreed, the hospital used one manufacturer for the devices except in rare cases. Many of the principles used by this hospital are demonstrated in Study 2 about a hospital system in the south of England. By coming together to standardize on products and demonstrating their commitment to implementing contracts, the Plymouth group was able to influence the market significantly.

A major aspect of market analysis is to determine market trends. Possible trends include changes in price, cost, current and emerging technology, new entrants in the market, and company consolidation. Progressive systems recognize that it is very difficult to track all market trends, so they rely on medical and other professional staff to be familiar with changes. Publications, consultants, and purchasing partners such as GPOs also provide important information for such decision making. Many of the materials used over the course of a hospitalization are captured within the global reimbursement schemes, such as diagnosis-related groups. Insurance companies currently appear to have little interest in directly influencing product selection. However, due to the escalating cost of materials, managers in progressive systems believe that it is just a matter of time before the insurance industry begins to assess products on the basis of costs and outcomes.

Interviewees in the ASU/CHMR study reveal that in order to obtain market information, they consult with colleagues whom they believe have a good

understanding of the market. As one manager said, "After being in this business
for so many years, a person just knows what is going on." Another manager said,
"A good way to understand the market is to talk to sales representatives or talk to
the docs who use the devices." While it may be true that a great deal of market
scrutiny occurs in such an unsystematic manner, progressive systems have put into
place much more disciplined methods for scanning the market. Technology officer roles and technology assessment committees provide systems with a structured
approach to scanning the marketplace and incorporating new procedures into the
care process. Unfortunately, there is not always a strong link between the technology and the purchasing functions. Through its over sixty value analysis teams,
Kaiser, a large, integrated delivery system, has developed a methodical, disciplined,
and prudent approach to buffering market complexity. These teams routinely
review new products and make recommendations to guide materials purchasing.
It is such recommendations that allow Kaiser to work closely with its GPO partner
to secure prices based on Kaiser's commitment to a high volume of brand
products.

Progressive supply chain organizations have a sophisticated understanding of
the importance of systematic market analysis. First, they believe that sales representatives provide limited and biased information. As one manager stated, "Their
job is to provide slanted information. This is not to say that it can't be valuable,
but it is not sufficient." Another reason is that it is extremely difficult to get accurate pricing information. A manager at a large system observed, "You can get pricing information from visiting with peers at other institutions, and you would be
surprised what you can learn by going to conferences." While such anecdotal
information has value, progressive systems recognize that it is no substitute for
rigorous research on cost and price trends that may be derived from market
indexes, government statistics, and materials and technology costs reports.

Strategy Development

After the product is analyzed in terms of cost and risk, the market is studied to
determine its complexity in terms of market structure, forces, and trends. The
results of these analyses then lead to the appropriate strategy for sourcing the product. A wide variety of sourcing strategies are available as described in the work of
Steele and Court[29] and Handfield and Nichols:[30]

- *Tactical goods strategy for low-cost goods in low-complexity markets.* These goods require
a tactical focus with a concentration on the reduction of transaction costs. Disposable
drinking cups are a good example of such a product. For these kinds of items,
progressive hospitals and systems use purchasing cards and allow vendors to manage

substantial aspects of their inventory. For highly competitive items, opportunities to reduce price may be minimal. Outsourcing supply management and sourcing functions through purchasing partners such as GPOs and distributors can reduce transaction costs and other aspects related to the total cost of ownership. Further product price reduction may not justify the time that hospital and system employees would expend with the hope of minimal returns.

• *Leverage goods strategy.* For high-cost goods in relatively low-complexity markets, it is important that hospitals develop leverage in the marketplace by aggressively finding value in the market. Because of low market complexity, however, it will be critical to understand the market thoroughly in order to find the best values. A typical strategy in this quadrant is to standardize products across divisions and then aggregate the purchase. In this manner, the entire system can have one contract for a product. This applies to both clinical and administrative items. A large system in the ASU/CHMR study used this approach for photocopiers. It found that it was spending over $2.5 million annually with four suppliers of photocopiers. When it standardized across hospitals and facilities to one type of machine, it was able to develop leverage and reduce the total cost by 20 percent. The general goal will be to leverage the hospital or system in order to obtain volume efficiencies and discounts. Leveraging may be accomplished by outsourcing aspects of purchasing through a GPO or other sourcing agencies. Short-term contracts may also be used to remain flexible as prices or costs change. At the same time, it is important to analyze the supply base to find new suppliers and assess the value brought through the GPO.

• *Critical goods strategies.* Low-cost critical goods frequently lend themselves to long-term contracts. A hospital in the ASU/CHMR study had a sole surgeon who conducted cochlear implant surgery. In this instance, the supply management team found it much more efficient to use the GPO and not question the price because product availability was much more important than price. This strategy seeks to ensure the presence of supplies and reduces the need to develop new sources for goods, thus reducing transaction costs.

• *Complexity strategy for high-cost and high-market-complexity goods.* This strategy requires a sophisticated supply effort over the long term. This is a multifaceted situation because the market is complex and the value of the product is high. In order to manage such goods, progressive systems develop strategic partnerships while seeking alternative suppliers and product substitutes.

Although the ASU/CHMR study did not carry out systematic scrutiny of how the hospitals or systems manage risk, it is estimated that approximately 20 percent of the hospitals and systems were not able to articulate any strategy that accounted for cost, market complexity, and risk. Even among the more progressive systems, the criteria for inclusion for each strategy are not systematically developed, and only the easiest commodities, such as linens and towels, are analyzed across units in the hospital or system.

Supplier Relationship Strategy

Supplier relationship strategy encompasses the nature and length of contracts, the number and mix of suppliers, and the mechanisms established to engage the supplier in a variety of relationships. The supplier relationship strategy largely depends on the previous three steps: the nature of the product including risk and cost, market conditions, and the supply strategy.

A good way to think about supplier relationship strategy is presented in Figure 2.4. On one end of the continuum is a transaction focus and on the other end is the collaborative focus. Strategies with a transaction focus generally have a short-term, arm's-length arrangement, and strategies with a collaborative focus generally have a long-term, highly interactive focus. Another way to think of the transaction focus is by referring to it as cash-and-carry, in that the goal is simply to complete the transaction.

Generally there tend to be a large number of suppliers for these products. However, because the organization may have low switching costs between suppliers, the amount of communication and the number of contracts that the organization maintains are frequently kept low. This could be used for such basic commodities as alcohol swabs and tongue depressors, capital items such as bed frames, and administrative necessities such as paper forms. The collaborative approach is much more involved and requires the parties to develop and maintain a continuing relationship. Here, the items are probably physician preference items

FIGURE 2.4. SUPPLIER RELATIONSHIP STRATEGY.

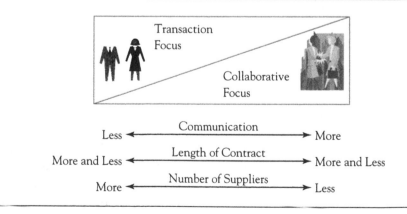

FIGURE 2.5. TRANSACTION AND COLLABORATIVE STRATEGIES.

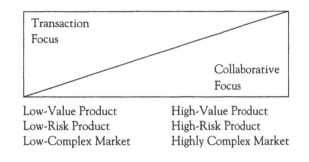

Low-Value Product	High-Value Product
Low-Risk Product	High-Risk Product
Low-Complex Market	Highly Complex Market

and high-cost supplies such as orthopedic implants, robotic surgical capital equipment, software, and temporary labor providers. Depending on the risks of the market and the number of suppliers, the organization will need to balance the number of relationships through depth and commitment.

The objectives that fit the transaction type of relationships (Figure 2.5) should be different from the goals for collaborative relationships. Products that fit transaction relationships generally have small profit margins, making it difficult to reduce the purchase price. Therefore, it is logical that the greatest savings will come from administrative and transaction cost reductions. At the other end of the continuum, it may be possible to obtain both large purchase price reductions as well as administrative and transaction cost reductions.

Figure 2.5 indicates when the appropriate focus is transactional compared to collaborative. Low-value, low-risk products sourced from a low-complexity market should have a transaction focus. Basic dressings, linens, and capital fit this classification. High-value, high-risk products from highly complex markets should have a collaborative focus. Robotic surgery devices fit this category.

There is no systematic research detailing how supply chain managers adjust their relationship strategy and goals to product and market differences. While many managers tend to use a transaction approach for all situations, it is interesting and important to note that these managers may also say that they are developing a partnership with the suppliers. This implies that they are using a collaborative approach. Yet the ASU/CHMR study hospitals and systems report that they had neither formal criteria for a partnership nor a systematic partnership selection process. In other words, they were simply using the currently popular term *collaborative* to rationalize their behavior without really knowing the implications of its practice.

On even further investigation, it became clear that for most of these organizations, the goal was only to reduce prices, and this was completed through distributive negotiation. What was being termed a collaborative approach was in reality a transaction approach. The conclusion is that many of the managers have not developed a systematic way to think about supplier relationships.

Supplier Analysis

A critical step in the strategic sourcing process is to identify, qualify, and select potential suppliers. In supplier analysis, the focus is moved from the product to the market and then to the supplier. As depicted in Figure 2.6, before it is possible to identify suppliers, it is necessary to clearly articulate the required specifications. In the case of services, such as specialized temporary labor, this is the development of a statement of work or, for products, the specification statement. Successful completion of this step requires extensive deliberation completed by a cross-functional team to ensure that both clinical and business perspectives are considered.

For the more successful systems in the ASU/CHMR study, the supplier identification stage often started during the market analysis. While reviewing the market, more than likely the major suppliers in an industry were identified as well as its competitors. The more advanced supply management groups used many sources to identify potential suppliers, such as Internet sites, catalogues, and

FIGURE 2.6.   SUPPLIER IDENTIFICATION AND SELECTION.

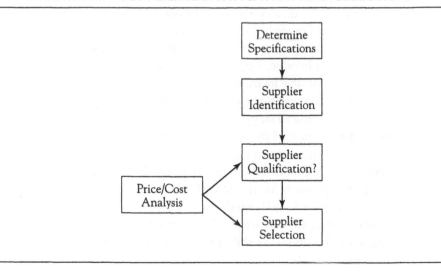

even discussions with competitors. The less progressive supply management groups used only the suppliers they had traditionally used or with whom they were familiar. Using only suppliers that are in the comfort zone did not always result in a highly competitive supply base.

After the potential pool of suppliers is identified, it is necessary to determine the best suppliers and qualify them to determine if they can meet the needs of the hospital or system. Compared to other industries, in only rare instances are formal requests for information (RFIs), requests for proposals (RFPs), or request for quotes (RFQs) sent to suppliers for desired goods. RFPs should be used as the health care supply chain professionals move directly to the RFQ. By not engaging in the RFP, RFI, or RFQ process, few hospitals or systems in the study used a total cost approach in selecting suppliers, as they had not collected adequate cost information.

The ASU/CHMR findings are consistent with research in other industries suggesting that the supplier selection process frequently lacks a systematic approach.[31] The process is influenced by individual bias and proclivities rather than a systematic process, as depicted in Figure 2.6. For example, one of the managers in the ASU/CHMR study believed that it was important to source syringes from a local supplier; another manager made a strong argument for a national supplier. Neither manager considered price or quality or a total cost model. Rather, both used only an emotional argument for and against a supplier. The desired specifications and qualifications of a desired supplier should have been identified prior to the actual selection, but this process was not followed. Failure to carry out supplier identification and selection precludes systems from effectively employing new technologies such as reverse auctions.

A question mark follows the term *supplier qualification* in Figure 2.6. The reason is that throughout the ASU/CHMR research, it was found that this was an extremely weak step for the hospitals and systems. Few hospitals or systems qualify suppliers in the earlier stages. Therefore, the subsequent step of supplier selection is weak. Unfortunately, supplier selection is often a matter of individual preference or a bowing to the political whims of an influential person within the organization.

Implementation risk (the risk that the incorrect products may be used) may be the greatest danger due to inferior service and price. Such risk can be offset by "trialing" products before switching suppliers and engaging potential users to score items to ensure that areas such as service, reliability, and quality are looked at in addition to price.

Price and Cost Analysis

Price and cost analysis is included in Figure 2.6 as if it is part of the previous step. However, it is presented as a separate step here because of its importance. Cost analysis implies the total cost of ownership, which is the sum of all the expenses and costs related to the acquisition and use of a service or good.[32] But it is more than just the purchase price. The analysis should include administrative and transaction costs that may be associated with the supply. Price analysis is the historic pricing of a product as well as the comparison of prices across brand names.

The benefit of total cost analysis is reflected by the purchase of an MRI in one of the systems in the ASU/CHMR study. When a system considered total costs as a result of its RFP, it realized that training was a major factor because one supplier was willing to provide training at a low rate while another supplier was charging a premium.

It is not uncommon to find that the purchase price represents only 50 or 60 percent of the total cost of ownership (Case 2.1), with large swings in cost savings existing for furniture as well as medical equipment. In one situation involving highly sophisticated medical operating room equipment, it was reported that maintenance and training alone accounted for nearly 75 percent of the total cost of ownership. Although total cost may be the most important analysis with capital purchases, it is imperative to realize that inventory and handling costs can also affect most types of goods and should be considered when making such purchases.

General total cost of ownership information can be obtained during the market analysis stage or during the RFP, RFI, and RFQ stages of the process. However, with few of the ASU/CHMR sites using RFPs, the critical information is not obtained. Informal supply and price analysis are the common modes. Although this is easier to conduct, it needs to be recognized that the same level of sensitivity of the differences between products or suppliers will not be obtained. When this occurs, the organization should not be surprised when it encounters the escalating costs associated with training and other incidentals, which have previously been included in the price of other supplies.

Fact-Based Negotiation

As a result of each of the previous steps in the strategic sourcing process, the cross-functional team ideally should have extensive information about the product, market, supply base, and cost and price. In a typical strategic sourcing process, this information should be put together in a comprehensive and fact-based negotiation brief.

Fact-based negotiation, which can result in distributive (win/lose) or integrative (win/win) outcomes, is generally advocated in strategic sourcing and differs from most traditional negotiation in four basic ways:[33]

1. Traditional negotiations are generally based on personal perspectives, opinions, and bias. Fact-based negotiations are based on facts derived from market analysis, supplier analysis, and other research. The strategic sourcing process leads to the negotiation.

2. In traditional negotiations, personal persuasion strategies are stressed. In fact-based negotiations, emphasis is placed on providing objective, factual evidence derived from extensive research. This research evidence is obtained through extensive preparation during strategic sourcing.

3. In traditional negotiations, the negotiators' personalities are stressed. Facts and evidence are more important in the fact-based negotiations.

4. As a result of these differences, traditional negotiation is more subjective, whereas objectivity dominates fact-based negotiations.

With a negotiation brief in hand, the sourcing team can clearly state its overall position including the Best Alternative to a Negotiated Agreement (BATNA). This is the sourcing team's alternative in the event it cannot obtain a deal with the first party. The negotiation brief also outlines the least acceptable alternative and the most supportable alternative, along with the point at which the initial offer should be set.

Fact-based negotiation can take either an arm's-length, competitive approach or a collaborative, problem-solving approach. The collaborative approach is generally best for high-risk, high-cost products (the upper-right quadrant of Figure 2.2), while the arm's-length approach would be best for low-cost, low-risk products (the lower-left quadrant of Figure 2.2).[34]

Summary and Conclusion

This chapter considers potential risks that exist in the health care supply chain and provides a potential strategic sourcing model observed in several ASU/CHMR study hospitals systems to manage risks and reduce costs.

This discussion may be summarized by returning to the discussion of risks confronting health sector supply chain management and assessing how the various strategies identified can be applied to manage and buffer risk (Table 2.2). Strategy risk can be buffered and averted by systematically and rigorously implementing the seven steps of the sourcing and market analysis processes discussed throughout this chapter. Many managers also indicate that the use of cross-functional teams and value analysis teams helps significantly in managing demand risk. Such risk is also better averted by developing effective information systems and engaging purchasing partners that have a comprehensive understanding of supply and demand. It requires managers who can learn from a broad-based group of clients about the factors that contribute to and provide relief from risk. Supplier analysis, inventory analysis, and outstanding operational staff provide important buffers for averting implementation risk. Table 2.2 provides an indication of risk-reduction strategies that can be achieved with purchasing partners.

TABLE 2.2. RISK REDUCTION SOUGHT THROUGH GPO AND DISTRIBUTOR ALLIANCE.

Characteristic of Risk	Definition or Description of Risk	Potential GPO Competency	Potential Distributor Competency
Capacity constraints (strategy risk)	The inability to produce an output quantity in a particular time period	X	
Cost reduction capabilities (market risk)	The act of lowering the cost of the same goods or services	X	X
Cycle time (strategy risk)	The time between purchase request to a supplier and receipt		X
Disasters	Any occurrence that causes great harm or calamity		
Environmental performance (strategy risk)	Activities such as selecting materials used, product design processes, and process improvement	X	X
Financial health of suppliers (market risk)	Profitability trends in cash flow and the existence of financial guarantees	X	
Inbound transportation (strategy risk)	Method to distribute, handle, and transport inputs		X
Information system compatibility and sophistication (strategy and market risk)	Information system capability of suppliers to transfer timely, accurate, and relevant information to buyer	X	X
Inventory management (strategy risk)	Supplier ability to manage raw materials, work-in-process, and finished goods and inventories		X
Legal liabilities (strategy risk)	Legal enforceable restrictions or commitments relating to the use of the material, product, or service	X	

Risk factor	Description		
Management vision (strategy risk and market risk)	Supplier management attitude and ability to foresee market and industry changes	X	X
Market price increases (market risk)	Trends, events, or developments that may increase prices		X
Number of available suppliers (strategy risk and market risk)	The existence of monopoly or oligopoly conditions in the supply market	X	X
Process technology changes (strategy risk)	The frequency of new ideas and emerging technology		X
Product design changes	The unpredictability of changes in product technology		X
Quality	The ability of suppliers to conform to specifications		X
Shipment quantity inaccuracies (strategy risk)	The gap between the actual demand requests and the quantity shipped	X	
Supply availability (strategy risk and market risk)	Availability of strategic materials in terms of quality and quantity and the relative strength of suppliers	X	X
Volume and mix requirements change (strategy risk)	Demand fluctuation in quantity and type of component or service	X	

Source: Adapted from Zsidisim, G. "Managerial Perceptions of Supply Risk." *Journal of Supply Chain Management*, 2003, 39(1), 16.

In addition to risk, costs can be managed within the strategic sourcing process. Early in this discussion, three types of costs were presented: purchase, administrative, and transaction. In many industries, activity-based costing is used to improve supply chain and purchasing effectiveness. There is a great deal of discussion for the potential of activity-based costing in hospitals and systems. The ASU/CHMR study did not study this, and it was not reported as a central supply chain feature. Given the extensive information technology necessary to carry out such costing, few health care systems have adopted this process.

The greatest opportunity for cost reduction would likely be determined at the category analysis stage. The type of costs best managed at the different stages depends on the product, market, and hospital or system. One progressive system found tremendous cost reduction during the supplier analysis stage when it determined that the supplier could better manage inventory than the system itself could. In another situation involving orthopedic implants, cost reduction was achieved through price analysis and fact-based negotiation, emphasizing that multiple strategies for managing risk are needed.

Case 2.2 demonstrates that strategic sourcing can reduce costs and risks. However, the fact remains that many systems are not using this potentially effective and efficient business process. Many systems scrutinized by the ASU/CHMR study have not implemented the seven steps presented in this discussion and do not understand how successfully completing one aspect of the supplier relationship process drives success at subsequent stages. These systems fail to recognize that the fact-based negotiation plan cannot be developed or the supply management approach devised until the earlier sourcing steps have been completed.

◆ ◆ ◆

Case 2.2 A Progressive System Director of Materials Management Describes the System Strategy to Reduce Risk

To begin to reduce risk our supply management team categorized the entire family of instruments on the continuum between capital and physician preference. We understood that many hospitals may categorize these items as operating expenses and put them in the commodity category. But we believed that a demand risk exists here and that some of the clinical staff have a high preference for a different brand or slightly different features.

Our next step was to work with a value analysis team to categorize the items using a matrix that allowed us to classify cost and risk. At this stage, the team realized that a market analysis was necessary to determine which of the products could be included in the family of goods. This reduced market risk and information risk. Information risk is included here because it was vital to aggregate the information on all of the related products. Strategy development was difficult also for the team. But we decided that if the item fit into a complex market and uncertain demand, it was necessary to manage the product aggressively. It is noteworthy that different members of the team thought that the product line had different characteristics. As a result, it was decided to have a supplier relationship that was a combination of collaborative and cooperative similar to that which is seen in much of the automotive industry.

The next step was to thoroughly analyze the key suppliers that could deliver the entire family of goods including sphygmomanometers, stethoscopes, laryngoscopes, replacement parts, and related instruments. It was important to know such things as the profitability for this line of business, how important volume was to the suppliers and other related characteristics so that a fact-based negotiation plan could be developed. A price analysis indicated that it was a highly competitive market but relatively high profit margins existed.

◆ ◆ ◆

Although risk will never be completely eliminated,[35] opportunities always exist for cost reduction.[36] It is critical that goals be established and achieved in order to make each organization more competitive and meet customer needs.

CHAPTER THREE

INTERNAL CUSTOMER RELATIONSHIP AND PERFORMANCE MANAGEMENT

Progressive hospitals and hospital systems are characterized by their superior ability to transform financial and human resource inputs into products and services to provide cost-effective and high-quality medical care. Effective management with internal customers allows health care supply chain managers to provide a controlled range and mix of products to meet patient demands. Achievement of this high level of management results from a combination of customer relationship management (CRM) efforts and customer preference management (CPM) efforts. The most observable, measurable, and valuable outcome of such management is product standardization and the cost savings associated with standardization. However, a host of other outcomes may be associated with effective CRM and CPM efforts, including improved clinical outcomes and employee and patient safety, better patient care processes, and strengthened alignment between physicians and the hospital or system. This chapter, read in concert with the evidence in Studies 1, 2, and 4, reveals the significant benefits associated with actively managing the hospital supply chain.[1]

This chapter provides an understanding of the importance of clinical preference standardization processes for materials in hospitals, clarifies the role of the clinician as a principal customer in hospital practice, provides a lens for assessing the contributions that physicians can make to the management of the supply chain, and scrutinizes factors associated with successful decision making and product standardization through formal and informal product value analysis processes and supplier influence. This last focus is due to the fact that the prevalent formal approach to standardization is value analysis as a "methodical search for systems and products that provide the greatest value in resources consumed toward the achievement of a desired outcome."[2] To the extent that value analysis is carried out in collaboration with clinician team participants and clinical leaders, the process and findings of value analysis teams constitute the foundation for effective CRM and ultimately CPM. The consequences of disciplined attention to products, as demonstrated in Case 3.1, are significant to hospitals and systems that are seeking to achieve improved financial performance.

◆ ◆ ◆

Case 3.1 What Happens When a Hospital Service Generates Less Revenue Than Expenses?

The push for standardization is not new. In scrutinizing the issues surrounding total joint arthroplasty (TJA), Richard Iorio and his colleagues observed that while there were striking decreases in the 1980s in the cost of the hospital room and other ancillary services, such as radiology, pharmacy, pathology and laboratory services, implants were not included in this attempt at cost containment. "As a result, the cost of total hip implants [THA] increased as a percentage of hospital costs, from 11% in 1981 to 24% in 1990. The cost of total knee implants increased as a percentage of the hospital costs from 13% in 1983 to 25% in 1991. . . . Essentially, the price increases of the implant in the above example negated the advances made through utilization control of goods and services. To make an impact, both the implant costs and service utilization need to be addressed."

"At Lahey Hitchcock Medical Center, a dual approach addressed the problem of rising costs and decreasing reimbursements. These strategies consisted of clinical pathways and utilization review combined with implant cost reduction." The success with this dual approach was substantial, with the algorithms leading to a reduced length of stay from 9 days in 1991 to 4.5 days in 1995. In approaching the implant cost issue, Lahey Hitchcock Medical Center negotiated a 5% to 10% reduction across the board in cost reduction by implant standardization and competitive bid purchasing. By engaging medical staff to clearly define specifications and engaging in competitive bidding, the center saved 25% on the average hybrid THA and 33% on the average all cemented THA compared to previous costs. Of significance, however, is the interaction between the two strategies with the pathway strategy actually reducing costs associated with other supplies including blood products, drains, antibiotics, and radiology services.

A similar program in 1994 at the Hospital for Joint Diseases analyzed the use of implants, developed a surgeon awareness program regarding the issues pertaining to costs, enlisted the participation of physicians in cost reduction, and engaged in standardization and a competitive bidding system. Here the total cost reduction between 1990 and 1991 was 14% for total hip implants and 24% for total knee implants. "Overall implant costs were reduced by an estimated $706,497 or 23% of the budget for implants for the previous year."

Source: Iorio, R., and Healy, W. "Economic Concerns in Total Joint Arthroplasty: Problems and Solutions." *Medscape General Practice Medicine,* 1999, *1*(1). www.medscape/iewarticle/408479_pring?WebLogicSession= Py1k1tMTfMh.

◆ ◆ ◆

The Case for Standardization

Medicine has been characterized as a profession with extensive autonomy over both the conditions and content of practice.[3] While managed care has frequently encroached on the physician's control over the workplace, physician control at the point of care has been to a large extent sustained. This high level of autonomy and discretion extends to the choice of materials, especially materials that are classified as physician preference items, such as implantable pacemakers, drug-eluting stents, and artificial hip implants. Progressive systems are characterized by clinicians who, in concert with their belief in clinical autonomy and commitment to providing appropriate products in the course of clinical care, understand product value and are adaptable in their choices to help the mission and resource strategy of the system. These organizations have a structure that facilitates collaboration and management and is able to develop strategies and organize formal and informal mechanisms to facilitate standardization.

Standardization is the idea of defining a common frame of reference associated with equivalence that, as demonstrated in Exhibit 3.1, benefits many different constituents; that is, all parties agree to a process of common practices, frames of reference, terminology, metrics, or materials. For the purposes of this discussion, standardization in supply chain includes narrowing the range of products used within the hospital that is applicable to any one procedure or achieving price uniformity across a number of products (or both).

Standardization through the reduction of the number of suppliers or items (stockkeeping units) frequently will allow the hospital or system to negotiate better prices. GPO pricing is frequently price tiered on the ability of a hospital to commit volume. Thus, standardization will allow a hospital or system to participate in a GPO's lower-priced tier. Materials standardization also ensures that physicians and nurses are familiar with items. This familiarity can reduce the chances of error in the delivery of care, improve safety, and contribute to better clinical outcomes. Supply chain materials managers in the ASU/CHMR study suggest that the case for standardization, beyond cost savings alone, is advanced by the

EXHIBIT 3.1. BENEFICIARIES AND BENEFITS OF STANDARDIZATION.

Clinicians
1. Error reduction
2. Improved clinical outcome
3. Improved safety and reduced risk
4. Improved quality
5. Reduced risk from litigation
6. Less time spent on decision making on a day-to-day basis

Materials management
1. Fewer contracting and product choice decisions day-to-day
2. Engage in strategy rather than transactions
3. Higher organizational status and leadership
4. Reduced staff
5. Increased ability to manage risk

Patient benefits
1. Improved outcomes
2. Improved safety
3. Reduced levels of uncertainty

demand for publicly published performance information.[4] However, the growing government and corporate interest in value purchasing and pay for performance for clinical services is only beginning to take into account the full range of factors contributing to outcomes, including product preferences. Creating an organization that can improve its performance through standardization will take great skill and understanding of the complex environment in which medicine is practiced.

Standardization through achieving price equivalency across suppliers allows physicians to choose products that are generally equivalent but have become their product of preference. Such preferences are developed in the course of training that begins in medical school and is carried forward into practice as a result of continued familiarity, support provided by suppliers in the actual use of the product and training associated with the product, and a variety of incentives associated with product use. While there has been increased scrutiny of the financial incentives provided to physicians by suppliers, physicians continue to benefit from fees associated with their speaking on behalf of a supplier, research grants, and consulting arrangements. Such practices have been increasingly scrutinized to ensure that they do not violate antikickback statutes associated with the practice of medicine.[5]

One of the persistent factors reported by progressive systems as contributing to physician collaboration with management is the level of trust that exists between physicians and their managerial counterparts. In nonprogressive systems, it is not uncommon for supply chain managers to point out the misalignment of

EXHIBIT 3.2.   CHARACTERISTICS OF PROGRESSIVE SYSTEMS I.

- Recognition of a window of opportunity for managers to bring together clinicians, under a flag of urgency, to join in inquiry into the role of standardization
- Recognition that the value of product standardization transcends cost saving on individual products (that is, improves outcomes and advances provider and patient safety)
- An understanding of the importance to manage relationships with suppliers
- Capitalizing on the collective knowledge that clinicians gain through continuing professional education, literature review, and interactions with manufacturers

incentives between physicians and management. A supply chain executive in a large academic health center pointed out that it was paradoxical that physicians with whom he worked were willing to entertain standardization efforts in the outpatient joint venture that existed between a hospital and an orthopedic group. Until early in 2005, sharing savings with clinicians as a result of their standardization efforts (gain sharing) has not been permitted. This has meant that the ability of supply chain managers to work to align organizational incentives with physician incentives has been somewhat limited. Management of the supply function in progressive systems, as detailed in Exhibit 3.2, has thus required managers who can understand and advance a wide range of stakeholders and forces affecting the delivery of health services.

In the spring of February 2005, the Office of the Inspector General in Advisory Opinion No. 05–06 (see Study 4) indicated that it would not, under certain circumstances, prosecute hospitals engaged in gain sharing (physicians sharing in savings achieved through changes in processes associated with care as well as savings associated with the selection of less expensive products). How such gain sharing will play out is not at all clear.

The "customer" for hospital products is rarely the patient; rather, it is a physician, nurse, or employee in an ancillary department. While all of these individuals must be satisfied with the products that are available to carry out their everyday work, the centrality of the physician to hospitals requires their participation in a targeted set of purchasing decisions. These decisions should be based on the contribution of the products to patient outcome and safety in the clinical experience. Progressive systems choose to involve clinicians intensely in the selection of products and monitoring product use for the benefit of both the patient and the organization.[6]

Not all hospitals and systems are equally successful in carrying out CRM- and CPM-strategic efforts with their medical staff. However, value analysis, which only five years ago was considered a well-kept secret in the health sector,[7] is now saving progressive systems across the nation hundreds of thousands of dollars. In 2004, one large system, spending in excess of $3.8 million in custom surgical trays, used value analysis techniques to reduce the budget by 10 percent. In the area of surgical gloves, an item where there are frequently strong clinician preferences, value analysis and standardization saved the same system over 15 percent of annual glove purchases.[8]

The key to this kind of success lies in finding the opportunities to engage medical staff that are consistent with their culture. If physicians in a medical group are data driven, the key to success is presenting comparative information on product performance. If there is strong physician leadership, the key may lie in persuading the leaders to endorse certain products. These observations regarding the management of standardization apply to hospital systems in other nations, including those where clinicians are actually system employees. It is instructive to recognize that the gains associated with value analysis are not limited to the United States. As detailed in Study 2, the Peninsula Alliance at Plymouth Hospitals in England was able to save 1.2 million pounds sterling and serve 10 to 15 percent more patients by consolidation and aggregation of demand in the area of cardiology. Similar organizations in other major systems in England are characterized by an enormous gap in collaborative ability between medicine and management. This precludes physician CRM and CPM in areas where supply management can make progress in the near future.

Hospitals and systems are characterized by unique circumstances that either facilitate or impede standardization. In searching for progressive practice organizations, ASU/CHMR scrutiny uncovered systems that have purposively decided to not closely manage the supply chain through standardization. These hospitals and systems tend to be reactive to the product and service demands of various customers, especially physicians. Such systems are also likely to seek purchasing partners (Chapter Four) that have policies that cater to their need for a wide selection of products.

The Clinician as Customer

Before examining the role that physicians play in materials standardization, it is important to look at their function as both a participant and a customer of the health care supply chain. The principal focus of internal supply chain management is the myriad of end users or customers. The hospital is an unusual organization that is characterized by very different "customers" at different points in the supply chain.[9] Patients, with virtually hundreds of different medical problems or diagnoses, are the downstream recipients of an incredible host of nonclinical and clinical products and services. While patients are the source of revenues and the recipients of the value attached to goods and services, traditionally they only marginally influence the upstream decisions that are made. Organizations and individuals act on behalf of patients as their formal and informal agents. These agents determine the nutritional balance of food, the supplies that shape the physical environment, and the clinically necessary products associated with direct medical and surgical treatment. While it is clear that a more patient-driven system is emerging as the result of direct-to-patient marketing and an interest in providing more patient-friendly services (such as customized gourmet meals), patients are actually in a position to express their preferences in only a minority of instances.

Recognizing that one of the hospital's principal customers is the physician (who frequently is not an employee of the hospital), Mark Pauley, an economist at the University of Pennsylvania, has referred to the hospital as the "doctor's workshop."[10] In reality, the hospital is a workshop for many different individuals who focus their attention on the care of patients. Supply chain managers, clinical department administrators, nurses, allied health workers, discharge planners, and of course physicians make decisions or directly influence the flow of supplies and services. The physician, however, has an especially powerful role. By determining 80 percent of hospital expenditures through their orders, physicians drive virtually every aspect of health care.[11] The continuous development of the hospitalist as a physician agent of the patient's community-based physician, hospital, or medical plan is an indication of the continuing physician-directed medical care model in the hospital.[12] The individuals working in the hospitals are the end users even though not the recipients of these products and services. Thus, a key aspect of internal supply chain management in the hospital is the development of strategies and processes that meet the needs of clinician customers and cost-effective management.

One of the very few surveys of physicians' concerns in the course of product selection (Table 3.1) reveals that surgeons rank price and hospital contracts at the very bottom of their list of considerations.[13] Thus, customer relationship management and customer product management take place in what was earlier described as a very difficult environment of autonomous physician practice.[14] The inability to influence choice is also associated with the lack of professional consensus and unbiased data regarding product superiority. The expertise that physicians gain in the course of using products, in concert with their relationships with suppliers around product service and research, shapes their preferences.[15] Even in clinical areas where evidence provides guidance to shape physician decision making, adherence to emergent standards is less than many have expected.[16]

TABLE 3.1.   RANK ORDERING OF SURGEON CONSIDERATION IN PRODUCT SELECTION.

Rank	Factor Considered
1	Clinical results
2	The ability to reproduce results
3	Ease of use
4	Familiarity with the product
5	Instrumentals
6	Representative services
7	Price
8	Hospital contracts

Cosmopolitans and Locals

Recognizing the role of physicians in product selection and evaluation, health care managers need to be aware of the level of participation that they should be able to expect from the doctors at their institution. As the ASU/CHMR study scrutinized the supply chain function in hospitals and systems, it found that a positive relationship between supply chain management and medical staff is consistently a feature that differentiates progressive systems. Supply chain managers in nonprogressive organizations characterize the physicians as dominated by attitudes and behaviors that are not supportive of their hospitals or systems. They define these individuals as uninterested in the operational issues facing the hospital.

The managers frequently point out "cosmopolitan" behavior characteristics, which are strongly grounded on professional norms and values that are external to the hospital or system.[17] They also feel that success in their collaboration is dependent on the efforts of the very few physicians whom they characterized as having a mix of "cosmopolitan" attributes and "local," or organization-focused, characteristics (Table 3.2).[18] While cosmopolitan characteristics are frequently attributed to individuals in academic health centers and large organizations, from the perspective of the supply chain manager, this characterization of medical staff seems to be as common in nonteaching environments as in academic health centers. Furthermore, the cosmopolitan versus local distinction is common in both large and small systems. Hospitals, unlike other organizations in which professionals are dominant in decision making, do very little to socialize physicians around the hospital or system value structure. They provide physicians with few incentives for participation in hospital management activities and develop few career ladders for physicians to participate in hospital or system affairs.[19]

TABLE 3.2.   CHARACTERISTICS OF COSMOPOLITANS AND LOCALS.

Cosmopolitans	Locals
Identify themselves more strongly with professional and functional specialty	Identify themselves strongly with the employing organization
More likely to be mobile	Career oriented with one firm
More concerned about their specialized skill or functional area	Committed and dedicated to the organization as an entity
Little concerned with internal details or politics unless they are inhibiting	More involved in and concerned about internal details and politics
Seek recognition beyond the company boundaries, for example, from peers in other organizations	Rely on getting recognition within the organization
Less tolerant and more vocal about job climate problems	More tolerant of and less vocal about job climate problems
Tend to have few—and relatively loose—ties with people in the organization	Develop closer and more extensive relationships with people in the organization
Have less influence because of less involvement	Tend to have more influence

Source: Alford, J. M. "The People Mix." *Air University Review,* May-June 1976.
http://www.airpower.maxwell.af.mil/airchronicles/aureview/1976/may-jun/alford.html.

Physician Relations in Progressive Systems

How do progressive hospitals and systems differ from their nonprogressive counterparts? Progressive system leadership does not buy into the idea that physician allegiance to their profession precludes their involvement in purchasing decisions. While they recognize that cosmopolitans have outside allegiances, they also recognize that cosmopolitans are attuned to the emerging best practices in the field and want to be associated with high-performing organizations. Also cosmopolitans, because of their wide-ranging networks, frequently have insider knowledge of competing and emerging materials. Cosmopolitans are furthermore influenced by data that compare their resource use and outcomes against other leaders in the field and are open to change.

The managers in progressive systems understand that while it is unrealistic to think that busy clinicians will devote extensive time to organize and manage ongoing standardization and supply chain activities, they are frequently disposed to assume ad hoc leadership roles. Physicians frequently participate in deliberations and influence their colleagues once decisions are made. Cosmopolitans can also support standardization by articulating the benefits gained by applying

TABLE 3.3.   CLASSIFICATION OF PHYSICIAN TYPES.

	Low Commitment to Resources	High Commitment to Resources
High acceptance of corporate values	D: Team Player—"Good Corporate Citizen"	C: Leader—"Strives on Behalf of the Whole"
Low acceptance of corporate values	A: Detached Clinician—"Uninvolved"	B: Independent—"Fights for Own Patch"

Source: Winkless, T., Pedler, M., and Mascie-Taylor, H. "Doctors and Dilemmas." In D. Sanderson and J. Brown (eds.), *Managing Medicine: A Survival Guide.* London: Financial Times Health Care, Maple House, 1997.

disciplined scientific thinking to product selection. In one of the more progressive systems studied, influential physicians even participated in visits to policy agencies, such as the Centers for Medicare and Medicaid Services, to advocate for reimbursement strategies that support their decisions to use certain products and advocate for special reimbursement for those products.

Assessing the Physician Customer

Progressive organizations find it useful to think more broadly about the medical staff in terms of their willingness to demonstrate concern for organizational resources and commitment to organizational values.[20] This allows managers to better anticipate physician potential for involvement in collaborative efforts, such as standardization. The depictions of physician types in Table 3.3 provide an important classification scheme for managers who want to understand the potential for physician involvement in clinical standardization efforts.[21]

Type A: Detached Physician. The detached physician, in the Winkless, Pedler, and Mascie-Taylor classification scheme, is generally uninvolved with the system, has a focus on one-to-one patient care and clinical management, and has minimal interest, awareness, or involvement beyond this level.[22] These are often attending physicians who may have privileges at multiple hospitals or may be employed through various agencies. Although they frequently have low knowledge and acceptance of the system's values or financial well-being, they collectively command substantial use of the organization's resources. The extent to which they affect organizational performance through use of resources depends on their specialty and frequency of interaction with the organization.

Assessment of how the Type A physician's behavior influences cost, outcome, safety, and market position will determine how vigorously to address the physician's behavior. Managers in progressive systems attempt to target Type A physicians, whose costly utilization behavior represents a threat to achieving goals, in these ways:

- Supporting physician programs for attending education programs that emphasize the benefits attached to participation in standardization efforts
- Involving attending physicians in organizational efforts to develop performance (cost and outcome) data that are relevant to their specialty
- Enlisting suppliers to help influence the attending physician's choice of products.
- Linking the detached physician with a respected "insider" colleague

Type B: The Independent. The independent physician, as depicted by Winkless, Pedler, and Mascie-Taylor, generally has a focus on his or her specialty.[23] These individuals are confident in their clinical abilities. They have strong political skills and are frequently entrepreneurial. There is great risk that the independent will be demanding of resources while having a fairly low acceptance of or interest in the system's strategy, culture, and values. The independent frequently has a low knowledge of and appreciation for management and believes that rules are to be broken. Traditionally, the independent would advocate securing preferred materials and may be unlikely to follow evidence-based directives. As outcomes and evidence-based standards emerge, these physicians may increase their levels of compliance due to colleague-related pressures or opportunities to participate in gainsharing. Such individuals are frequently rapid adopters of technologies.[24] This attribute has important implications for materials cost and control because they are able to adapt to new technology more easily than their colleagues can. Independents may be employed by the system, but many are physicians with attending privileges, frequently admitting a small proportion of their patients to any one hospital.

The independent is less likely than others to be able to advance his or her own agenda in an environment that has strong formal systems in place. At the same time, an excess of rules may lead the independent to withdraw from practicing in the organization. Strategies that incorporate and recognize the independent's input are likely to reap the rewards of the independent, working vigorously to ensure that the position to which he or she has committed is operational.

Type C: The Leader. Leaders, in the Winkless, Pedler, and Mascie-Taylor classificatory scheme, strive on behalf of the whole organization and have a strong commitment to it.[25] Leaders are also characterized by their broad vision while engaging in strategic thinking. They may be politically astute and influential, act as change agents, and have very good interpersonal skills.

It is important to be sure that these are individuals who are not seen by their colleagues as having sided with management and no longer represent the interests of the larger medical staff.[26] From a clinical perspective, these individuals may be either cosmopolitans or locals, but the most valuable among them will be the cosmopolitans who have developed a strong appreciation for the organization's goals and understand how clinical excellence can move the organization ahead. The cosmopolitan who has attained leadership skills and perspective will provide the most value to the success of management efforts in improving supply chain performance.

Progressive organizations have placed leaders in positions that incorporate managerial and clinical thinking to ensure that they become the thought leaders in the organization. Organizations that have a deficit of such individuals may want to consider applicants' leadership characteristics as they engage in recruiting new clinical affiliates.

Type D: The Team Player. Team players are good corporate citizens who advise rather than lead the organization. These individuals are posited by Winkless, Pedler, and Mascie-Taylor to be economical with resources, participative, cooperative, loyal, and supportive.[27] They may be more likely than other physicians to express local rather than cosmopolitan values and can be highly effective when they collaborate. Team players who are not respected for their clinical excellence, however, may not be as useful as others in moving the organization to engage in value analysis and standardization.

Medical Staff Mix. Hospitals and systems are characterized by a mix of these four types of physicians. There has not been an attempt to systematically carefully classify medical staff into these types. Thus, it is difficult to specify what mix leads to best performance. The ASU/CHMR study observations are consistent with studies suggesting that progressive systems build committed medical staff participation by (1) involving physicians in supply chain standardization processes over long periods of time, (2) involving physicians early on issues pertaining to product selection emerge, and (3) and carefully considering physician concerns.[28] Progressive systems also realize that nonphysician clinicians, such as nurses, are key to working with physicians to achieve standardization in the supply chain. HCA, a large investor-owned health care system that is actively working to manage the supply chain across several hundred hospitals, employs large numbers of nurses to influence standardization. This strategy is consistent with research findings that even physicians who do not participate in formal standardization processes frequently accept decisions when nurses have formally represented the physicians' preferences.[29] The nurse in this instance often serves as an ambassador who is able to integrate across organizational units and ensure vertical linkages in the organization.[30] In progressive supply organizations, managers recognize the potential for placing physicians, nurses, and others in linking-pin roles as facilitators, liaisons, and orchestrators of change through communication, information management, evidence-based management, and pressures associated with colleague influence and control.

The Role of Value Analysis Teams

Value analysis provides hospitals and systems with a tool to achieve savings with both commodity and clinical preference items. For systems that are disciplined in this effort, savings are reported in the range of millions of dollars on an annual basis.[31] However, the ability of hospitals to develop such programs, especially as they relate to the most expensive clinical preference items, is highly uneven.

Prescription for Team Success

Successful value analysis teams (VATs) are highly disciplined, translate their common commitment into performance goals, and seek out measures to assess their performance.[32] Successful teams, in considering the factors identified in Table 3.4, (1) establish urgency by demanding performance standards and direction, (2) pay particular attention to the commitment by the organization to the teams' importance, (3) establish roles for behavior to help achieve common team goals, (4) challenge the group through the infusion of new information, (5) spend necessary time together, and (6) provide positive feedback, recognition, and reward.[33] Successful teams are also characterized by the inclusion of both senior management and physician representatives, determination of specific annual goals for cost savings

TABLE 3.4.   PRINCIPAL VALUE ANALYSIS FACTORS.

Factors Considered by Value Analysis Teams

1 Technical properties and performance
2 Safety and risk to patients and health care workers
3 Efficacy and effectiveness
4 Economic attributes
5 Acceptability to patients and clinicians (comfort, ease of use, utility)
6 Risk of liability
7 Potential for standardization
8 Impact on market share and competitiveness
9 Requirements for facility modification and work flow
10 Manufacturer reputation and support
11 Capacity of vendor to provide sufficient and reliable supply

from the committee's efforts, and provision of concrete, quantitative analysis and follow-up to ensure that benefits are realized.[34]

The development of effective teams requires the establishment of high levels of trust between the various stakeholders and team members. Katz, in studying project teams, has pointed out that team-building performance increases over the initial period of team formation. Performance increases as members understand "each other's capabilities, contributions, and working styles."[35] His observation of sustained performance over the first few years of a team's life cycle and subsequent deterioration requires attention in the health supply arena.

GPOs and Value Analysis

Depending on the configuration of the systems and the structure of the medical staff, the engagement of physicians in standardization and GPO affiliation seem to affect how hospitals and systems engage in value analysis. The options include:

- Internal and active engagement through systemwide committees
- Internal and active engagement through individual system member committees
- Outsourcing the engagement through consultants
- Outsourcing the engagement through the GPO
- Passive engagement through the distribution of information provided by GPO and other sources
- Some combination of these options[36]

Curiously, not all hospitals or systems value or participate in these GPO services.[37] In addition, systems that are very active in GPO standardization efforts almost always carry out their own value analysis and drive to collaborate in product selection for GPO purchasing. When GPO contracts do not supply the products or cost these systems can achieve on their own, these organizations are likely to purchase outside their GPO contract or engage the GPO to work closely with them to secure desired products and prices. Others seem very anxious to follow on selections made within the GPO process that frequently rely on member and client representatives.

Commitment to Customer Relationship and Customer Preference Management

The ASU/CHMR study reveals that health care systems differ in their commitment to achieve standardization. Variation in commitment can be viewed as related to structural, cultural, and managerial differences that characterize systems. There are a number of important barriers to managing customer relationships and preferences.

Structural Barriers

Structural barriers to managing customer relationships and preferences include system centralization, size, and marketplace domination.

System Centralization. The practice of centralization has the potential for an integrated delivery network to manage a variety of members with a common set of standards and practices (Chapter Five). In many of the progressive systems examined in the ASU/CHMR study, successful centralization improved the chances for product standardization. These systems capitalize on the collective knowledge that clinicians gain through continuing professional education, literature review, and interactions with manufacturers during professional meetings and direct-to-clinician marketing sessions. Through centralization, they also build collaboration with physician leaders in various system locations.

The ASU/CHMR study also recognizes that variation across geographically dispersed hospitals within a system poses obstacles to centralized standardization efforts. This is consistent with research findings that centralized administrative control can serve as a barrier to the alignment of incentives and goals between physicians and a system.[38] Clinician participation on a systemwide VAT and involvement in dissemination of VAT decisions can counter the problematic aspects of centralization. Buy-in at various local levels is important. It is also important that physicians understand that standardization does not prohibit products to meet the full range of patient needs from entering the system and that there will be ample opportunities to consider new products.

One of the progressive systems studied convened its systemwide surgical VAT monthly. (This frequency of meeting, even at times when no major changes in products were being entertained, is consistent with the idea that team members require frequent interaction.) While this system used its meeting to entertain queries by physicians and others across a wide range of products, it was clear that an incredible amount of time had been used prior to the meeting to develop comparative product data. Such data include information pertaining to physician preferences and relationships with suppliers, information pertaining to outcomes and safety, and costs associated with product standardization and change. Information was distributed to team members prior to meetings, and concerns were addressed as individual team members raised concerns or anticipated questions. This pre-meeting work consistently paid off by allowing the use of a consensus agenda that ensures that meetings are brief and focused on decision making. The minutes from one monthly meeting, which operated on a consensus agenda, included the following items and resolution:

- *Item.* Entertain the report from an ad hoc group of surgeons to reduce the number of vendors for a product.
  Resolution. Follow up with report to form the team.
- *Item.* Consider a new scrub product that was being evaluated by a group of surgeons at one of the principal hospitals.
  Resolution. Approved.
- *Item.* Consider the request for a relatively expensive technology product that reduces the use of blood for implant surgery.
  Resolution. Invite presentation at next meeting.
- *Item.* Request product to auto-transfuse blood back into the patient.
  Resolution. Approved.
- *Item.* Consider evaluation of new cement. Report on outcomes is negative.
  Resolution. Denied.

For each of these considerations, there was careful input from both clinicians and supply chain management staff—with conspicuous physician committee leadership. Key, however, was the support given to these physicians in preparing data on cost, clinical efficacy, patient acceptance, and market considerations.

System Size and Marketplace Domination. Both large and small systems in the ASU/CHMR study report that GPOs assisted in educating the clinical staff about products. Systems of different size also use GPOs for securing a wider range of products. One executive indicated that in his relatively small system (two hospitals), staffed by many attending physicians who practice "geographically all over the community," there was no articulated strategic effort to achieve standardization. While he hoped that the clinical staff was provided advisory recommendations in order to influence physician product selection by the GPO's VAT, the system had no intention of directly soliciting physicians to conform to internal or external standards.

A very large system with small, geographically dispersed hospitals echoed the small system's lack of aggressiveness in physician engagement. Common to both systems is the absence of a strategy to manage physician product selection. In addition, fears exist that attempts to shape physician choice would cause more problems than gains for the system. Perhaps it is fair to say that such systems do engage in CRM by providing medical staff with the products of their own choice. The ASU/CHMR study did not characterize such systems as progressive in their practices. These systems are rarely distinguished by efforts to better manage other supply chain functions such as distribution, cost management, or risk reduction.

The previous discussion addresses a continuing reluctance on the part of managers to engage medical staff in standardization processes. When questioned about this reluctance, they report that standardization efforts in areas where there are virtually hundreds of products that can serve multiple functions for many different clinicians (for example, suture reduction) are too sensitive an area for clinical engagement. Many attitudes appear to be grounded in stereotyped views of clinician behavior. The managers articulating these sentiments have generally been in the field for a good number of years and perceive a fairly insurmountable gap between the cultures of medicine and management. They also have invested little effort or few resources in building physician leadership and have no strategies for taking advantage of that leadership within the system.

As suggested above, reluctance to engage the medical staff on standardization is frequently based on the assumption that product restriction will lead physicians to shift admissions to other organizations. Health supply chain managers frequently report that physician loyalty to the hospital is very fragile and based on noninterference. This impression is found in the continuing belief among materials managers that medical staff continue to be "uncooperative" when it comes to the intersection of medicine and business. One materials manager explains that physicians are indifferent to costs and other nonclinical aspects of product selection that result in standardization and committed purchasing. The ASU/CHMR study observations reveal that progressive system managers do not fully support this position. Progressive systems work consistently to alert their medical staff to differences in product costs, quality, and possible clinical outcome variations.

A recent study suggests that it is generally a myth that physicians will shift their admissions to other hospitals if their preferred products are limited.[39] It has also been found that those who do leave improve the hospital's cost per case ratio due to their more costly profiles. Managers who believe that active engagement of clinical staff will have negative effects on the organization are not very likely to develop strategies that include standardization.

Cultural Barriers

Hospitals and health care delivery systems are frequently characterized by organizational cultures that are focused around individual departments or specialties.[40] While some departments defer decisions to the autonomy of the individual professional workers, forward-looking organizations are characterized by "atomized" units that allow flexibility and decision making that benefit the broader organization.[41] Such atomized organizations frequently bind various parts of the organization "like molecules into a strong corporate whole through the shared corporate ties that define what the company of the future is all about."[42]

Kaiser Permanente is a good example of such organization. It has long been recognized for its culture of physician participation through its group practices. Consistent with this effort, Kaiser, which is unique in its structure in the United States, is characterized by over sixty specialty product teams. These teams report to the National Product Council, which reflects a culture with a commitment to excellence in practice, effective use of limited resources, and bringing value to Kaiser's members. The Kaiser teams are staffed by executive medical directors and other experts who consider evidence on safety, efficacy, cost, effectiveness, quality of life, system impact, and legal and social implications.[43] The Kaiser physician groups have a strong alignment of incentives, both clinical and financial, to the health plan. As the CHMR/ASU study considered other systems with strongly aligned physician incentives, there was no consistent pattern of success in value analysis and standardization. This suggests that organizational culture may be more important than physician employment in achieving standardization.

Discipline in approaching standardization is not restricted to extremely large systems. BJC HealthCare (St. Louis) and Swedish Medical Center (Seattle) pride themselves on having built a culture characterized by commitment to working with clinicians across the system to achieve consensus on materials. Since Swedish Medical Center does not belong to a GPO, it cannot rely on GPO processes to aid clinicians in product selection and sourcing. It carefully manages the clinical standardization process internally. Exhibit 3.3 documents a number of the characteristics demonstrated by progressive systems in this important area.

Culture expresses itself in many different ways in regard to product selection and standardization. Some items are defined as "emotionally charged" in the eyes of medical staff, while others are treated as prime items for standardization. Hospitals and systems in the ASU/CHMR study report both opportunities and barriers in selecting products that are candidates for standardization. A survey of CEOs and materials managers found that opportunities for standardization include both commodities (such as lab supplies and gloves) and physician preference items (such

EXHIBIT 3.3. CHARACTERISTICS OF PROGRESSIVE SYSTEMS II.

- Collaboration with their medical staff to consider clinical preference items as well as commodities for standardization and committed purchasing
- An understanding that they have leverage in working with the medical staff and that medical staff are responsive to information relating to their own behavior
- Belief that physician allegiance to their profession does not preclude their involvement in clinically oriented deliberations that would benefit the system
- Placement of leaders in positions that incorporate managerial and clinical thinking to ensure that they become the thought leaders in the organization
- A consistent strategy for physician stakeholder engagement

as orthopedic and spine implants).[44] The ASU/CHMR case studies reveal that there are differences in opinion, within and between systems, in what actually constitute appropriate items for standardization. One major system (BJC HealthCare in St. Louis) experienced great success in reducing the number of suture stockkeeping units. Other systems report that they are unconvinced that such standardization can be achieved due to physicians' preferences for particular sutures. This can be true even if the only difference between a competing product is the thread length.

Physician relationships with suppliers, which provide a wide range of services for surgeons and other specialists, make standardization very difficult. In many instances, these representatives provide technical assistance regarding specialty products in the operating room. Such collaboration is most common in orthopedics and cardiology, where new technologies are quickly emerging and the half-life of products can be fairly short. Supplier representatives provide physicians with access to products that may not be stocked in the hospital by bringing them into the hospital on the day a procedure is to be carried out. Finally, physicians frequently have preferences for items in which they have had a role in developing. While such preferences may represent conflicts of interests for the physicians themselves, physicians believe that their performance is dependent on such products of choice.

Managerial Barriers

Physicians involved in VATs of progressive systems are willing and able to participate in and lead standardization efforts. At one of the ASU/CHMR study sites, VAT meetings were designed around the strategic engagement of physicians on four areas: (1) product selection, (2) vendor service, (3) research implications related to product selection, and (4) the differences between emergent products. Managers interviewed stated that such collaboration relies on strong trust by clinicians that management will carry out the general will of the medical staff. Trust is built by working closely with physicians on all relevant issues, inclusiveness of all relevant physicians on a given issue, recognition that different physicians will have different concerns (for example, research versus nonresearch), and a commitment to excellence in clinical facilities as a consequence of achieved savings. Physicians are consistently brought together to identify areas where exceptions are important for improved clinical outcomes.

Success with VATs

Success with VATs, especially in the area of clinical preference items, appears to vary significantly on the basis of the (1) organization's culture, (2) mix of physician types, (3) mission pertaining to excellence, (4) past relationships with physicians, (5) ability of the system to demonstrate need, and (6) the willingness of the organization to manage the relationship of the physician with suppliers. The CHMR/ASU study respondents frequently reported key accomplishments in standardization and associated them with savings. However, consistency in strategy and the sense that efforts could be replicated and made easier or extended as a more strategic process as learning progressed was not present.[45]

Leadership organizations even learn from their mistakes and anticipate opportunities. Progressive VATs consider both the opportunities missed in achieving reduced prices in order to gain experience for future deliberations. The ASU/CHMR study respondents reported that they needed to be forward looking in their deliberations. Discussions included strategies for managing a therapy that appears to be approaching its half-life and on how to manage the emergence of a new therapeutic class that would have competition in the near future.

The Changing Landscape of Customer Relationships and Customer Preference Management

Perhaps it is best to think of the health industry as containing a web of customer relationships and preference management strategies. In the most progressive systems, materials managers and physicians work closely together to achieve the most favorable conditions for purchasing their desired products. Progressive systems understand that it is important for them to manage their relationships with suppliers. Effective management at the hospital and system levels requires an understanding of how those with allegiances upstream from the hospital or system work to shape the movement of products and how these suppliers work to sustain their marketplace position. Effective management also requires understanding how purchasing executives can best spend their time to engage the manufacturers themselves—either individually through their system or in collaboration with purchasing partners.[46]

Progressive systems strategically manage supplier relationships. The discussion of suppliers was focused principally on the system's need to sustain clinician loyalty and the various strategies they employ. While suppliers may have special relationships with "cosmopolitan" physicians, it is important to stress that supplier relationships extend throughout the clinician community. Suppliers bring value by providing mechanisms for physicians to remain aware of the latest developments in materials. They also assist physicians to become proficient in the use of new technologies and provide needed information for both the physician and the system to engage in product selection. A principal goal of suppliers is to move transactional contact to a more committed relationship.[47]

Progressive organizations recognize that supplier relationships must be managed to ensure excellence in value chain performance. It is not clear if many systems understand what drives the decision making of physicians on clinical preference items. In addition, they infrequently recognize the extent to which the patient, as a result of direct-to-patient marketing, may occupy a new role in the equation for the purchase of such items. Managing the power relationships between suppliers and health care systems is critical if systems are to reduce their costs through achieving better prices.[48] To accomplish this, progressive health care systems structure their environment to build buyer dominance and capitalize on the interdependence between buyers and suppliers. This includes linking favorable price to high levels of product purchase commitment.

Systems are frequently uncertain about the conditions of contracts that best fit their strategy. They recognize that when there is an increase in commitment to suppliers, they are able to gain supplier support and improved pricing. They also are aware that sole- or dual-source contracting can place them in a dependent position with suppliers over time. One consequence is less-than-desirable pricing and the inability to convert to emergent products. Buyers recognize that suppliers also differ in their strategies. Some are committed to cutting-edge and unique products, which frequently carry high price tags. Others provide products at lower costs that meet specifications, hoping to accrue volume. Strong management-clinician collaboration is necessary to ensure an understanding of the marketplace for goods.

Suppliers benefit from an environment in which there is little real knowledge by end users of the cost associated with products. They also benefit from the extent to which physicians value, if not rely on, supplier collaboration in both practice and research. Physicians who have strong commitments to suppliers cannot be expected to play value-free roles in product evaluation and standardization decision making. For ethical reasons, physicians with such conflicts should be excluded from some product selection deliberations or, at the very least, declare their involvement with the supplier.

One progressive system in the CHMR/ASU study tightly controls the presence and flow of supplier-held inventory into the operating room. It has a strict policy of not paying for any product that is not approved by the value analysis process. This includes "upgraded" products that are of higher cost. The result of this policy and enforcement is a substantial reduction in costs for goods not under contract.

Study 2 demonstrates that increased physician understanding of the profit structure surrounding the supplier industry. The study indicates that transparency in supplier relationships and pricing may lead physicians to take a stronger interest in resource use. This is no different from the processes used by some GPOs that, through VATs, secure high levels of signed commitment from its clients.

Suppliers and the Clinician Customer

Relationships between physicians and suppliers are grounded in a wide variety of factors that include (1) early exposure to products and preferences developed by clinicians in the course of training, (2) research relationships (physicians themselves are innovators as well as involved in the trials of pharmaceuticals and products), (3) the introduction of products in the course of continuing education, (4) one-on-one physician office visits, and (5) product introduction through consignment to the hospital of materials that may not even be under contract.[49]

A recent study of orthopedic surgeons helps us understand how physicians value supplier relationships and identifies some of the factors pertaining to the mismatch between physician, supplier, and purchaser relationships.[50] Table 3.1 revealed that although product choice is based on a range of factors that materials managers would see as important, such as price and existing contracts, these factors are not foremost in clinician thinking.

When spine surgeons were asked what factors influenced their use of spinal fusion cages, patient care issues were ranked high; cost issues ranked substantially lower. Given the substantial differences in price for many clinical preference materials, this is a critical finding. Clinicians increasingly recognize that failure to select the most clinically appropriate product puts them, and perhaps even the patient, at considerable risk. To reduce risk, over half of the respondents to the survey reported having changed their selection of materials due to a fear of lawsuits. In this regard, clinicians recognize that materials matter. Progressive systems, as indicated in Exhibit 3.4, will take advantage of the tensions that clinicians perceive around product selection issues to engage clinicians.

Surgeons in the study expressed doubts about (1) the actual need for certain products, (2) difficulties in linking parts of various pieces of technology, (3) problems visualizing how the product could be placed, (4) problems placing the product, and (5) difficulties in integrating different company products. When asked to state what characterizes the best companies, surgeons, not surprisingly, ranked the quality of service and representatives as paramount in their assessments.[51]

EXHIBIT 3.4. CHARACTERISTICS OF PROGRESSIVE SYSTEMS III.

- Engagement of clinicians in product choice by taking advantage of the tensions that clinicians perceive around product selection issues
- A recognition that although it is not in their interest to disintermediate the relationships built between physicians and suppliers, it is important to strengthen the relationship by establishing strategies for physician and system to collectively engage suppliers
- Value analysis of and collaboration on product selection for GPO purchasing

This presents an interesting paradox as surgeon preferences are considered. On the one hand, surgeons speak of clinical results and patient outcomes as important influences in their product decisions. On the other hand, although price may not be the most influential factor in a surgeon's choice of product, it remains foremost in their minds. Spine surgeons reported having lost income as a result of a cost-conscious environment. In this sense, their most frequently spoken message to manufacturers is related to lowering costs. Again, this is a tension that can be of use as hospitals and systems work with clinical staff to secure best prices as a result of product negotiations.

A report by VHA, an alliance of a large number of hospitals across the United States, suggests that the direct relationship between the physician and supplier, based on physician preference and supplier support, results in a lack of coordination, inefficiencies, high costs, and contentious relationships. Change will require that hospitals and systems "proactively seek physician involvement and work to address the historically strong relationships between physicians and suppliers."[52] The VHA study reinforces the importance and impact of the structure of the relationships between physicians and suppliers both within and outside the hospital. It stresses the importance of understanding the nature of value-added services provided by the supplier and specification of the hospital-suppler relationships. Progressive systems, however, have not placed themselves between the clinician and the supplier in a contentious manner. Rather, through active collaboration with the clinical staff through VATs, progressive systems use the medical staff to meet the supplier on a more level playing field. In Study 2, the system demonstrates physician-system collaboration by having the chief of medical staff sign all requests for purchasing. This memorializes the intention of the medical staff to use the product if it is secured at a reasonable price.

Few hospitals or systems clearly articulate their policies to suppliers. Progressive systems have given substantial thought to this area and have developed and enforced rules to ensure effective management of the supplier-physician relationship. These systems recognize that it is not possible and not in their interest to fully eliminate the relationships between physicians and suppliers. Supplier representatives assist in ensuring that needed products are available for surgery by acting as distributors for their own products and bringing a range of potentially useful products into the operating room. They also provide assistance to physicians in the course of the physician's carrying out a procedure. While this may come a shock to the layperson, who assumes that the physician is the sole repository of clinical knowledge in an environment characterized by highly complex and frequently changing technical products, a teaming between those who manufacture and those who apply products is a feature of practice in many fields. Nevertheless, the control of these relationships is important. University Community

Health in Tampa has assembled policies that structure the relationship between suppliers, physicians, and the hospital:

- All sales representatives must make an initial contact with the buyer in purchasing prior to an initial visit.
- Sales representatives must register with the materials management department at the facility before visiting.
- All product samples and trial equipment must have approval from the materials management department.
- Community Health will not assume responsibility for samples, supplies, or equipment left on the premises without prior approval.[53]

In many instances, major systems refuse to pay for any material used in a procedure that is not included in an existing contract.

Suppliers and the Patient Customer

One needs to watch television for only a few hours to realize the investment in direct-to-customer (DTC) advertising by pharmaceutical companies and, increasingly, medical companies supplying high-cost implantable items such as hip and knee prostheses. Leadership in hospitals and systems has not identified DTC advertising as affecting system supply management strategies. The orthopedic surgeon survey discussed previously reports that the vast majority of surgeons have had at least one patient who inquired about specific procedures (93 percent), specific techniques (84 percent), and specific company products (37 percent). Fifty-six percent of the surgeons indicated that the number of patients making such inquiries was on the rise.[54] The publicity around the approval of drug-eluting stents has led to patients' gaining awareness of brand names for cardiology implants and the opening of the door to a whole new era of patient demand. One of the more progressive systems in the study confirmed that patients were being provided with information on spinal cages and that the information was shaping practice.

As systems engage in standardization processes, management needs to help structure clinicians' responses to patient expectations. Information packets that help patients understand why clinicians may choose products other than those seen on television need to be developed. In an environment where patients have product awareness, the physician is the key to educating the patient to accept equivalent products, recognize that certain advertised products may not fit a specific case, or make the patient aware of payer policies that do not allow a specific product. When there is physician and patient demand for a product not normally

TABLE 3.5.   WHEN PATIENTS DEMAND PRODUCTS.

	Positive Physician Preference	Negative Physician Preference
On system formulary	Meet patient expectations	Threat of loss of patient (need for physician education)
Not on system formulary	Threat of loss of case and provider on case (need to consider exceptions)	Threat of loss of patient (need for patient education)

available in a given hospital or system, policies must be in place to determine how exceptions should be managed to reduce dissatisfaction by end users. It is, however, too early to assess if patient demand for products will lead to the loss of patients to alternative hospital settings. Internal and external VATs will find themselves pressured by physicians advocating for products that reflect patients' demands. Multitiered strategies, such as those developed by the managed care industry to allow patient choice in pharmaceuticals, may not be appropriate for the acute care product marketplace. As demonstrated in Table 3.5, managing both physician and patient preferences is a key to success in the changing environment of product selection.

Summary and Conclusion

Physicians, who frequently have very strong preferences for brand products and the services associated with branded products, may be reluctant to accept alternative products, even in the face of evidence regarding equivalencies. This is especially true for high-cost clinical preference items in cardiology and orthopedics. As value analysis processes reveal equivalences among product configuration and outcomes as well as substantial discrepancies in prices for equivalent products, managers find themselves increasingly supported by physicians (despite their strong desire for branded items) in negotiations with suppliers over price reductions. Thus, the outcome of value analysis may be standardization (or a cap) on price paid for a certain time, if not the reduction of branded products.

Standardization efforts for both commodities and clinical preference items are the key to achieving increased savings according to a broad consensus.[55] Both physician and nurse involvement and leadership in product analysis is necessary for standardization success. VATs routinely consider low-technology and low-cost items, such as surgical gloves and sutures, which cumulatively have a high cost impact on hospitals and systems. Products are subject to scrutiny at multiple levels. A lower-cost item to replace a frequently used plastic specimen jar might be found unacceptable to a clinician if it regularly failed to seal and led to spills of potentially dangerous contents. Thus, standardization efforts must also consider the linkages among clinician, product selection, cost, and outcomes as accomplished through VATs within systems and GPOs.

Assuming that items provide desired outcomes, the outcome of VATs may well be information supplied to negotiators, who can counter supplier claims for superiority of products. The result is the ability of the purchaser to influence the entire market price for a given product. The function can be the accommodation of both the clinician's desire for choice and the hospital or system drive for cost containment. In considering clinical preference items, materials management executives require a sophisticated understanding of the factors physicians consider in making product decisions. While the medical device manufacturers as well as pharmaceutical industries have studied this topic carefully, the sparse research on factors that drive clinician preference hampers effective managerial action.

Through standardization efforts, progressive hospitals and systems consider how products contribute to the strategic direction of the organization. Indeed, good VATs become value management teams by demonstrating value in relation to the system's overall goals, including cost reduction (Chapter Two), safety, and outcomes.

Part of a successful hospital and system strategy for implementing standardization will depend on providing metrics pertaining to products and their relationship to the performance of the supply chain. As the ASU/CHMR study progressed, items relevant to value analysis, as proposed by health industry groups (such as VHA, B&D, and the Health Industry Group Purchasing Association), were summarized and served as guidelines for assessing hospitals and systems. Over the course of the ASU/CHMR study, many benchmarks and indicators used by GPOs, suppliers, trade organizations, and hospital systems were identified that were seen as critical for building a value management scorecard. A number of these are found in Exhibit 3.5. Exhibit 3.6 provides a series of indicators developed over the course of the study that reflect the high-level balanced scorecard for system performance.

The ASU/CHMR indicators provide feedback to managers who have an interest in understanding how their supply chain is performing within the environment of competing hospitals and systems.

The demand for new technology will continue due to the aging population, highly informed and proactive consumers and clinicians, and a strong and competitive economy. Some technologies are reaching the stage of becoming commodities; others continue, through innovation, to have multiple uses, off-label

EXHIBIT 3.5.   BUILDING A VALUE MANAGEMENT SCORECARD.

1. Build a compelling case for change
2. Develop a data and information tool with a focus on:
   a. Reduced cost
   b. Forecasting
   c. Cost
   d. Infection rates
   e. Case time
   f. Product equivalent
   g. Progress toward commoditization
   h. Inventory turns
   i. Number of lines in inventory
   j. Product differentiation
   k. Safety and risk to patients and workers
3. Build senior management involvement
4. Manage physician involvement
5. Manage supplier involvement
6. Understand incentives
7. Clearly defined system (steps) for standardization and use of VATs
8. Commitment to error reduction
9. Vendor capability analysis
10. Improved logistics
11. Information systems sophistication
12. Increased team-based environment resulting in self-directed activities by clinicians, administrators, finance, and materials management
13. Better managed supply as an investment
14. Attention to consequences including:
    a. Improved alignment between providers and the organization
    b. Cost reduction
    c. Inventory reduction; share responsibility across stakeholders
    d. Improved awareness of key strategies
    e. Make analysis a routine and systematic process

applications, and linkages to outcomes that do not lend themselves to rigorous evaluation. In this robust technological environment, progressive systems, with the assistance of their supply chain partners, find the need to improve decision-making skills to evaluate new technologies, make contractual decisions, and lead change at a pace that may make contemporary contracting models obsolete.

In progressive systems, physicians are valued team members who collaborate in value management for achieving standardization and cost management. Yet physicians are rarely prepared to assume such roles. Inclusion of knowledge and skills related to resource use is rarely part of medical and postgraduate training. Progressive systems look toward medical staff with an eye to selecting physician

EXHIBIT 3.6.   FOCUSED ASU/CHMR INDICATORS.

1. Metrics applied to:
   a. Clarity of specification in measurement of goals.
   b. Developed strategies regarding cost reduction.
   c. Successful specification of the relationship of supply chain goals to the larger enterprise goals.
   d. Articulates appropriate use of reward and incentives.

2. Supply chain relationship management to:
   a. Develop a clear understanding of how to manage cost, information, and improved efficiencies with manufacturers, GPOs, and distributors.
   b. Ensure an understanding of relationship among units within a system or network.
   c. Identify facilitators and deterrents (enablers and barriers) to value management efforts.

3. Organizational dynamics:
   a. Provide value management solutions to recognize how unique culture affects decisions and outcomes.
   b. Evidenced by leadership at the corporate or system level.
   c. Evidenced by leadership at the hospital level.
   d. Counter constraints relating to organizational structure (facilitators deterrents).
   e. Successfully nurture physician relationships.
   f. Successfully engage physicians in standardization.
   g. Ensure a consistent and effective model of change management.

4. Information flow as evidenced by:
   a. Progress toward integration of cost, clinical, and charge systems.
   b. Recognition of what types of information systems do and do not work (facilitators and deterrents).
   c. Achieved internal communication of goals and missions.
   d. Achieved integration of distributors' information with internal systems.
   e. Provided point-of-use information-data-integration.

leaders who understand the importance of preserving resources, improving outcomes, and exercising leadership. Without such individuals and what they can contribute in VATs, systems will not be in a position to collaborate with their GPO partners (see Chapter Four) to select materials better. In turn, this will create and sustain an environment that values the role of materials, increased safety, and improved outcomes. Progressive systems also develop service line manager roles (frequently occupied by nurses) to serve as linking pins between the supply chain management department and the clinical staff. The occupants of these roles have not been systematically studied to understand exactly what it is that they do to lead to success in standardization.

Progressive systems understand that their progress cannot continue in an environment in which soft links, due to physician claims for autonomy, characterize the relationship between the system and the physician in product selection.

Executives contemplating improvement in the value management process must exercise leadership in a manner that will capture the motivations of multiple constituents. Effective VATs will contribute to the reduction of risk for various parties residing toward the end of the value chain: the clinician, patient, and the system.

Managers contemplating a comprehensive value analysis program should develop their strategies around key components of supply cost reduction, including (1) recognition of a "burning platform," (2) demonstration of need and opportunity, (3) the creation of a vision by senior management, (4) buy-in from representatives and the identification of physician champions, (5) profiling of existing and potential suppliers, and (6) identification of incentives and perspectives.[56] Research on physician leadership has demonstrated the importance of change management and the ideas of teams working effectively in the supply chain health arena.[57]

Rapid change in technology requires that VAT strategy and structure recognize and lead change. Yet with so few hospitals and systems having a clear mission statement regarding materials and the broader supply chain, this is frequently difficult. As new technologies rapidly enter the marketplace, managing the marketplace becomes increasingly difficult. Products that appear to be state of the art sometimes prove to be less effective than anticipated following their use with larger populations. Commitments to suppliers on the basis of current knowledge must be made with great caution. At the same time, there are systems that have engaged in sole-source contracts with manufacturers for technologies that appear to be at the forefront of the field—at the expense of sustaining relationships.

There is growing consensus that success in securing physician participation is dependent on incentives that relate to quality of care and preservation of physician autonomy as well as the presence of financial incentives. In studying physicians in groups, Conrad and Christianson point out that a variety of financial incentives must be considered as groups work to achieve improved quality and better outcomes in an environment that is focusing on health care improvement.[58] Their work draws heavily on the Institute of Medicine's report, *Crossing the Quality Chasm*, which associates alignments with the ability to both the provision of fair payment for good clinical management of different types of patients and the opportunities for providers to share in the benefits of quality improvement.[59] In discussing physician participation in VATs and other quality improvement activities, directors of purchasing consistently pointed to the legal issues associated with any cost sharing that might result from cost savings associated with product standardization in the hospital. In systems where there was less success than others in achieving standardization, directors of purchasing frequently reported that specialists seemed to have no problem restricting their choice of products when practicing in outpatient clinics in which they held some ownership equity. While they pointed to their ability to improve physician amenities, they felt that the degrees of freedom to manipulate rewards were too narrow to be effective.

The ASU/CHMR study reveals that progressive practices pertaining to customer relationship and customer preference management are dependent on the presence of medical staff who are characterized by a willingness and ability to exercise leadership with colleagues, the design and use of internal committees, and external resources and partners to create an environment that values the role that materials can play in improved outcomes as well as cost savings. This chapter has demonstrated that supply chain management requires that leadership play many different and complex roles. There must be a concerted effort by hospitals and systems to articulate and manage a vision of the strategic importance of the supply chain and build necessary competencies to engage strategically in customer relationship and customer preference management.[60]

Finally, progressive systems enter the procurement process with medical staff product use commitment. As a result of effective internal VATs, those that belong to GPOs are sometimes able to manage with their GPOs or independently engage the market themselves in product selection and procurement. These systems also recognize that physicians have very strong relationships with their suppliers and can help the system engage suppliers on cost issues.[61] As internal VATs become more common, GPO models are adopting new business models to work with their members to meet their objectives. They are allowing custom contracts within the GPO as well as providing services, such as the reverse auctions discussed in Chapter Two, to their participants to engage the marketplace independently.[62] Value analysis indeed provides the information platform for significantly changing the relationships between buyers, sellers, and purchasing partners throughout the health sector.

CHAPTER FOUR

GROUP PURCHASING ORGANIZATIONS

Shaping the Health Materials Marketplace

Hospitals and systems face the enormous task of sourcing and contracting for over sixty thousand products to accomplish their clinical and non-clinical goals. Failure to meet the needs of internal customers can, as demonstrated in Chapter Two, expose the hospital to substantial risk. Progressive managers seek information and strategy to assess and counter risk. In the complexity of the hospital and hospital system, such assessment must be conducted within the context of deciding whether risk-related problems can best be solved through internal supply management or one of a variety of outsourcing options.[1] While a significant focus of health sector supply chain management is on the internal aspects of satisfying customer needs, including customer relationship management (CRM) and internal customer management, such needs cannot be fulfilled without careful attention to sourcing, which includes product identification and contracting.

Group purchasing organizations (GPOs) are designed to fill this sourcing need and avert a variety of market, strategy and demand-related risks, as discussed in Chapter Two. Yet there is great variability among the ASU/CHMR study participants about the extent to which they felt comfortable relying on the GPO to manage any one kind of risk. This chapter details the variety of factors associated with decision making regarding outsourcing of supply functions, develops an analytical understanding of GPO characteristics, assesses how GPOs contribute to hospital and system strategic purchasing, and scrutinizes the value that purchasing alliances, such as GPOs, bring to the marketplace.

The chapter focus is on purchasing partner management and strategy, as revealed by the ASU/CHMR research site respondents. It is important to remember that the purpose of the ASU/CHMR study was not to scrutinize the variety of GPO strategies, but rather to focus on strategies that contribute to progressive hospitals' and systems' success in supply chain management. The study identified and analyzed the ways progressive systems weigh the advantages and disadvantages of strategies associated with product selection, negotiating for contracts, and other product procurement functions.

Since the summer of 2002, GPOs have been under constant scrutiny for many of their business practices by both the U.S. Senate and the Federal Trade Commission. Although a full review of the issues surrounding the GPO inquiry is outside the scope of this book, their implications for hospital and hospital systems' ethical behavior in the purchasing process are considered at the end of this chapter.[2]

How GPOs Bring Value

From the perspective of the hospital or system manager, GPO involvement is best thought of as an activity that requires skillful supplier relationship management and purchasing partner management. Partnerships imply reciprocal relationships and appropriate relationship management from both parties. Thus, to ensure hospital and system satisfaction and compliance with GPO purchasing contracts, GPOs engage in extensive CRM activities with the hospital and system. National GPOs provide staff at the regional and even hospital level to assist hospital systems in procurement management and build relationships with their clients across a large nation. GPOs sponsor annual meetings at which their members and clients can share best practices and bring together their members with a variety of suppliers. While GPOs provide such services to benefit their broad membership, the hospitals and hospital systems attempt to gain advantage by their own skillful customer relationship management with end users of clinical and nonclinical products (as discussed in Chapter Three) and with suppliers. Hospitals are increasingly reporting increased success in working with suppliers to achieve their mutual goals with both commodities and clinical preference items.

GPOs Offer Procurement Solutions

Hospital procurement operations have several different approaches available to them. Nollet and Beaulieu contend that a procurement strategy:

- Identifies the area more likely to generate potential savings and then uses the approaches that make it possible to do so.
- Specifies the extent of group negotiations.
- Contributes to the organization not only by reducing costs but also by adding value through better operational links with suppliers.
- Distinguishes competitors by assessing product quality.
- Shortens lead times.[3]

Hospitals and hospital systems expect GPOs to assist them by outsourcing some part of the purchasing function to (1) purchase effectively and efficiently (by consolidating volumes and engaging in aggressive negotiations), (2) buy better (by optimization of services and increasing service), and (3) bring about better product use (through standardization of products and specifications).[4]

At the most basic level, hospitals seek alliances with GPOs to carry out exchange functions associated with product sourcing, supplier negotiations, and the contract development and management functions associated with procurement and materials management.[5] The value analysis function, elaborated on in Chapter Three, is one potential GPO benefit. Since GPOs are external to the hospital or system (see Appendix 4A), the services they provide must be considered a collaborative exchange model designed to achieve best price and other purchasing goals. Goals beyond price may include bringing value to a larger community of GPO members (for example, a cluster of nonprofit or church-related systems), assisting a set of hospitals and systems committed to a given value (for example, purchasing environmentally superior products), or improving the general well-being of association or affiliates (for example, academic health centers).[6] In this sense, a GPO should be assessed by the value it brings to a hospital or system and the various benefits and vulnerabilities that it represents. At the very least, GPOs must deliver reduced transaction costs.[7] According to a recent report by the Lewin Group, GPOs:

- Save their institutions an average of 10.4 percent on supply costs, which includes savings on goods purchased through GPOs, patronage dividends from GPOs, and labor costs avoided by using GPOs.
- Offer flexibility and commitment with contracts.
- Save the average system approximately $198,000 annually in avoidance of direct costs of adding purchasing staff.

- Have a "Wal-Mart effect" in the health care supply chain, which means that the GPO's best price makes prices lower for products not on GPO contract.[8]

The fact that so many hospitals and systems continue to carry out their purchasing through GPOs attests to the relatively high level of satisfaction with these organizations. GPOs apparently demonstrate their advantage to both senior management and supply chain managers. Of the progressive systems participating in the ASU/CHMR study, only one system, Swedish Medical Center in Seattle, is not a GPO member.

GPOs Draw Together Substantial Volumes

GPOs are an outsourcing strategy for over 90 percent of U.S. hospitals, and GPO contracting remains the dominant force for "going to the market" for health services provider organizations. This is accomplished by consolidating volume to engage the suppliers of health care goods and services. The vast majority of hospitals and hospital systems in the United States use GPO contracts to secure their materials.[9] In addition, it is estimated that 72 percent of hospital purchases are done through a GPO contract. With these purchases accounting for the second-largest dollar expenditure in hospitals,[10] the GPO market for hospitals and nursing homes is estimated at between $148 and $165 billion annually and is projected to grow to $257 and $287 billion, respectively, per year by 2009.[11] The Health Industry Group Purchasing Association (HIGPA) estimates that over six hundred organizations in the United States act in some form of group purchasing. Of these, two companies, Novation and Premier, handle purchasing for over 60 percent of the hospitals in the United States.

GPOs Are Heralded as Price Reducers

GPOs are formally constituted entities designed to reduce prices for medical material by aggregating spending, thereby benefiting not only hospitals but also all of those who purchase health care (consumers, employers, and insurance companies).[12] The Center for Advanced Purchasing Studies at Arizona State University found average GPO annual dollar savings of 13.43 percent.[13] This translates into group purchasing saving of $12.8 to $19.2 billion, or 10 to 15 percent of total purchasing cost.

GPO Value: Historical Context

GPOs historically have served many functions. They brought together executives to engage in both formal and informal exchanges about the state of health care delivery. This helped to satisfy the affiliative needs of individuals in a large industry who hoped that the strengths of an affiliative relationship would lead to lower costs. GPOs also provided advice and services on topics as diverse as facilities development, process engineering, and nursing recruitment. They are continuously redefining their mission as being substantially beyond contracting and providing the best product for the least cost. New offerings include consulting-related services such as revenue recovery, facilitating benchmarking, managing the value analysis process, human resource management, and information management. A review of the proceedings of the agenda for a national meeting of GPOs and their members indicates that standardization, price, and cost reduction activities continue to be the primary "wants" of GPO members. Systems are attempting to see GPOs as their strategic partners that can provide information, communication services, information on patient safety initiatives, and increased services pertaining to system standardization.[14] GPOs are also characterized by extensive involvement in clinical review processes in the areas of "monitoring and improving 'breakthrough' and other novel technologies."[15] Such diversity suggests that GPOs are becoming mixed-mission organizations.

Outsourcing product selection of contracting has a long history in the United States. The first GPO was created in New York in 1910. By the 1970s, the U.S. health care system had experienced extensive growth that resulted in over six thousand hospitals serving a nation with a growing population and highly dispersed hospital system. Small and rural hospitals seemed to be especially vulnerable to supplier pricing strategies in a marketplace characterized by inequities in knowledge, money, and managerial skills. With hundreds of thousands of supply-line items in multiple product categories,[16] GPOs were seen as an important strategic option to assist hospitals and hospital systems in achieving their purchasing goals.[17]

In 1986, GPOs were granted immunity (what is referred to as a "safe harbor") from federal fraud and abuse rules and were allowed to collect limited fees from suppliers and manufacturers. While this opportunity makes GPOs less reliant on hospitals for their revenues, many GPOs from their inception secured funding in a variety of ways from their hospital and system purchasing partners as well as from suppliers. As a result, GPOs have continuously been enmeshed in a complex and controversial set of business and strategic relationships regarding their ability to act as the agent of their members. GPO positioning in the marketplace requires that they engage in CRM activities with the hospitals and systems customers. They must also engage in PPM activities with suppliers on which they rely to provide products and services to their customers. (Appendix 4A provides the opinion of the Office of the Inspector General regarding the scope of GPO activities and their relationships to the organizations for which they act as agents.)

Today GPOs find themselves working with hospitals in an environment that no longer is characterized by a large number of independent hospitals scattered across the nation. Mergers and consolidations have created large hospital systems that themselves bring purchasing power to the marketplace. Even so, these same hospitals and hospital systems have largely failed to maximize the operational improvements and cost reductions they were designed to deliver. Many of the barriers to alignment of incentives with physicians in order to achieve discipline in purchasing clinical items (as detailed in Chapter Three) persist. The benefits that many associated with increased size and affiliation have been slow to materialize due to differences stemming from a lack of sophistication in information technology, variation across systems in and hospital medical staff composition, and cultural differences associated with system and individual hospitals. Perhaps this partially explains why the vast majority of progressive hospitals and hospital systems continue to see GPO alliances as one part of their strategy to improve marketplace performance. GPO membership, for the industry as a whole, continues to grow, "countering the belief of several years ago that large integrated delivery networks were poised to abandon their GPOs and strike out on their own."[18]

Deciding When and What to Outsource

Activities that are central to the operations of an organization should not be outsourced, but it is often difficult to develop a list of what should be outsourced across different hospitals and hospital systems.[19] Insourcing and outsourcing decisions are among the most difficult decisions that an individual hospital or system must make as it seeks to become an "integrated value system."[20] In assessing this outsourcing strategy, hospitals and systems examine a number of issues:

- The investment the hospital or system needs to make to be its own purchasing agent (either fully or partially)
- The extent to which the benefits of outsourcing allow for further specialization and provide an opportunity for achieving cost and price objectives[21]
- The extent to which insourcing or outsourcing increases flexibility in terms of the size of the organization and achieves an opportunity for managing through contracts and contractual relationships
- The extent to which insourcing and outsourcing affect transaction costs

Oliver E. Williamson, the eminent analyst of transaction costs, has pointed out that "there is no one, all-purpose, superior form of organization. Transactions vary in their attributes; governance structures vary in costs and competencies; efficient alignment is where the predictive action resides."[22] Study 1 reveals there is a duplication of supply functions and transaction costs associated with hospital system and GPO purchasing. Hospitals and systems must clearly understand their competencies and weaknesses and organize accordingly in order to bring transaction cost thinking into alignment with organizational strategy and to reduce redundancies in a variety of costs.[23]

Outsourcing and Core Competencies

Table 4.1 looks at GPO-hospital engagement on a matrix of involvement. The left column represents organizations that have high reliance on GPOs for both contracting and product selection. These organizations have chosen to reduce transaction costs as much as possible and have confidence in their system dealings. The right column represents systems where GPOs are key to reducing transaction costs associated with the business of purchasing and contracting, but where their GPO influences product selection in a minimal way. The left column is populated by systems that use GPO prices and product identification as reference points for product selection but frequently enter the market on their own to engage in purchasing. Finally, the right column reflects systems that fail to engage their medical staff or others in product selection and are likely to enter the marketplace on their own.

Progressive systems generally fall within a zone of collaboration using GPOs and their own supply chain resources. Frequently their individual efforts are carried out with the knowledge and support of their GPO partners. This raises the question of what purchasing functions should be outsourced by an organization. The extent to which that progressive systems appear to answer this question in very different ways gives credence to the point made in the Introduction that health sector supply chain managers must take a contingency approach to their jobs,

TABLE 4.1. MODELS FOR HOSPITAL AND SYSTEM ENGAGEMENT WITH GPOs.

	High GPO Involvement in Product Selection	Low GPO Involvement in Product Selection
High use of GPO contracts	GPO-dominated purchasing	Strategic outsourcing of contracting
Low use of GPO contracts	Strategic manipulation of purchasing	Purchasing dominated by integrated delivery networks strategic outsourcing of technology assessment

deciding how the organizational culture, structure, and other key organizational factors affect strategy selection.

Reducing Outsourcing Risk Through GPOs

Hospitals are service agencies that provide care by employing finished materials to achieve clinical goals. Since no hospital or outpatient practice is designed to produce products from raw materials, it is conceivable for a hospital or hospital system to decide to fully outsource the purchasing, distribution, and warehousing of its materials and even services without even taking ownership of the goods.[24] But outsourcing is a difficult decision. Christine Harland and Louise Knight at the Centre for Research in Strategic Purchasing and Supply at the University of Bath carried out an extensive literature review pointing "clearly to the lack of alignment between initial objectives and eventual outcomes of outsourcing decisions, for the public sector and various industrial sectors, resulting from the failure to monitor and act upon the cumulative impact of outsourcing decisions."[25] Rigorous analysis of the consequences of outsourcing in the U.S. health sector has not been forthcoming. Thus, managers face significant uncertainties as they confront a wide variety of outsourcing opportunities, including purchasing options.

As hospital systems seek to achieve cost reduction and improved performance through standardization, they look to GPOs for some of the needed competencies associated with managing physician stakeholders. There are also a number of such systems that have sought GPOs to assume responsibility for their contracting and purchasing function with the hope that their committed purchasing, compounded with the purchasing of other systems, will lead to even further price reductions. The challenge for management is to understand the variety of materials outsourcing options. There are three principal questions regarding outsourcing:[26]

- What kinds of services should an organization purchase from outside suppliers?
- What criteria should be used for choosing activities to outsource?
- What contingencies make outsourcing desirable in one situation but not in another?

The ASU/CHRM study did not identify leading systems that fully outsource both the purchasing and distribution functions. Interviews were completed with hospitals and hospital systems that participate in an outsourcing model that involves purchasing virtually all of their goods through the GPO. Similarly, interviews were completed with hospital and hospital systems that outsourced the distribution function to suppliers. However, only a minority of hospitals or systems

FIGURE 4.1. THE ZONE OF STRATEGIC FIT.

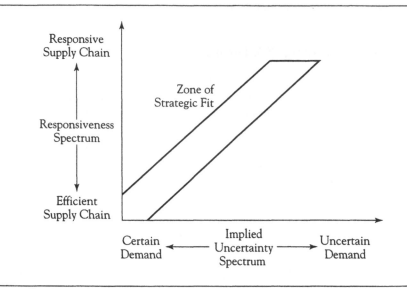

Source: Chopra, Sunil, and Meindl, Peter, *Supply Chain Management* (2nd ed.). © 2004. p. 38.
Reprinted by permission of Pearson Education, Inc., Upper Saddle River, NJ.

seem willing to take either option, believing that it is important for them to retain a larger involvement in the management of the supply chain.

Progressive hospitals and systems assess GPOs by the extent to which they serve their market and reduce risk as they react to the demand for needed products. While few hospitals or hospital systems articulate this process in a formal manner, it is clear that progressive systems seek purchasing partners that position them in a zone of strategic fit. As Figure 4.1 shows, the more uncertainty involved in a process, the more responsive the GPO needs to be.[27] The GPO's ability to fit its business practices into this zone of strategic fit is an important factor when making the decision to outsource purchasing activities.

Hospitals and hospital systems continually test the extent to which GPO pricing is superior to their own pricing. This results in a wide range of buy-versus-make options regarding sourcing and contracting functions. But how such decisions are made, even across progressive systems, is far from uniform. In some systems, the decision to outsource purchasing on commodity goods, where price is the principal outcome measure, is quickly relinquished to GPOs. Such systems are comfortable making the assumption that GPO pricing is sufficiently low to avoid the transaction costs associated with their own scrutiny of the marketplace. Other systems have identified items that are worth pursuing on their own or in a unique partnership with the GPO. In such instances, the GPO may bring its expertise in techniques such as reverse auctions to the system or negotiate on the system's behalf.

With clinical preference items accounting for an inordinately large and increasing percentage of a hospital's materials costs, the ability of hospitals to manage the acquisition of these products, with or without GPOs, is critical. GPOs recognize that their ability to bring the hospital or system cost and price reductions and improved service on such items will differentiate the GPO in the marketplace. Evidence of this is the degree to which GPOs are touting their success in working with their customers to achieve standardization on clinical preference items and reduce costs.[28]

Hospital-GPO Alliances

GPOs serve multiple hospital systems by bringing together many purchasers under an umbrella that is designed to pool the demand power of the participants to favor their purchasing goals. In this sense, GPOs are alliances between hospitals or systems and purchasing entities.[29] GPO business models, however, are increasingly heterogeneous, including revenue generation from membership fees, revenues generated on the basis of achieved savings on purchased items, and even fee-for-service revenues based on the use of specific GPO services or contracts. Some GPOs treat all of their participants as equal partners. Others have developed strategies to attract or segment only those that hope to benefit from the features of a price exchange based on their high level of committed volumes. Still others bring together members of a community of hospitals such as a group of hospitals associated with a religious group. University Health Consortium, for example, recognizes many of the unique characteristics of academic health centers as it brings together teaching hospitals to engage the marketplace in purchasing. Newer GPOs are much more eclectic in their membership: they bring together academic health centers, investor-owned systems, nonprofits, and large, integrated delivery systems under one roof. Health Trust Purchasing Group is the GPO purchasing arm of HCA, the largest investor-owned system in the United States, but it is also open to other members seeking GPO services.

Some GPOs have advanced new business models and service lines to differentiate themselves from their competitors on the basis of strategy rather than affinity. These models, and the observation of modest churn (members changing GPOs) in the GPO marketplace, are challenging GPOs, as discussed later in the chapter, to carry out due diligence and consider the value associated with their organization. Increasingly such value is related to objective purchasing goals rather than to the power associated with affiliation with other hospitals and systems.

GPO members recognize that GPO-sponsored activities, such as process or resource management and value analysis teams (VATs), provide added value

(Chapter Three). Some analysts believe that GPOs have been overly focused on new services rather than the achievement of better prices. Price differentials in the marketplace are not so large as to be the driving criteria in GPO selection. Thus, while GPOs attempt to distinguish themselves through a range of new service offerings, they must be mindful that they are participating in a marketplace that is the domain of a much wider set of consulting organizations. Since these businesses have many years of experience in providing services that the GPOs are moving to offer, it is not clear that such lines of service will emerge as major GPO competencies.

As hospitals and hospital systems consider GPO affiliation, they must be mindful that GPOs have become businesses that exist to achieve their own financial goals as well as to support the goals of their members. This succession of goals may not benefit alliance participants. As hospitals and systems scrutinize potential GPO alliance partners, it is important that they find ones that match up to their own needs, goals, and cultures.

Assessing the GPO

The hospital-GPO relationship is a special and changing kind of organization. The GPO serves as a hospital or hospital system "agent" to the host of suppliers that provide goods and services.[30] However, the GPO also has its own goals and objectives that may not necessarily be aligned with those of its members. Unless the GPO provides improved focus as a result of value gained, GPO participation will be limited. How do progressive hospitals and hospital systems assess strategic GPO alliances? These agents must be evaluated by the extent to which they contribute to the hospital or system's risk-reduction strategy to transcend a narrow price-per-product focus. Evaluation criteria include the capability by the GPO to (1) improve enterprisewide spending, (2) improve market information, (3) build a deeper understanding about supplier capabilities, and (4) help the hospital or system to improve overall supply management capability.[31] The ASU/CHMR study suggests that GPO-hospital alliance development conforms fairly closely to other supply chain alliance processes in other industries:

- Alliance conceptualization. Alliance conceptualization begins when a hospital becomes interested in a purchasing partner or changing a purchasing partner and engages in internal discussion and review and assessment of alliance performance for similar hospitals and systems.
- Alliance pursuance. This begins when the hospital or system decides to form an alliance or seek a new alliance and establishes a set of criteria associated with selection of a GPO or other type of purchasing partner.

- Alliance selection. Alliance partners are reviewed, and one or more potential partners may be asked to provide proposals that include clarification of alliance membership criteria, business plan specification, and expected alliance benefits, including price savings expectations.
- Alliance implementation and continuity. Strategies are devised to monitor the alliance relationship with feedback mechanisms to continually administer and assess performance to determine if the alliance will be sustained, modified, or terminated.[32]

Within this context, successful alliance partners appear to use a feedback mechanism to assess alliance effectiveness and consider sustaining, renegotiating, or abandoning the ongoing alliance.[33] Such assessment must be carried out with an understanding of how GPOs bring value to the system.

Purchasing Competencies and Progressive GPO Practices

Progressive systems enter into GPO relationships with the understanding that the decision to outsource aspects of sourcing and contracting necessitates extensive purchasing partner management. Long-term relationships are dependent on the ability of the GPO to meet the hospital or hospital system's expectation for savings and service, as well as expectations that the relationship will be carried out in a trusting manner. This is especially important as GPOs seek to gain a competitive advantage in a business environment.

Achieving Competitive Advantage

Achieving a competitive advantage requires developing a trusting relationship with partners.[34] Trust can be defined as "the willingness to be vulnerable to the actions of another party based on the expectation that the other will perform a particular action important to the trustor, irrespective of the ability to monitor or control that other party."[35] For the hospital or system to transfer purchasing power to the GPO, there must be the belief that the risks of vulnerability are minimal. For such a transfer of confidence to be effective, trust must exist not only between the individuals within the group but also in the integrity of the organizations involved.[36] Handfield and Nichols have identified five ways to gain trust: reliability, competence, goodwill, vulnerability, and loyalty.[37]

Reliability is defined simply as the ability of a company to "follow through on [their] commitments and act predictably."[38] Most are aware that actions speak louder than words. If a hospital or hospital system has had good business relationships with a GPO, then it will be more inclined to stay with that GPO. But if the GPO is unable to deliver on promised claims, customers will find it unreliable. In many cases, reliability corresponds to integrity: "the extent to which a person repeatedly acts according to a moral code or standard."[39] Integrity leads to reliability, which then advances toward the trust necessary for a supplier-consumer relationship.

Competence is established as the system increasingly understands that it can allow the GPO to act as its agent without continually reviewing GPO behaviors. Competencies are frequently shared by a hospital or system and a GPO. In such instances, as trust develops and there is reduced fear of incurring risks associated with purchasing, it seems important that the hospital or system relinquish some of these shared competencies to the GPO, if for no other reason than the opportunity to reduce transaction costs.

Goodwill or affect-based trust is established through emotions of benevolence (Is the supplier working for the good of its consumer?) and openness (How comfortable does each party feel sharing information with the other?).[40] These two characteristics are important in that they express how a customer feels that the actions of the GPO are in its behalf. This is one of the greatest areas that GPOs need to work on, as there are allegations that GPOs lack transparency (in distribution rebates and other benefits) and are not working for the good of their customers.[41] Therefore, it is extremely important for GPOs to show that their actions are in the best interest of their consumers and are truly providing value.

Group Purchasing and Progressive Hospitals

For many hospitals, materials management, while not defined as a core competency, is retained as a system function and is associated with the system's success.[42] In contrast, Swedish Medical Center in Seattle, which does not belong to a GPO, has structured its purchasing function into the organization as a core competency. Swedish Medical Center is a unique organization in its dominant position in the Seattle marketplace. It recognizes that suppliers want to have their products used in the community and that their size, positioning, and reputation can lead to favorable prices. Other organizations believe that their endorsement of a product carries a great deal of prestige that tips the balance of power between supplier and purchaser toward the purchaser.

One of the consequences of outsourcing supply functions is the recognition that one no longer has core competencies. This can lead hospitals and systems to feel vulnerable to risks associated with having entered into an agency relationship with a GPO. But when trust is present, such vulnerability gives ways to the positive feelings associated with having developed alliances.

Loyalty is a reflection of successful trusting relationships. Increasingly, with new GPO business models entering the marketplace, hospitals and systems have engaged in due diligence to assess their ongoing supply partner relationships. Such due diligence must be seen as an important business competency rather than a sign of potential disloyalty. It allows hospitals and systems to build depth in their trusting relationships. Having made decisions, acts of disloyalty include not keeping one's commitments to a purchasing partner or a GPO purchasing partner to a hospital or system. Such feelings of distrust will add to a system's belief that it is vulnerable in the marketplace and can lead to increased scanning of the marketplace by hospitals and systems for new purchasing partners. GPOs with many different kinds of members may act in ways that favor one of their member categories (such as large organizations) over some other category of membership. Such behaviors may be seen as acts of "disloyalty" by the less favored category of members. It takes a trusting relationship to understand that the GPO may not be able to act in ways to favor all members all of the time. It is important that GPOs progressively are more likely to develop strategies to partition members in their best interests (for example, assisting them to individually carry out a reverse auction on an item where there is already a GPO contract for all members). Finally, GPOs increasingly recognize that transparency in their behavior with hospitals and systems is key to success.

A CEO's belief about GPO value and his or her overall goals for the supply function is a principal determinant of GPO use. Organizations range from those where CEOs are committed to high levels of GPO contract purchasing to CEOs who believe that GPO pricing is considered the ceilings from which negotiation outside the GPO should begin. These CEOs were willing to experience much higher costs in the purchasing process than those who were willing to take GPO pricing as acceptable. CEOs frequently identify GPO added-value services as having great importance. Perhaps Nollet and Beaulieu are correct in their contention that "value-added benefits protect GPOs from a threatening environment."[43] Paradoxically, few purchasing managers even accurately identify such services.

ASU/CHMR research identified eight characteristics of progressive hospital system/GPO practices:

1. *Leadership that is willing to manage with the GPO.* Progressive systems are characterized by leadership that sees GPO membership as a strategic option and is committed to "manage with" the GPO. This is especially important for systems that allow the GPO to assume a wide range of the purchasing platform for the system. It is critical to monitor the extent to which GPO actions bring value to a wide range of stakeholders, including clinicians, finance officers, and materials managers.

2. *Selectivity based on knowledge about the culture of the hospital or system.* As suggested in Exhibit 4.1, progressive systems recognize that all GPOs are not alike and all

EXHIBIT 4.1.   PROGRESSIVE PRACTICES.

- Progressive systems participate on GPO value analysis councils and committees and strive for leadership roles in these arenas.
- Systems are increasingly strategic in their choice of a GPO.
- Progressive systems seek GPOs that will provide opportunities for bringing together the commitments they can bring to the table and at the same time will accommodate the system itself as it engages in aggressive marketplace behavior.
- Progressive organizations recognize the value of data, information, and knowledge management.
- Progressive systems report regularly assessing their relationship with their GPO, considering new entrants into the GPO market, and reassessing their expectations for the GPO.
- Progressive systems are data driven.

will not be a good fit for their system's culture. They are able to communicate what is important about their culture to the GPO. A hospital system that has a culture designed to allow each of its operating unit leaders to determine a separate materials policy will find success with a GPO that provides flexibility by differentiating prices for different levels of product commitment or system wide pricing.

3. *Recognition of the value of transfer of transaction costs to the GPO.* Progressive systems reduce the size of their purchasing departments as a result of GPO membership and understand what functions they would have to carry out if the GPO were not there. These hospital systems can account for the costs that would be accrued to the organization if specific kinds of purchases were internal. Progressive organizations understand the level of outsourcing they can best manage.

4. *Identification of competitive edge gained by GPO participation.* Supply chain analysts have pointed out that although competitive benchmarking is an easy concept to comprehend, "it is difficult to achieve effectively as few direct competitors are willing to reveal the secrets of their success to other competitors."[44] Through GPOs, hospitals can obtain information by which to benchmark their own practices. While supply chain leaders in progressive hospitals and hospital systems participating in the ASU/CHMR study report that they independently follow the market closely to assess prices, they frequently contend that this is a practice that is restricted to higher-risk products characterized by complex markets. They recognize the value to be gained by strategically managing products that have the potential to make a substantial difference in the organization's performance as well as the value to be gained by confidence in their purchasing partner's ability.

Progressive hospitals and systems seek GPOs that can accommodate their level of committed purchasing. They also recognize that GPO competencies in sourcing, negotiating and contracting can be of value to them in their efforts to engage the market beyond the GPO contract. This is reflected in their offering a new range of member services, such as carrying out reverse auctions for individual systems[45] and thus reducing a member's transaction costs and perhaps achieving a lower price for a small group of member hospitals.

5. *Recognition that hospital systems should not fully outsource value analysis and strategic decision making.* Health care delivery systems are characterized by a wide range of physician-organization relationships, serve different populations, and experience different levels of risk in attempting standardization. Progressive hospitals and systems communicate to the GPO the ways in which the GPO can contribute to the alignment of organization-physician incentives and goals. Hospital and hospital systems that cannot stipulate the requirements that their physicians seek in products cannot expect GPO value analysis activity to bring satisfaction to the medical staff.

6. *Relationship assessment and management.* Progressive hospitals and systems regularly assess their relationship with their GPO, consider new entrants into the GPO market, and reassess their expectations for the GPO. These organizations recognize that the best GPOs work to meet client demands for services and provide custom financial relationships with clients around demands for specific products, price, and savings targets. They also recognize the costs associated with exiting one GPO relationship and entering a new relationship. These costs lead progressive systems to work to sustain productive relationships and build trust with their GPO.

7. *Understanding that supplier relationship management is critical to success in working with GPOs.* Suppliers target their marketing to a full range of parties involved in decision making, including hospitals, systems, clinicians, and GPOs. The services that suppliers offer, especially for clinical preference items, include education, research, and assistance with product use at the point of service (including the operating room). While suppliers introduce new and expensive products directly into the practice and operating setting, progressive organizations (as discussed in Chapter Three) have developed policies to limit the introduction of unapproved products. These organizations work closely with both their physicians and GPO representatives, who also have relationships with suppliers, to clearly articulate their policies.

8. *Knowing success when you see it.* Progressive systems are data driven. They have developed a set of metrics that allow them to monitor the cost of supplies and understand the extent to which their success relates to meeting the conditions set out between the hospital system and the GPO. These systems also know that managing within the individual hospital and the hospital system is critical to success in their overall purchasing and GPO involvement.

Hospital executives are increasingly engaging in strategic thinking as they consider their organization's engagement with a GPO (Case 4.1). Systems are taking what they see as strategic value from their GPOs and making decisions as to when and how to engage in their own contracting, value analysis, and strategic sourcing.

◆ ◆ ◆

Case 4.1 Strategy at Trinity Health and Consorta

Trinity Strategy

Trinity Health is a member of Consorta. When deciding whether to participate in a Consorta contract, Trinity Health enlists the aid of stakeholders and clinicians to check a list of eight to 10 strategic criteria. It may go its own way for a number of reasons, including moving market share, compliance, contract length, firm pricing or discounts. On the other hand, "If we feel we'd be leaving money on the table without the GPO, but [find that] its portfolio doesn't meet our needs, we'd do a custom contract using our Consorta model," Lou Fierens, then vice president of supply chain at Trinity, stated: "If we have reasons to contract totally outside the GPO relationship, we do that."

Now in its second year, the contracting program has yielded "double-digit millions" of dollars of savings and administrative fees for Trinity Health. The IDN is on track to achieve its five-year goal of $110 million in savings.

Two other Consorta shareholders have followed Trinity Health on this path. And others are doing similar things outside of a compliant GPO relationship. Fierens' advice for them is simple: "It's absolutely key to have top leadership support, and to truly understand that it will be a three- to five-year process to build the infrastructure and change the culture."

Consorta Strategy

Consorta president John Strong explains that the customized contracting program isn't for everyone. "You have to be a certain size and have a certain amount of contract volume to make this profitable," says Strong. "I think all three shareholders would like to do custom contracts in areas of high clinical preference where it's been historically difficult for a GPO to do that and extend real meaningful value back to the members. And they would like to do it in cases where they believe they can be more committed to one or two suppliers themselves than the rest of the group collectively is willing to be. In those cases they feel they can get a better cost advantage by doing a separate contract." Strong goes on to argue that customized contracting is really "customized complexity."

"I think the reason you don't see a lot of people doing it right now is because it requires a fairly significant amount of sophisticated management tools," he says. For example, Trinity's electronic catalog may include all of the Consorta contract portfolio as well as its own custom portfolio, but the rest of Consorta shouldn't have access to the custom information. The same holds true for Ascension and CHI.

Managing customized contracting portfolios concurrent with the general contracting program takes a lot of behind-the-scenes management coordination, too, says Strong. "We need to know whether someone's going to opt in or opt out of a contract before we go to market as Consorta the GPO," he says. "We don't want to tell a supplier that everybody's in if somebody's planning on doing a custom contract on their own. All three shareholders have been particularly mindful of the impact on the other shareholders if they opted out of a certain contract. I think there's a considerable amount of genuine interest in doing the right thing to ensure that the group isn't harmed for the interest of a single shareholder."

Sources: "Trinity Strategy": Richter, S.M.R. "Trinity Health's Hybrid Contracting Model." *First Moves, 11,* July–Aug. 2003, at http://www.medicaldistribution.com/rep/Rep_2003_August/Rep_8202003112266.htm. "Consorta Strategy": Barlow, R. "Consorta: Straight Shooter." *FirstMoves,* http://firstmoves.com/view_magazine.asp?id=236.

◆ ◆ ◆

The Future of GPOs

GPOs face many challenges in the health care arena of the early twenty-first century. New technologies applied to purchasing challenge GPOs' transaction-focused services. The increased ability to purchase through various Internet Web sites reduces many of the transaction costs that hospitals could not attack on their own. While there is research to demonstrate that the total cost of purchasing and ownership is important in understanding the value brought to the delivery system by GPOs,[46] many purchasing managers, as well as policymakers and critics of the GPO, continue to evaluate GPO success on the basis of purchase cost only.

The political environment continues to dispute how GPOs have leveraged their power in the marketplace. Since 2002, there has been an aggressive attack on the safe harbor legislation and increased scrutiny of ethical issues surrounding GPOs. A number of small manufacturers continue to argue that "anticompetitive practices in the hospital supply market by the nation's largest group purchasing organizations threaten the quality of patient care by stifling medical innovation."[47] As a result of inquiries conducted by the Senate, the Federal Trade Commission, and the Justice Department, GPO strategies to secure hospital and hospital system business, such as sole-source contracting and bundling of materials, have been reconsidered. Yet even if the use of such purchasing strategies is diminished, such strategies, including sole-source contracts, guaranteeing commitment, and seeking various rebates, are duplicated by hospitals and systems as they seek, on their own, advantage in the purchasing marketplace.

Few believe that hospital-GPO collaboration in purchasing should (or could) be abandoned. Health care is an industry where an extraordinary range of skills is needed to engage in sophisticated product selection. Also, a wide scope of supply management talent is needed to source and contract for goods and services. Suppliers recognize that GPOs streamline the number of transactions that they have with hospitals and systems across the nation.

How strong is the case for hospitals to engage the market through GPO outsourcing? The jury is still out on the extent to which GPOs are successful in offsetting the negotiating power of suppliers, especially with physician preference items. In other industries, target pricing allows end users, working closely with suppliers, to achieve product costs that contribute to the profitability of their manufactured goods and services and "continuous cost reductions throughout the product life cycle."[48] Such an accomplishment requires extensive sharing of information, collaboration, and high levels of trust. The health environment is characterized by high levels of investment and risk associated with new product development that make it difficult to assess a price based on costs associated with manufacturing, including labor, materials, administrative, selling, and other related expenses.[49]

A Government Accountability Office (GAO) study found that price savings to hospitals and systems differ by the size of the hospital, with large hospitals (more than five hundred beds) often obtaining lower prices than the GPO contract price. In contrast, medium and smaller hospitals were more likely to realize savings through GPO contracts.[50] It is interesting that in one metropolitan U.S. market, the GAO found that GPO contracts resulted in considerably better prices—up to 26 percent better than hospitals not using GPO contracts for some models of a pacemaker. However, this savings was not consistent for all pacemaker models. For other models of pacemakers, GPO contract prices were higher—on one occasion, 39 percent higher. Overall, the GAO study found that the median GPO-negotiated price was higher than the median price hospitals paid without the GPO contract for all six safety needle models examined and over 60 percent of the forty-one pacemaker models that were in the study.[51]

In many ways, the GAO findings can be seen as a sign of a diverse and competitive marketplace where hospitals and systems have multiple purchasing options. Purchasing managers for large hospitals and systems often report they find it advantageous to use the GPO quoted prices as the ceiling from which they can enter into negotiations with other GPOs and suppliers. Another reason often cited by hospitals for not using purchasing groups is that the availability of shorter contracts allows them to take advantage of falling prices.

GPO and hospital and hospital system interests are not always fully aligned. GPOs attempt to buffer themselves from their members' engaging in non-GPO purchasing by encouraging members to make commitments to purchase through the GPO contract. Both GPOs and hospitals seem to recognize that in the health care industry, sole-source contracts may reduce leverage and agility in the marketplace for products. However, savings must be understood in a context that takes into account nonprice factors associated with transaction and administrative costs (as discussed in Chapter Two). By purchasing through the GPO, the hospital will save money by not having to employ the necessary support staff to test, research, negotiate, and purchase items on their own.[52] The GAO study found a disparity in the GPO saving of the two products they studied, pacemakers and safety needles. To consistently find the best price, the hospital would have to employ personnel to compare prices of every model available. As new models emerged, hospital system employees would have to assess the value of the new models, the costs of converting to new models, and any changed clinical outcomes. For most organizations, the increased overhead might not justify the savings that could be obtained by buying through the GPO contract.

While there has been no systematic study of GPO financing and manufacturer rebates, GPO profits remain a controversial topic. Any decision in determining the economic advantages of buying through a GPO contract must also take into account the profits returned to its members by the GPO. Reported revenue sharing ranged from 20 to 70 percent for a number of large GPOs. At least one GPO returns all rebates directly to its hospitals, incorporating these funds into a model of accountability for the individual units.

The GAO study of purchasing prices through GPOs has also been criticized for its methodology and focus on a relatively small number of items. A study supported by HIGPA reports substantial savings as a result of group purchasing.[53] The study found that implementing additional restrictions on the GPO business model would result in an increase in expenditures in both private and public health-care-financed programs. For every one percentage point decline in the rate of GPO-generated savings, HIGPA made these estimates:

- Medicare—Expenditures would increase by an additional $540 million to $641 million.
- Medicaid—Expenditures would increase by an additional $395 million to $468 million.
- Department of Veterans Affairs—Health care expenditures would increase by an additional $61 million to $73 million.

- Department of Defense—Health care expenditures would increase by an additional $36 to $73 million.
- Workers' compensation—Health care expenditures would increase by an additional $32 million to $39 million.

Given research methodologies and in some instances the affiliations and sponsors of studies, it is difficult to assess the accuracy and levels of bias in existing research on costs associated with GPO purchasing. HIGPA contends that providers and payers, and ultimately consumers, will pay more for products and services purchased through GPOs if their ability to negotiate on behalf of their providers is curtailed by additional restrictions on the GPO contracting processes. This general contention is supported by observation of the outcomes of negotiations by both GPOs and hospital systems.

Codes of Conduct for Ethical Purchasing

Scrutiny of codes of professional responsibility across a variety of industries reveals a series of issues that address various professions in regard to their clients and the behavior of individuals within the organizations in which they work.[54] A report from the Human Rights Research and Education Centre by Mendes and Clark identifies five generations of corporate codes of conduct.[55] Ethical business conduct is one of the leading issues transcribed in the code of ethics due to the overwhelming public interest and how "ethical business practices help protect the company's reputation and ensure fair competition."[56] Codes of conduct appear to go through five "generations": (1) conflict of interest, (2) business/commercial conduct, (3) employee and third-party concerns, (4) community and environmental concerns, and (5) accountability and social justice.[57] Topics to be considered in regard to health sector materials purchasing include (but should not be limited to) statements ensuring:

- Accountability and responsibility. Purchasing agents must see their role as providing the best product, at the best price, in a timely fashion. Depending on the reimbursement models by which the organization secures revenues, the outcome of purchasing can reduce risk from losses from various high-cost materials over the course of a hospitalization. Overall, effective purchasing can mean the difference between organizational solvency and insolvency.
- Advocacy role on behalf of clients. Purchasing agents serve multiple clients: the system, the patient, and the clinician. They must recognize when the interests

of each of these strategic constituents take precedence and ensure that each client's needs are served. This is a delicate balance that requires honesty, trust, and candor.

• Antitrust or trade regulation compliance. When organizations dominate a market, their purchasing behavior may exclude new entrants. Purchasing agents should be mindful of how their contracting behavior affects local and national markets.

• Commission, rebate, fee splitting, gifts, favors, or financial incentives compliance. Purchasing partners should establish and enforce clear policies regarding commissions, rebates, fee splitting, and financial incentives in all purchasing agreements. Policies should extend to undisclosed and contingent fees and unreasonable benefits to any employees.

• Misconduct reporting (whistle-blowing). Policies should encourage employees to report instances of misconduct or other violations of the law or ethical principles without fear of job loss or other penalties.

The GPO industry, in response to the several criticisms discussed earlier in the chapter, has used HIGPA to craft and put into place an industrywide code of conduct that is attentive to the issues discussed above. In addition, many GPOs have developed their own codes of conduct that include the GPO industry criteria. The code of conduct requires that all GPOs implement internal policies to correct questionable business practices to create "peer pressure with other suppliers in the [system], essentially creating a 'shame factor' for low-performing suppliers."[58] Because hospital systems themselves engage in purchasing for several members that might be conceptualized as constituting a group, it is important for hospital systems, like their GPO counterparts, to create strategies designed to ensure ethical business practice.

The development of the GPO code of conduct is an important first step in articulating expected behaviors along the health care supply chain. Given the diversity of partners in the supply chain and the tendency of employees to not truly understand ethical issues, it is important that the code is developed in collaboration with vendors and other supply chain partners. The code provides attention not only to conflict of interest and disclosure issues but to the processes related to health system improvement, including safety, cost reduction, and diversity.

To monitor compliance to the code of conduct, hospitals and systems, as have their GPO counterparts, should appoint an ethics compliance officer. In addition, the director of purchasing should declare in his or her annual report that the purchasing function is complying with the principles of the code.

Summary and Conclusion

Hospital systems occupy a critical position in the health sector as they collaborate with their clinical staff in the selection of materials. Both patients and staff expect that the process will produce safe products that contribute to excellent outcomes. In an environment characterized by technological change and a large number of competing products, sourcing and choice are difficult. To the extent that clinician users of the products vary in their preferences and have established relationships with vendors, the selection process is even more complicated. Finally, there are an enormous number of transactions involved in bringing the full range of necessary products to the system. Outsourcing some aspects of this process is necessary for organizations that see their core competency as the delivery of patient care. Even the one system that had no GPO made the decision to engage in group purchasing for pharmaceuticals. This was an area in which the system did not feel it had the full range of competencies or need to engage the marketplace directly.

Purchasing activity can be linked to broader systemwide goals, such as improving safety and outcomes, to move purchasing beyond "being 'just' about contracting and distributing."[59] At the October 2004 meetings of the HIGPA, a panel of leading GPO executives reported on emerging GPO business activities that included a focus on environmentally friendly products as well as products characterized by their ability to crate a safe working and patient care environment.

Effective management of a hospital or hospital system purchasing clearly requires partners, such as GPOs, that can help to reduce the number and cost of transactions. The ethical issues raised regarding GPO purchasing extend to hospital and hospital system purchasing behavior. GPOs are driven by the goals of their members and clients. Hospital management has the responsibility to ensure that their purchasing practices meet the criteria of good ethical practices. The professional groups pertaining to materials management can be helpful in raising issues regarding ethical behavior. Hospital and hospital system purchasing ethics need to be part of the broader mission of the organization.

The choice of materials is increasingly being recognized as critical to clinical success. Products require careful evaluation and assessment within the broad context of safety, outcomes, and organizational performance. There is a growing recognition of the value that purchasing brings to the organization and recognition, throughout the system, that materials matter. At the same time, systems seem content to position materials at a notch below the executive suite. Unless aspects of materials management are recognized as a point of strategic intersection for information pertaining to the cost of materials and their effect on the broader performance of the hospital, it is unlikely that materials will migrate into positions of broader responsibility.

Appendix 4A: Legal Analysis Regarding GPOs

The anti-kickback statute makes it a criminal offense knowingly and willfully to offer, pay, solicit, or receive any remuneration to induce the referral of business covered by a Federal health care program. Specifically, the statute provides that:

Whoever knowingly and willfully offers or pays [or solicits or receives] any remuneration (including any kickback, bribe, or rebate) directly or indirectly, overtly or covertly, in cash or in kind to any person to induce such person—to refer an individual to a person for the furnishing or arranging for the furnishing of any item or service for which payment may be made in whole or in part under a Federal health care program, or to purchase, lease, order, or arrange for or recommend purchasing, leasing, or ordering any good, facility, service, or item for which payment may be made in whole or in part under a Federal health care program, shall be guilty of a felony.

Section 1128B(b) of the Act. In other words, the statute prohibits payments made purposefully to induce referrals of business payable by a Federal health care program. The statute ascribes liability to both sides of an impermissible "kickback" transaction. The statute has been interpreted to cover any arrangement where *one* purpose of the remuneration was to obtain money for the referral of services or to induce further referrals. *United States v. Kats*, 871 F.2d 105 (9th Cir. 1989); *United States v. Greber*, 760 F.2d 68 (3d Cir.), *cert. denied*, 474 U.S. 988 (1985). "Remuneration" for purposes of the anti-kickback statute includes the transfer of anything of value, in cash or in kind, directly or indirectly, covertly or overtly. Violation of the statute constitutes a felony punishable by a maximum fine of $25,000, imprisonment up to five years or both. Conviction will also lead to automatic exclusion from Federal health care programs, including Medicare and Medicaid. This Office may also initiate administrative proceedings to exclude persons from the Federal and State health care programs or to impose civil monetary penalties for fraud, kickbacks, and other prohibited activities under sections 1128(b)(7) and 1128A(a)(7) of the Act.

A number of statutory and regulatory "safe harbors" protect certain arrangements that might otherwise technically violate the anti-kickback statute from prosecution. *See* section 1128B(b)(3) of the Act; 42 C.F.R. § 1001.952. Safe harbor protection is afforded only to those arrangements that precisely meet all of the conditions set forth in the safe harbor. The relevant safe harbor here is the group purchasing organizations ("GPO") safe harbor. *See* 42 C.R.F. § 1001.952(j).

Source: Office of the Inspector General, Advisory Opinion 98–11, September 14, 1998.

The GPO safe harbor provides protection for payments by a vendor of goods or services to a GPO (the "GPO fee"). For purposes of this safe harbor, a GPO is defined as an entity authorized to act as a purchasing agent for a group of individuals or entities who (i) are furnishing services for which payment may be made in whole or in part under Medicare or a State health care program and (ii) are neither wholly owned by the GPO nor subsidiaries of a parent corporation that wholly owns the GPO (either directly or through another wholly-owned entity). The GPO fee must be paid as part of an agreement to furnish goods or services to the group of individuals or entities for which the GPO is the authorized agent.

The GPO must have a written agreement with each individual or entity that will purchase items or services from the vendor. The agreement must accurately reflect the amount of the GPO fee by satisfying one of the following two conditions. First, the agreement may state that the GPO fee will be three percent or less of the purchase price of the goods or services sold by the vendor to the individual or entity. Second, if the GPO fee is greater than three percent, the agreement must state the specific amount of the fee, expressed either as a fixed sum or as a fixed percentage of the value of the purchases made from the vendor by the members of the group under the contract between the vendor and the GPO. If the amount of the GPO fee is not known at the time the agreement is signed, the agreement must state the maximum amount to be paid to the GPO by the vendor. In addition, where the entity that receives the goods or services from the vendor is a health care provider of services, the GPO must disclose in writing to the entity at least annually, and to the Secretary upon request, the amount received from each vendor with respect to purchases made by or on behalf of the entity. *See* 42 C.F.R. §1001.952(j).

CHAPTER FIVE

INVENTORY AND DISTRIBUTION PROCESS

The Search for Strategy

From a systemwide perspective, "supply chain management is a set of approaches used to efficiently integrate suppliers, manufacturers, warehouses, and stores so that merchandise is produced and distributed at the right quantities, to the right locations, and the right time in order to minimize systemwide costs while satisfying service-level requirements."[1] Such an orientation has been very difficult in an industry where health care has not traditionally viewed distribution and inventory as an expense for which value is clearly defined or as part of their strategic investments. Nevertheless, it is an investment due to the extent of assets involved. Recent studies have shown that tremendous cost savings and potential revenue can be generated with strategic management of distribution and inventory. Wal-Mart and Dell Computers have become industry leaders because of their distribution and inventory processes. This is not to say that a hospital or system will make these processes their core competencies. However, it is a strong argument that distribution and inventory can become a strategic force.

At the time the fieldwork for this book was initiated in 2000, research on the hospital sector projected that a hospital could reduce its total expenses by about 2 percent through better inventory and distribution processes of finished medical materials.[2] While some very large suppliers and manufacturers, such as Johnson and Johnson, manufacture many different products, many suppliers manufacture only one or two unique items. As Burns and DeGraaff have pointed out, "There are 12,000 medical device manufacturers. Most of these manufacturers are small. Eight hundred members of the Health Industry Manufacturers Association (HIMA) reportedly generate 90 percent of the revenues."[3] The complexity of the environment is amplified by the need to assess the way a hospital or system should use multiple distributors as well as by the fact that not all suppliers choose to use distributors. This is the case for many suppliers of high-cost physician preference items, such as implantable materials, where supplier representatives both maintain inventory and assist clinicians in the actual choice of product at the point of service.

Given the $125 billion that providers spend annually on supplies and pharmaceuticals, an efficient supply chain inventory and distribution process could substantially provide savings to health care delivery in the United States.[4] Paradoxically, few of the ASU/CHMR study participants (even those that had made major advances in reducing inventory and distribution costs) articulated inventory management as a critical variable in achieving excellence in managing the supply chain. The real work of supply chain, in the eyes of many managers, is achieved through a focus on securing lower prices for products.[5] Although major companies outside the health sector attribute a significant proportion of their savings and improved performance to advances in inventory and distribution efficiencies, health care managers are skeptical about what concepts will transfer across the "sector barrier."[6] Also in other industries, vertical integration provides organizations with some of the components needed for achieving finished products. Hospitals, however, produce little of what they consume. Furthermore, hospital materials managers rarely view goods sourced and received as an asset; rather, they view them as a liability.

This chapter emphasizes the lessons learned from progressive system materials managers in the course of the ASU/CHMR study regarding inventory and distribution. In functional terms, the combined purpose of inventory and distribution is to get the goods to the right place at the right time with little or no waiting for delivery. Throughout the chapter, *inventory* refers to the product in some stage of postmanufacture "holding." *Distribution* is employed as a more fluid term, referring to the movement of the product along the supply chain. Inventory may be held at a variety of points: hospitals, distributors, and even suppliers themselves. Moving and storing goods costs money; thus, inventory and distribution management needs to be done as cheaply as possible without losing availability of the desired supplies. In health care delivery organizations, where demand is uncertain and many finished products are consumed in the course of treatment, inventory is necessary because it is not always possible to get the goods immediately from the manufacturer in a timely manner.

One of the principal reasons that hospitals have come together into systems is to gain the advantage of integration, allowing them to purchase larger quantities at lower prices. At the same time, each hospital requires materials on a daily basis, with demand being driven by patients, clinicians, and the variety of system sourcing strategies. This means that attention to inventory and distribution should be present at the micro (point of use such as a hospital nursing service or surgical suite), meso (hospital or other operating unit), and macro (system) levels of analysis.

Supply chain researchers point out that "volatility of demand and inventories in the supply chain tend to be amplified as one looks farther 'upstream'—that is, away from the end user."[7] Hospitals and hospital systems are characterized by a high level of uncertainty for many kinds of products and relative consistency in demand for others. This bimodal feature of product demand in the sector makes managing the internal supply chain difficult for hospitals. Products and processes in health care that are characterized by increased rate of change, predicting demand further up the supply chain, is even more difficult. For example, when drug-eluting stents were introduced to the market, there was still uncertainty about their intended use by surgeons. This made it difficult for suppliers to forecast demand. Anticipation of demand is made even more difficult as surgeons develop new, off-label applications for products. When these stents first came onto the market, some hospitals reported difficulty in securing any quantity of the product, while competing hospitals, some of which had long-standing relationships with the manufacturer, enjoyed ease of access.

The volatility of demand for supplies is described as the "bull-whip effect" or, more recently, as "volatility amplification."[8] This phenomenon leads suppliers to use distributors to buffer (by holding inventory) them against the demands at the hospital or other end use level. At the same time, clinical end users, faced with process-related increases in the processes surrounding their work (or what Fine describes as clockspeed amplification),[9] rely on distributors to develop communication systems that provide accurate product demand information to suppliers. This collaboration is critical to ensure a smooth working environment through effective inventory management. Such distributors may be distinct organizations (for example, Cardinal and Owens and Minor) or the supplier's own distributor organization efforts.

The Role of the Distributor Organization

Over twenty thousand suppliers, spread out across the world, manufacture health care materials.[10] It is noteworthy that purchasers, distributors, and hospitals exist in an environment where there are multiple suppliers for similar items (especially commodities). Distributors assume a stabilizing role by linking hospitals to the many suppliers.[11] For hospitals and systems, 80 percent of materials flow through distributors. Service offerings can be judged by the range of products offered and the satisfaction associated with moving products to the hospital or system (including frequency of delivery, repackaging of goods, and provision of information technology to track use and demand). Just as GPOs manage relationships between purchasers and manufacturers for product selection, price negotiation, and contracting, the purpose of distributor organizations is generally to manage the inventory issue by taking control of many supplies and moving the supplies from the manufacturer to the users.

Few systems are in the position to influence supplier control production schedules and to move sufficiently large quantities of supplies to the hospital. Therefore, the distributor has taken on this role in order to aid in the placement of products and to smooth the demand for goods. The traditional role of the distributor is to:

- Aggregate supplies from many manufacturers
- Customize orders to meet customers' needs
- Dispense or deliver the product to the consumer and move it within the facility

The decision to use a distributor is one of the strategic alternatives that comprise supply chain strategy for both suppliers and for hospital and system buyers. Few suppliers, however, want to take on the distribution function. Systems theoretically could purchase a significant proportion of their goods directly from manufacturers and take ownership and move goods from the manufacturer to the point of service themselves. However, the incredible number of potential partners and items constitutes a daunting task for the supply chain management function. Thus, the vast majority of systems outsource some aspect of their inventory and distribution to one or more of the several large distributors serving hospitals in the United States. To the extent that hospitals and systems develop strong relationships with some of the distributors, hospital distribution relationships take on the features of alliances discussed in Chapter Four.

Level of Distributor Penetration into the Organization

There is significant variance in how progressive hospitals and systems balance their own participation in distribution and inventory. Many of the ASU/CHMR participating hospitals and systems have significant stores and strong distributor relationships. They also believe that it is not in their best interest to manage the hundreds of invoices or to receive the thousands of goods directly themselves. However, a number of systems studied by Burns and DeGraaff engaged in "disintermediation": the elimination of distributors as middlemen firms in their supply chains.[12] Their motivation was to (1) increase flexibility in contracting, (2) leverage manufacturers' willingness to underprice national buying groups, (3) generate new sources of revenue, and (4) reduce the cost of supplies.[13] The regional service center developed by LeeSar Health Trust Partners has a fifty-thousand-square-foot distribution center that allows it to couple self-distribution and self-contracting in order to insource both distributor and GPO functions. But such regional cooperatives have been difficult to form, and they require, beyond a strong business plan, an incredible level of trust and institutional commitment.

Consistent with the discussion of strategic fit in Chapter Four, the ASU/CHMR progressive hospitals and systems seek a mix of distributor services that best meet their circumstances.[14] A number of progressive systems at the time of this study were considering extending their warehousing and internal distribution capabilities. The decision to take on this function adhered to the extent that insourcing of the function would allow them to save transaction costs and better meet predicted demand. Paradoxically, other progressive systems were interested in the idea of more fully outsourcing aspects of distribution and developing strong distribution alliances. While many articulated a fear of losing part of a hospital or system's competency, there appeared to be a growing view that inventory and distribution management might not be a hospital's core competency. The University of Nebraska Medical Center (discussed later in some detail) was the only system visited that can be characterized by a comprehensive inventory and distribution outsourcing strategy.

Figure 5.1 describes the flow of items from manufacturer or supplier to the hospital floor. As detailed in Table 5.1, inventory can be held or manipulated by the distributor and the level of distributor of penetration into the hospital (levels 00 and 0) or distributor (levels 1 to 4). Levels 00 and 0 distribution actually pertain to products where the supplier holds inventory at its own stores or at its own sites or its agent's site near the hospital. The penetration of distributor services into the hospital varies considerably in progressive systems. It is noteworthy that level 1 and successive levels are characterized by functions that are frequently additive. Thus, in level 1, the distributor receives the item from the manufacturer and generally holds the item for some period of time in a warehouse and distributes quantities to the hospital warehouse or stores as needed. Level 4 distribution involves the full assumption of inventory and distribution functions by the distributor's employees.

FIGURE 5.1.   A SIMPLISTIC VIEW OF THE FLOW OF MATERIALS.

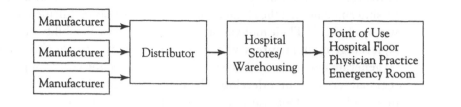

TABLE 5.1.   LEVELS OF DISTRIBUTOR FUNCTION.

Level	Distributor Function	Hospital Function
Level 00	Supplier-held and -managed products through supplier-employed distribution agents.	Hospital frequently does not take ownership of such goods or goods enter into hospital accounting and inventory system after they have been used.
Level 0	Supplier-held and -managed products through third-party logistics companies to reduce transportation costs and management and to better connect to suppliers and distributors.	Hospital acts as a receiver of the product and deploys the product into use or inventory.
Level 1	Distributor brings ordered goods to hospital warehouse.	Hospital employees break down orders into quantities that are transported by hospital employees to individual hospitals in a system and onto floors for storage.
Level 2	Distributor breaks down orders into quantities needed on different floors and brings ordered goods to hospital shipping dock.	Hospital employees transport goods to floors and stock goods into floor stockrooms and dispensing systems.
Level 3	Distributor carries out levels 1 and 2 functions and transports goods to the floor.	Hospital employees place goods into floor stockrooms and dispensing systems.
Level 4	Distributor carries out levels 1, 2, and 3 tasks and places goods into floor stockrooms and dispensing systems.	Hospital employees have minimal role in transporting goods and servicing dispensing systems.

At a minimalist penetration level (level 1), hospitals and systems use distributors to bring goods to the hospital warehouse. From there, hospital-employed distribution teams take ownership of inventory and manage its transportation to the point of service. Successive levels are characterized by distributors' transporting goods to the point of service on the hospital floor. This amounts to a partial outsourcing of the distribution function.

Level 2 distributions may include products that have passed through both the distributor and hospital warehouse but are now delivered in quantities that are relevant to their eventual destinations. In many progressive hospitals, one can observe containers that have been delivered from a distributor or hospital central store and are now awaiting someone to move the product to the point of use.

Level 3 distributions involve the distributor's employees actually delivering products to the floors. This is an advanced alliance in which the agents of an outside entity are carrying out an internal function. It requires that the distributor hire individuals who have both the technical skills necessary for such a role as well as the ability to be "guest workers" within the hospital. This level of distributor penetration requires a major investment in information systems and personnel. Hospitals are in business twenty-four hours a day every day of the year, and the demand for products is continuous. Level 3, when carried out effectively, serves all hospital shifts and is characterized by a service focus that is compatible with the hospital's own personnel and expectations. As "guest workers" in a hospital, a distributor's employees must understand the hospital's culture and variable demands that will be made on stores at different times.

The most extreme example of distribution penetration and alliance development is level 4, which is characterized by the outsourcing responsibility for the holding and movement of a good with the distributor, which actually retains ownership of materials to the point of use. The University of Nebraska is a level 4 organization; it has outsourced virtually its entire materials management function to Cardinal Health. It has reported savings of $1.2 million per year due to less inventory shrinkage, better product mix, and more efficient inventory management.[15] Some of the benefits associated with such outsourcing include the freeing up of capital to invest in new ventures, reduction in the need for the hospital to directly supervise a large number of supply management employees, the ability of those who are employed by the hospital to engage in strategically focused activities, and the opportunity to continuously improve the inventory and distribution function at a state-of-the-art level. In addition, the hospital appears to benefit significantly from the presence of distributor staff who continuously provide consultation to the hospital on its use of materials. These benefits must be assessed in relationship to the fees paid to the distributor, the transaction costs involved in managing the relationship between the distributor and the hospital, and the hospital's true benefit from not having funds tied to inventory.

Distribution, Inventory, and Their Associated Costs

As hospitals strive to serve their customers and avoid stock-outs, they present themselves as a complex mix of inventory and distribution models. While predicting the need for linen and laundry is not very complex and easily outsourced to a distributor or local laundry organization, many hospitals have their own linen stocks and carry out their own laundry functions. A hospital that carries out a significant amount of orthopedic surgery might have a high level of comfort that distributor-held inventory in a very competitive local market can reliably serve the hospital's needs. A hospital with a similar volume of surgery in a market that it dominates might find it much more convenient to demand that a supplier provide the inventory on an owned or consignment basis. What all of this complexity means is that it is very difficult to assess the cost or return on investment of inventory strategy and inventory-related technology.

Inventory Owned by the Hospital. A traditional way to assess a hospital's inventory is to assess the quantity of a material being held in its own warehouse, in operating unit storage rooms, or on hospital floors themselves. The average inventory and the rate of inventory turnover are a function of the reorder quantity. Smaller replenishment order quantities result in a lower average inventory. Several factors affect average inventory and order quantity, including the shelf life of products, purchasing discounts, minimum order and lot sizes, storage requirements, transportation economies, and a willingness to manage the inventory.

The capacity to track inventory and replenishment strategies determines inventory and order quantity. In the health sector, as in other industries, an exact order quantity policy can be determined by balancing the cost of ordering and the cost of maintaining average inventory. Given the tens of thousands of items available to an average hospital, under conditions characterized by uncertainty regarding demand, ensuring that the correct products are available at the correct time, and for the lowest price, has been challenging. A hospital or system that has invested in extensive technology to track inventory and report use, both internally and to a distributor, will enjoy a wider range of inventory options than a hospital or system with inadequate information. In addition, inventory options are affected by geographical factors, including proximity to a distributor's warehouse and the dispersion of hospitals in a system.

Inventory Held by Others. To the extent that costs incurred along the supply chain are passed on to those who pay for care, costs associated with inventory that is not owned by hospitals are paid for as part of total price and must be considered as part of inventory and distribution costs. In the health sector, as in other industries, suppliers and distributors themselves take on the responsibility of managing a part of the hospital's need for inventory. Some of these inventory stores may be close to where products are manufactured, but many are characterized by products held close to their point of use. Suppliers of highly specialized clinical preference items, for example, employ individuals who work closely with clinicians, bringing products directly from a local supplier-owned storage site into the hospital on the day of a procedure. Understandably, some of these items may never be logged into a hospital's inventory system. Therefore, hospital or system costs associated with local storage, transportation, and services are not being accurately accounted for.

Inventory Technology and Strategy

While there is little formal research related to return on investment (ROI) for health sector supply chain technology and innovation, a wide range of technology-related information is providing improved transactional efficiencies and, in many instances, lowered operating expenses.[16] The use of automated inventory control cabinetry systems, such as Cardinal's Pyxis, provides inventory control including inventory updates and automatic billing records. Such technology allows hospitals and distributors to track product use and reorder status. Cardinal's use of its own systems at the University of Nebraska Hospital provides value to the outsourced relationship and reduction in costs. While progressive systems report that over 80 percent of their transactions are electronic, with a continued decrease in the orders processed using fax and telephone, many hospitals and systems continue to hand-process many orders to their distributors.

Different Environments, Different Strategies

Progressive systems are not consistently characterized by any one level of inventory and distribution management. This is consistent with the central idea associated with contingency management as emphasized throughout this book: that there may not be one solution for all circumstances or products. Two of the Mayo Clinic sites (Rochester, Minnesota, and Scottsdale, Arizona) provide an interesting example of a progressive system that has centralized a number of its supply chain leadership and operations functions, but employs very different distribution and inventory strategies and tactics. The Mayo Clinic Scottsdale hospital, which is relatively small (just over two hundred beds), uses sophisticated computer technology that monitors inventory on each nursing service and communicates, based on preestablished levels, replenishment orders to the distributor. Its point-of-use scanning technology guides a just-in-time (JIT) inventory system that allows the hospital to be characterized by minimal warehousing and storage of materials within the hospital. By definition, JIT "means that components and raw materials arrive at a work center exactly as they are needed . . . providing the right part at the right place at the right time."[17] One of the expected outcomes is that the average inventory in this hospital is extraordinarily low, and inventory turnovers are extraordinarily high when compared to hospitals that do not use the JIT program. In addition, the predetermination of replenishment levels dramatically simplifies the planning and control function.[18] Traditional inventory management metrics, such as number of inventory turns, may not describe the performance of hospitals with JIT systems. Such hospitals may want to look closely at how companies such as Dell, which holds inventory for very short periods of time, benchmark their own performance.

Hospitals that effectively use JIT inventory models are frequently able to achieve their goals because they are in markets where distributors that serve multiple hospitals in the market have fairly deep stores at the regional level and are able to respond quickly to the information that is received on a fairly real-time basis. Hospitals in a more isolated market, with the same technology, might have much larger inventory in order to buffer itself against the cycle time between posting an order and actual delivery.

The Mayo Clinic in Rochester, Minnesota, a complex multihospital system in a relatively isolated geographical area, has a substantial warehouse and distribution system. Between St. Mary's and Rochester Memorial, the home site has over two thousand beds. Mayo's centralized supply management leadership recognizes that variability in circumstances determines differences in strategies and tactics. Other hospitals within Phoenix and similar markets have not invested in electronic inventory systems to ensure JIT delivery. Such hospitals are characterized by larger orders at different points of inventory depletion. They must be judged on their ability to manage a low-cost warehouse and distribution system based on factors such as bed size and labor costs. Thus, the appropriate average inventory is truly a product of marketplace, resources, and overall strategy.

Systems and even hospitals within systems find themselves in very different operating and geographical circumstances. A rural hospital cannot expect the same level of distributor response as an urban hospital where a distributor is using inventory to service multiple customers. Thus, a low-level inventory approach may be useful in one setting but not another. This means that while a system may have a strategy that attempts to integrate its cost-containment goals, policies, and action sequences into a cohesive whole, tactics may differ.[19] Because of this, no one approach to inventory and distribution improvement in the progressive systems in the ASU/CHMR study was revealed.

Improving Inventory and Distribution Systems

Frazelle has identified five initiatives that lead to both increased return on inventory and inventory availability: (1) improved forecast accuracy, (2) reduced cycle times, (3) lower purchase order and setup costs, (4) improved inventory visibility, and (5) lower inventory carrying costs.[20] Few of the systems in the ASU/CHMR study were engaged in systematically profiling their organizations on optimal decision variables associated with these initiatives (such as economic order quantity, unit fill rate, optimal safety stock levels, reorder points, or order up-to-level points).[21] Rather, the progressive systems tended to articulate their inventory and distribution systems as a series of trade-offs and tactics around availability and cost.

Progressive systems assess the trade-offs between availability and costs of materials as well as plan and carry out supply chain tactics to meet their goals for supply chain performance. Perhaps of greatest importance is the ability of managers in such systems to manage the uncertainty of demand and assess the advisability of employing different tactics, such as overnight shipping, to ensure the seamless operation of the hospital.

Trade-Offs Exist Between Availability and Cost

In general, the greater the availability of a good for immediate use, the greater is the good's cost. The trade-off is the service that a product's availability brings to the hospital or system and the revenue generated by the product's availability. In general, a product should generate revenue greater than the cost. When inventory is reduced, cost is reduced, but customer service is potentially sacrificed. Therefore, there must be a careful management of these trade-offs.

A number of factors significantly affect how ASU/CHMR materials managers view trade-offs across and for unique portions of their systems. Systems in major metropolitan markets are able to take advantage of stockpiles by distributors within a geographical environment and work to approximate a JIT environment. The strategy is much more problematic for hospitals in more geographically remote areas. Systems that engage in extensive standardization find that problems with securing goods are significantly streamlined. This is especially true when compared to their counterparts with a wider range of clinical preference items that must be made available on demand.

Asset return in organizations is frequently seen as a function of risk management, with hospitals and systems attempting to deploy their assets in a manner that will create the greatest returns with the smallest risk. As discussed in depth in Chapter Two, in the health arena, risk of overpaying for inventory exists in order to ensure availability. The trade-off to overpaying would be suffering loss of clientele due to poor customer service, inferior clinical outcomes, and decreased revenue when the asset is unavailable.

Reimbursement models that limit the amount of compensation to a fixed amount, such as diagnosis-related groups and capitation, provide incentives for the system to engage in efficient purchasing. Consider an example where medical device A costs $500 and device B costs $1,000; both lead to similar outcomes. The amount of reimbursement, no matter which implant is used, is fixed. Therefore, using a higher-cost device will lead to reduced revenues for those under such global reimbursement schemes.

The hospital materials department traditionally manages the availability-cost trade-off by having an extensive safety stock, maintained in order to protect against demand uncertainty. The focus on average inventory is built on a formula of average demand plus a percentage of added safety stock. This is used as a risk-averse strategy but could also be construed as a poor use of assets. In one of the ASU/CHMR research sites, the added percentage for most products was a 50 percent safety stock. Yet no formula for determining the appropriate level was available for review. In the Scottsdale Mayo hospital, par levels are established and inventory replenished as such levels are depleted. Hospital evaluation of risk in the distribution environment, trust established with distributors, and ability to manage demand all influence how hospitals will approach the issue of safety stock.

Economic Order Quantity Models

Economic order quantity (EOQ) models in many industries provide a specific order quantity that balances availability and cost components. Management is then able to identify the minimal total cost of inventory by determining the EOQ and dividing it into annual demand (the frequency and size of replenishment orders).[22] The issue in health care is that annual demand is irregular, which makes it difficult to determine the EOQ. In addition, irregular circumstances, such as a multiple train-car accident or act of terrorism, are significantly beyond the capability of everyday models employed by hospitals. Yet these models, when applied in health care, help to identify the appropriate levels of buffer inventory necessary to prevent stock-outs. Perhaps it is best to think of "buffer level" as that level of stock that reduces risk and turns what is apparently irregular into a better level of predictable material.

Effective management of inventory requires that simulation models and other statistical techniques are appropriately applied to the health sector. However, the "complexity of probabilistic models increases greatly when lead times, usable quantities received, and inventory shrinkage rates, and so on, also vary under conditions of uncertainty, when nonnormal distributions are observed and when the variations change with time."[23] However, few health care materials management departments employ individuals who can effectively calculate and strategically use the findings of such simulations, let alone carry them out.

Inventory carry cost, the expense associated with maintaining inventory, is calculated by multiplying annual inventory carry cost percentage by average inventory value. Inventory carry costing includes obsolescence and storage. The cost of obsolescence occurs when the product ages beyond a recommended sales date or a new product replaces the need for an old one. Storage costs are the facility expenses related to the product.

The inventory issue is especially acute with hospitals due to economies of scale. Few hospitals are large enough to have an inventory function that can carry all of the diverse product lines. Imagine the thousands of products that a hospital consumes in an average month. Standardization assists in reducing the number of items to be carried in inventory. Progressive systems, for example, have identified areas for such reductions (such as sutures) and find dramatic cost savings associated with their actions.

Greater challenges stem from the complexity and uniqueness of clinical specialty products or rare pharmaceuticals with a short shelf-life. One solution, observed in virtually every hospital in the United States today is the use of overnight shipping, or drop shipping. These shipments are costly and frequently represent the inability of the system to manage demand and the distributor to manage client's needs.

Hospitals must also consider the chance that prices will increase over time and develop strategies to meet increases. Long-term contracts, which specify the range of allowable increases, are one strategy. Other strategies include the actual purchase of additional inventories and the costs incurred by such decisions.[24]

Swings in product demand, frequently described in the supply chain management literature as the "bullwhip effect," influence the availability of goods and the efficiency of manufacturers.[25] Distributors buffer inventory problems by carrying substantial quantities of goods in warehouses. The inability of their hospital customers to predict product demand leads, as in many other industries, to a wide range of upstream inefficiencies. As the inability to predict demand intensifies and as orders transmitted from end user to supplier remain unpredictable, suppliers may engage in relatively irrational manufacturing patterns to meet perceived (if not real) demand.

The costs of these irregularities in the health sector remain relatively unexplored, but there is a strong belief that the robust distributor and hospital warehouse systems create "a buffer between the supplier and hospital or system trading partners."[26] Burns and DeGraaff suggest that "direct contracting between buyer and seller," or what was discussed earlier as disintermediation, "continually confronts any wholesaler/distributor."[27] *3PL* is a term that refers to the use of outside carriers that transport items to a business. Hospital loading docks are characterized by a constant parade of delivery trucks moving goods, principally directly from the supplier to the hospital. It has been pointed out that such firms offer value to hospitals and hospital systems. According to one analyst, a medium-sized system can spend $500,000 a year in both inbound and outbound small package delivery. Manufacturers estimate that a twelve-hospital system can spend up to $800,000 a year in overnight shipping.[28]

In many instances, the use of 3PL is an efficient response to meet needs that are difficult to anticipate and for goods that are too costly to maintain in a warehouse situation. Interviews with one of the nation's largest suppliers, Johnson and Johnson, suggest that in many cases, however, 3PL deliveries represent a breakdown in the ability of hospitals to manage their own inventory needs efficiently. Greater study is needed to assess the costs and benefits associated with 3PL. However, the increased sophistication and reliability among 3PL systems has enhanced the ability of the health care system to reduce inventory, meet demand, and satisfy a number of clients.

Strategic and Tactical Questions

Progressive materials managers use a strategic approach in the development and management of inventory and distribution within a complex supply chain. These individuals scrutinize their assets (time and money) to obtain the greatest value at the lowest cost. On the basis of this discussion, a series of strategic and tactical questions assess value, control, and power in the management of the supply chain. (Readers are cautioned that these questions cannot uniformly be answered in a way that will meet the needs of all systems.)

Strategic Questions

Different strategies are needed to maximize assets, system structure, geographical constraints, and clinical strategies.

What Do Inventory and Distribution Value Mean? During the ASU/CHMR case studies, it was found that most managers have difficulty defining value for inventory and distribution. It may almost be true that the phrase *adding value* has become a cliché that is used to fit nearly everything. To quote a long-term observer of the health care supply chain, "The term 'value' has become so over used that it has created an interesting paradox."[29] The reason that it means almost nothing or has created a paradox is that most health care executives, while invoking "value" as an attribute of a relationship or transaction, do not have a definite meaning and measurement for it.

The strategic value of inventory is to both increase service and decrease costs. However, trade-offs exist in a rather contradictory manner. While the strategic value of an item determines the trade-offs, the attributed value of a product will determine how much a system is willing to pay for the service being provided by inventory.

The strategic value of a distributor must be assessed by the efficiencies achieved in the movement of goods and strategic advantage gained through distributor information such as market intelligence. Distributor value is also related to the financial services associated with distribution and product ownership.

In the absence of clear definitions pertaining to value, it is not surprising that few systems have a scorecard to assess each of the value proposition items. However, the service acquired from the distribution may help to define the expected value.

How Important Is Control over Inventory and Distribution? As discussed in Chapter Four, strategic management theorists question the extent that "a non core competency could become a competitive advantage among its peers."[30] If all systems are outsourcing their distribution and inventory to third parties, could a competing system develop a differential advantage by developing greater in-house capabilities?[31]

As hospitals and systems consider distribution options, it is important to conduct a total cost analysis of all insourcing and outsourcing alternatives. In this process, systems must consider the current cost of insourcing and how those costs compare to additional costs that might be incurred through switching to outsourcing. The costs must be weighed against potential monetary savings.

Distribution and inventory may not be core system competencies; however, assessment of the hospital's knowledge regarding the value of inventory and distribution should be considered in system strategic development. Figure 5.2 suggests that there is a continuum of strategic locations for managing distribution and inventory. Each type of partnership can result in different value propositions. A variety of partnerships can flourish in contract outsourcing, as demonstrated by the success of newer GPOs. It would appear that such partnerships rest on trust, relationship customization, retention of intellectual property, determination of strategic direction, and recognition that partnerships cannot be translated into abdication for responsibility.

FIGURE 5.2.   CONTINUUM OF DISTRIBUTION CONTROL.

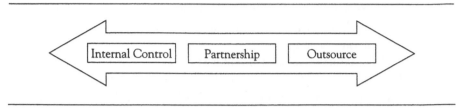

Distribution is not a core competency of a health care provider, but when a process is outsourced, some level of control over both expenditures and customer service may be lost. The hospital is essentially hiring an agent for its distribution and inventory; however, the agent is also managing many other customers. The hospital must assess the extent to which its agent will express an appropriate level of concern for internal and external customers.

Management needs to consider the strategic relationship that exists between control and intellectual property. When a process is completely outsourced, the related knowledge is outsourced as well. Eventually it makes it difficult to evaluate the service obtained.[32] It is important to fully measure the internal intellectual capability necessary to continually assess those areas that are outsourced. One of the key observations from examining one system that engaged in a great deal of distribution outsourcing was the difficulty it experienced in assessing the value of services provided by the distributor.

While organizational culture, availability of managerial talent, and interest in building strategic advantage must guide decisions regarding distribution and inventory outsourcing, it is important that systems develop a sufficient understanding of the outsourced functions to assess performance on both a day-to-day and a long-term basis. At the University of Nebraska Hospital, which has outsourced a significant portion of its inventory and distribution, the system has retained strong internal leadership with such capability. Outsourcing a function does not give a system authority to stop managing the function; rather, it should monitor its relationships and ensure that it continues to sustain advantage.

What Is Your Power Within the Supply Chain? Research has indicated that equal collaboration is seldom, if ever, present in a supply chain. One party generally has a dominant level of power.[33] One way to visualize the distribution process and power in the health care supply chain is within an hourglass that is extremely large at both ends (Figure 5.3). Hundreds of manufacturers and thousands of hospitals seek distributor partners. Yet a very few distributors control the flow of materials and information. Both hospital systems and distributors are

FIGURE 5.3.   HOURGLASS MODEL.

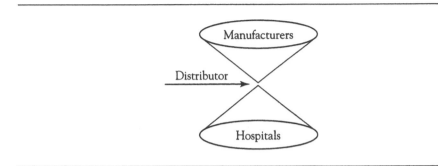

characterized by their power to influence the health care supply chain, but the power balance differs from one situation to the next. Although distributors and manufacturers exercise power by presenting a unified face to the hospital,[34] increasingly there are tensions between suppliers and distributors. Suppliers, for example, have resisted paying fees as distributors find their avenues for income reduced and hospitals and systems have sought new services for affiliation with distributors. Thus, it is not clear if the hospital system or the manufacturer can be classified as more important and having more power with the distributor.

In the health sector, distributors seek fees from both hospitals and suppliers. Distributors believe they are providing valuable services to both groups and generally have established a comfort level with the subsequent tensions that arise in working with an organization that has gain from both its suppliers and its customers. Perhaps this is because the distributor is actually serving two sets of very fragmented markets. Any service provider likes to serve fragmented markets because the customer generally has less power. While this may be the ideal situation that any service provider desires, distributors continue to operate on fairly low margins. Suggested reasons for this include intense rivalry among distributors and that distributors have not clearly distinguished themselves with a new set of either added- or needed-value products.

Progressive systems closely follow the opportunities afforded by changes in distributor and supplier relationships and work to secure supplier services to assist in their management of the supply chain. If the system does not receive service, it can seek an alternative distributor. The hospital system can also pursue structural or operational changes to make it more attractive to a distributor partner. The system might, for example, ask the distributor to distribute not to the hospital loading dock but to provide added service by delivering materials directly to the floor. Alternatively the system might invest in better software to give the supplier a better understanding of the system's utilization and demand patterns.

What Strategies Can Systems That Lack Leverage with a Distributor Use? Not all hospitals and systems appear to have great leverage with distributors. Some, for example, have not brought great discipline to their purchasing and order relatively low quantities on an unpredictable schedule. Distributors have worked closely with these organizations to improve performance, not always with success. Small hospitals, by their very nature, have difficulty providing distributors with the kind of volumes they prefer to manage for any one customer.

Among the possibilities are these:

• Local alliance formation to improve power with distributors. One system took the approach of forming a partnership with a large, freestanding hospital in another city. Because the two cities were relatively near each other, they could form a viable inventory system that was not seen as a competitive threat.

• Collaboration with distributors. A small network formed a close collaboration with a large distributor. It gave up much control in order to make itself an attractive partner. When the distributor took over the system's inventory management, it offered value to the system by serving as a model in its promotional efforts.

• Insource-selected distribution functions. An example of becoming equal partners is provided by two systems that individually lacked power but were able to gain power by forming a collaborative inventory and distribution system that could compete with the distributor. Because of their increased volumes, the two systems could generate much additional power in their negotiations with the distributor and they formed a viable partnership.

Building Partnerships. An important note here is that for many years, business experts have advised manufacturers to treat their distributors like partners in revenue creation.[35] Unfortunately, the same has not been strongly advocated for health care providers, as they have generally abdicated their business control to the distributor. Analysis of the ASU/CHMR study sites indicates that strategic questions revolving around value, control, and power are infrequently addressed by health care executives. However, before it is possible to improve distribution and inventory, it is necessary to define strategic value. Then it is imperative to determine the extent of control the executive team wants over the expenses and services represented in these processes. In addition, the depth of desired knowledge must be determined. Also, the power within the supply chain must be assessed. The information provided from these strategic issues, in addition to

EXHIBIT 5.1.   TACTICAL QUESTIONS TO IDENTIFY DISTRIBUTION AND INVENTORY STRATEGIC IMPROVEMENTS.

Can you identify and classify all externally acquired goods and services?

What is your inventory turnover?

What is your percentage of inventory waste?

What is the cost of a stock-out or a poor fill rate?

To what extent can an integrated and centralized distribution and inventory system be used for the system?

How effective are your standardization efforts?

What are your distribution and inventory information capabilities?

What are your distribution and inventory personnel capabilities?

---

the following eight tactical issues, will develop a strategic approach to the supply chain.

Tactical Questions

Strategy is implemented with tactics. The current state and maturity of tactical efforts, however, help determine appropriate strategic directions. The eight tactical questions or issues addressed in this section and summarized in Exhibit 5.1 provide directions for strategy development.

Can You Identify and Classify All Externally Acquired Goods and Services?
Distribution and inventory strategy must be considered within the context of individual products and product portfolios. The average hospital makes about fifteen thousand annual purchases of pharmaceuticals, medical devices, surgical supplies, and capital equipment. This is in addition to other operational services and supplies, such as office supplies, cafeteria services, and janitorial services. Expenses resulting from external expenditure quickly add up.

To understand the external acquisition, movement, and inventory of goods, it is helpful to classify goods in several different ways, such as by dollar, service, and criticality. The dollar value is probably the easiest classification to develop, but even this can be difficult. In hospitals and systems, a spend analysis may be difficult because different suppliers use different product numbers and brand names for similar products. In addition, the same system may use different information systems in various hospitals, making it difficult to determine the aggregate spend. To complicate the situation even more, in even the most progressive systems there is purchasing of many contracted items through noncontractual sources. In the area of office supplies, for example, a major hospital business unit, located close to a retail office supply company, purchased many supplies through the local unit rather than using the existing contract. This not only leads to paying different prices for many items, but it leads to many avenues for items to enter the hospital. Even in the face of such difficulties, it is important for a hospital or system to determine the aggregate spend for a product or class of products in order to know if it is possible to establish a separate distribution process for a product. If the spend is high, the manufacturer may be much more willing to discuss alternatives for direct distribution.

A classification system also clarifies the importance rate by which an item is replenished (the fill rate). Availability is more vital for some items than for others. If availability is important, it may be more justifiable to pay extra for the inventory than if the service is less critical. A highly related question asks about the ultimate user and the value of the item to the user. Even when the identity of the user is known, the nature of that user is often not known.

A hospital that does not know how much it is spending on an item or a family of goods cannot develop a strategy. Most of the hospitals in the ASU/CHMR study are beginning to form a spend analysis. However, the major issue was that items were difficult to classify because each company would put a slightly unique attribute on an item so that it would appear to be different. The goal of marketing is to make products appear differentiated even if they are similar. Meanwhile, the goal of the hospital's supply management is to identify the product commonalities and standardize them. This creates a conflict of interest between the two parties, making it difficult to use advanced supply chain purchasing tactics.

In summary, all inventory and distribution analysis depends on the classification of items and a family of goods. Organizations that fail to conduct a strategic analysis of distribution and inventory often fail at this first critical step.

What Is Your Inventory Turnover? This question could be stated another way: What is current inventory costing you? The ASU/CHMR research indicates that hospitals have only a general idea about their inventory costs. An important note is that inventory can officially be classified as materials that are in a warehouse or central inventory area. However, it may also be stored near an operating room or other distributed locations. These areas are relatively easy to monitor. Inventory may also be in a "cache" such as a nurses' station, where it is no longer found in the hospital's records or officially classified as inventory.

An example of unofficial inventory was seen in an emergency room where many supplies were there "just in case," but nobody had any idea how much was there or how long the supplies had been there. One indication of mismanaged inventory was that large packets of gauze discontinued over six months ago could still be found along with gauze from the new supplier. This was a symptom of both poor inventory control and understanding of the inventory turns. For large systems, this is not a trivial issue. If the inventory turnover for individual supply or a class of supplies cannot be determined, neither can its cost or value. Furthermore, it is not possible to determine how to improve a process when the current state cannot be identified.

What Is Your Percentage of Inventory Waste? How much inventory comes through the front door but is never used? Some items are not directly charged to a patient account, and other items simply disappear. In an academic health center, a materials manager explained how many personal toiletries disappeared. He assumed that the residents took them for personal use. When asked about the cost of this, he simply explained that it was considered "a cost of doing business." When considering the total cost of supplies, these toiletries are not a large expenditure; however, it is a symptom of poor controls.

Waste occurs when unused but still viable products are thrown away for no reason. For example, when walking through a storeroom, a materials manager supervisor took an item from a table and threw it in a wastebasket. When asked what it was, he explained that it was returned from a floor because it had mistakenly been opened.

The greatest waste probably occurs when only a small portion of a surgical kit is used and the remainder is either returned or discarded. When asked about this issue, another materials manager replied, "I know there is a lot of money walking out the door in these situations, but I don't know what we can do about it. It really isn't anything new." This is a difficult situation but again an example of poor inventory and distribution control. This may be one of the greatest opportunities for immediate cost reduction.

What Is the Cost of a Stock-Out or a Poor Fill Rate? The irregular demand cycles for most hospital supplies make stock-outs an especially difficult issue. Therefore, the place to start with managing the cost of stock-outs is to develop a clear understanding of demand cycles. This should be done in combination with the product profile mentioned above. For some of the items, a 100 percent fill rate may be extremely important and a stock-out costly. Unfortunately, an accurate assessment of the inventory service cannot be determined unless the items are evaluated in a quantifiable manner.

It is difficult to determine the cost of a stock-out because it is an attempt to quantify an intangible attribute: service. However, it can be accomplished with different levels of accuracy. One system developed a method for putting dollar values on stock-outs that provided concrete feedback to the distributor and top-level management. Although the accuracy of the system could be debated, they saw this as a first effort to quantify service levels. In another situation, an effort was made to calculate the amount of labor required to expedite an item when it was not in inventory. The main finding was a surprisingly high number of expedited items and high labor expense. This labor cost subsequently justified hiring an inventory management professional.

To What Extent Can an Integrated and Centralized Distribution and Inventory System Be Used for the System?

While there has been much speculation about the advantages and disadvantages of centralization of services through a system, many have not been recognized.[36] The assumption is that centralization of distribution services and inventory management within a large, integrated delivery health care system would lead to economies of scale and scope.[37] Chopra and Meindl identify a variety of advantages related to the economies of scale, including the ability to exploit fixed costs, the exploitation of quantity discounts, and short-term discounting. As volume increases, it would be possible to rationalize a larger number of services and manage inventory over more items.[38] The application of quantitative methods for forecasting demand in larger systems, such as queuing theory (which considers the entry and exit of numerous demands into the system), explains why large hospital systems can carry smaller inventories as a percentage of sales than smaller systems to maintain a fixed rate of stock to avoid outages.[39]

The potential value of centralization depends on several things. First, it is important that there be centralized coordination of four systems: control, information, inventory, and distribution. It would be of no value to have a centralized information system if no centralized control exists. Also, it will not be possible to have any centralized distribution and inventory without a centralized control and information systems.

Second, it is important to understand the extent to which common supply needs exist across the system. If each unit has highly dissimilar needs, economies of scale will be more difficult and the power of centralization limited. The importance of a centralized standardization process therefore is important to determine the extent of common supply use.

The third consideration is geographical proximity. It will be much more difficult to develop economies of scale and scope as the units become more geographically dispersed. Centralized distribution and inventory is probably more likely for a system situated in an urban environment than one based in a rural area.

How Effective Are Your Standardization Efforts?

A purpose of distribution is to aggregate products from different manufacturers and deliver to one point of use. However, the possibility exists that highly similar products are being obtained from two different manufacturers. If they were being purchased from the same manufacturer, it would not be necessary to aggregate across manufacturers. In addition, if volume was great enough with one manufacturer, it may be possible to work directly with the manufacturer rather than a distributor.

It was not the purpose of the research reported here to identify precise cost savings amounts. However, other research indicates that an estimated savings of 5 to 6 percent can be experienced with the average standardization program and 5 to 7 percent on substitution programs.[40] This is regardless of the model used, such as a vendor direct to the hospital or a distributor. The hospitals in this study recognize the potential in standardization and are attempting to develop, as with pharmaceuticals, a materials formulary. HCA, with its several hundred hospitals, has moved in this direction. In most other systems, however, standardization in even most commodity items is not being realized. As one executive in the ASU/CHMR study said, "At times there seems to be no common grounds between great ideals and basic implementation." Standardization is a basic implementation that must be achieved for any distribution and inventory strategy to be successful. Even when it is accomplished, systems seem to slip back to having numerous items for those that were formally standardized. The logical explanation is that many institutions still do not recognize the importance of standardization. As a result, in many instances, adequate personnel resources are not being dedicated to the process.

What Are Your Distribution and Inventory Information Capabilities? Information technology is identified as the number one facilitator of supply chain improvement.[41] While there is an accelerating adoption rate of online exchange opportunities, enterprisewide supply chain systems, and other Web-based applications, they have not yet become the most influential dynamics in the distribution market and have not led to distributor disintermediation.[42]

A 2001 consulting study on the value of e-commerce in the health care supply chain concludes that value can be created in the range of 1 to 3 percent of total provider supply costs of fully using e-commerce capabilities.[43] This conclusion was based on the following information:

- Electronic data interchange (EDI) use is only about 31 percent of the total possible electronic invoices.
- An e-commerce solution could reduce processing errors by as much as 52 percent (accounts payable rework and invoice reconciliation).
- Providers can overpay suppliers by 2 to 7 percent.
- Extensive time is spent on manual processing of transaction.

To quote an executive from a major, highly respected system, "Technology is the next item on our agenda. We have just begun to look at this issue." This statement seems to summarize the situation for many providers. A number of reports indicate that health care lags in technology expenditures, and supply chain information technology is still looking for a clear direction.[44] To quote a white paper from a major consulting firm, "Supply chain integration requires significant IT investment." But to quote a CFO from a case research site, "Show me the money!" A definite conflict exists.

Progressive systems carry out due diligence in assessing distributor information capabilities associated with market demand, point-of-use information, the speed and clarity of information, and electronic interchange ability.

The adequacy of market information about the changing nature of products, pricing trends, and use changes. In the current environment, many distributors promote the value of their information for their hospital customers. However, the extent to which distributors provide market information must be questioned. Their ability to provide in-depth, unbiased analysis is limited because they are being paid by the manufacturers as well as the hospitals. The distributor may not be motivated to conduct penetrating research on the price trends that could make a manufacturing customer look less competitive than others in the industry.

Major distributors have been developing point-of-use inventory management systems. These handheld scanners allow caregivers to gather and record supply use information through bar codes. The systems have met barriers, such as clinician acceptability, that many new technologies may face. However, as the barriers are overcome, the result is an accurate inventory record. The problem is that many hospitals have not fully implemented a bar coding system, and although there is substantial improvement in code standardization, full industry standardization is still on the horizon, albeit nearer.

EDI and other forms of interchange can be characterized by the accuracy, clarity, and speed of communication between the distributor and the manufacturer.[45] While a great deal of attention has been given to the ability of hospitals and systems to engage in electronic exchange in the process of ordering materials, much of the focus is on providing valuable information for distributors rather than the suppliers themselves. It is difficult to estimate how information has been transmitted upstream and how such information has affected production schedules, stockpiles, and costs. Distributors have frequently purchased large quantities of goods at relatively low prices to be able to increase their profits and buffer themselves against supplier price increases. Better forecasting models have the potential to lead to cost and price reductions in the health sector only if there is transparency of information across the entire supply chain.

The capability of the EDI system for managing all invoice and payment term information accurately and in a timely manner appears to be limited in even the most progressive systems. In fact, in 2001, 40 percent of buyers' time and 68 percent of accounts payable time was spent on the manual processing of transactions.[46] Although there has been radical improvement in reducing the number of nonelectronic exchanges, the opportunity exists for some radical improvements.

What Are Your Distribution and Inventory Personnel Capabilities? As the previous questions were addressed, the need for improved technical competencies in hospital inventory and distribution personnel emerged. Supply managers who find it difficult to hire competent distribution and inventory personnel were the most likely to consider outsourcing of inventory and distribution functions. It appears that this is compatible with the strategic direction that distributors are attempting to generate as they put tremendous resources into the development of new business services such as the activity-based costing systems offered by Owens and Minor, one of the larger distributors. Such competencies are difficult for hospitals or systems to match with their current level of professional expertise.

When outsourcing is seen as the strategic alternative, health care providers' employee expense is simply being transferred to a different operational expense category. Therefore, the ultimate decision should be based on whether outsourcing this human resource is providing greater value. What would it cost to hire the personnel necessary to manage the entire process rather than outsource it? Would it be possible to select current personnel for these positions? These are basic questions that must be addressed when developing the strategic options.

Managerial Understanding of Inventory and Distribution

While the real and potential savings associated with inventory and distribution are recognized by management, there continues to be uncertainty regarding their real purposes and impact on the health care organization. Management recognizes that failure to have the appropriate product at the time of demand subjects the system, the hospital, and the patient to a wide variety of risks. And they also understand that having a surplus of materials is another kind of risk: the system is not effectively using its financial assets. But they have not attached a strategic value to improved financial performance as a result of supply chain efficiency.

Perhaps the situation described is attributable to the fact that hospital inventory is not seen as constituting "value." Manufacturing, retail, and other service industries are able to turn inventory into cash by using inventory for the development of new products or reducing inventory by offering special pricing for immediate purchase. Surpluses of hospital materials are not easily managed outside the confines of disease-related patient demand, which is frequently difficult to predict. Materials, in the eyes of health care executives, do not equal assets. Thus, as new processes improve inventory performance, top managers tend to see that a costly area is "now under control." However, management rarely sees the greater value these processes bring to the organization and its future performance. Managers also observe that lean shelf stock is frequently backed up by stores residing in the warehouses of distributors or the system. This means that the trade-offs between system costs and low inventory levels at the point of service are not well understood. What is frequently described as just-in-time inventory distribution in the health delivery sector is actually an approach to replenishment of point-of-use materials to reduce shelf stock.

The few instances where inventory is recognized as part of an organization's asset portfolio were generally related to the association between materials and a center of excellence where materials are a significant portion of the procedures involved. In cardiology or orthopedics, for example, senior management recognizes opportunities to organize materials and distribution around certain product lines, thus transforming materials from being an expense to a part of the asset repertoire necessary for success. Managers in the ASU/CHMR study point out that specialty hospitals, due to their focus on few procedures and their ability to standardize, were able to think much more strategically about their use of materials. This led them to make better-informed decisions about inventory and distribution options and made them more effective negotiators with both suppliers and distributors.

Senior managers also point out that the day-to-day pressures associated with their jobs do not push them to think about inventory and distribution. Progressive systems have achieved working levels of product availability and distribution that do not jeopardize the system's operations. As a consequence, there are few instances where materials outages are a factor in being unable to deliver services.

Senior management start to think about inventory and distribution as they and their supply chain managers consider the balance of insourcing versus outsourcing for inventory and distribution functions. Some systems have stock delivered in bulk to their central warehouse. Others have stock delivered by the distributor to each hospital's loading dock within the system. Yet other systems have distributors bring stock to the floor and even shelve it. Progressive systems increasingly consider outsourcing the inventory and distribution function: working closely with the distributor to ensure that the goals for outsourcing are met and that the system derives the benefits associated with the transfer of function.

Summary and Conclusion

This discussion began by asking how to improve distribution and inventory services. The answer can be looked at in a simplistic manner. It is a trade-off between service and costs. In fact, all strategy may be considered a matter of economic trade-offs.[47] Progressive managers continually evaluate their behavior by considering if the trade-off between services and costs can be improved with distribution and inventory processes? If the answer is yes, increased attention to inventory and distribution is warranted, as well as additional investments in technologies that will make these areas work to the benefit of the hospital or system.

Hospitals and systems have too frequently viewed distribution and inventory as an either-or question pertaining to insourcing versus outsourcing. The two potential answers are to completely outsource the processes or manage it all internally.[48] However, based on the ASU/CHMR case studies and observations across the field, it appears that a more finely tuned approach must be taken in which the economic values of trade-offs must be considered. It must be determined which distribution and inventory process improvements can create revenues through greater economies of scale and scope. Finally, if one side of the either-or question is taken and the processes are completely outsourced, the outsourcing must still be monitored and managed to ensure that workers from the distributor organization fit into the organization where they are "guest workers."

This chapter was designed around the observation that most hospitals and systems do not strategically look at both sides of the trade-offs. As a result, the different variables associated with distribution and inventory are not being analyzed. The hospitals are looking at either the cost or the service issue and do not recognize what they should be examining in the processes.

For senior management to effectively provide leadership in the materials aspects of their organizations, they must address the issues of value, control, and power within the supply chain. The answers to these questions will vary from situation to situation depending on the distributor and the structure of the system or hospital.

Strategy is a matter of selecting the correct options in order to take advantage of existing assets. For inventory and distribution to become strategic, it is first necessary to determine their expected value. In addition, it is vital to establish the amount of organizational control desired over the processes because potential weaknesses exist by having to share company-specific information. For example, if the processes are completely outsourced, there is a possibility that intellectual property could be lost.

The value that most systems seem to be seeking in their deliberations regarding inventory and distribution is total dollar savings. As they approach the determination of savings, they do not consider the alternative use of dollars accrued or the costs associated with bringing an outsourced function back into the system. Finally, few systems systematically calculate the total cost of ownership of goods but tend to focus on one discrete aspect of the contracting, distribution, and inventory process.

Inventory and distribution within systems and hospitals is complex due to a number of unique conditions, such as product proliferation, irregular demand schedules, and high customer demands. Senior management has frequently seen inventory and distribution as areas to be efficiently administered, not critically managed. Materials managers need to be hired who have the skills, competencies, and capabilities to cope with the intricacies of a system's materials challenges rather than providing leadership necessary to move to a more strategic level of development.

The purpose of the ASU/CHMR study was not to study the wide range of products and services offered by distributor organizations. Broadly, distributor selection should be on the basis of the ability of the distributor to add value[49] and match customer value with the services provided.[50] Distributors have found that it is necessary to provide more value than just movement of goods. As Crawford and Mathews suggest, "To succeed a company needs to be dominating in one attribute, differentiate itself on another, and be adequate in all of the rest, but not below that."[51] The health care distributor has greatly increased its role to include support services for the movement of supplies and the development of new technologies for deployment of the supplies in the hospital. These services typically include:

- Communication among members of the supply chain, such as sending and receiving orders and resolving customer issues
- Billing, including sending invoices and receiving payments
- Financial issues, such as assuming the risk of future payment and activity-based costing systems
- Sales and marketing support, including demand analysis and use

To quote a supply chain manager interviewed in this study, "When I used to think of report generation and market information, I thought of a truck moving goods. Today I think of a total business service." Distributors appear to be successful in creating models that provide value to the hospital end users and, in turn, to the hospital and the system. At this point, it is unclear if it will be the distributor, the GPO, or another information technology provider that will provide the data to reflect the hospital's use of products and process.

A number of keen observers of the field of supply chain management have observed that there are four basic ways for a firm to ensure that logistics functions are completed: (1) internalizing the processes, (2) acquiring capability, (3) engaging in arm's-length transactions, or (4) strategic alliances between partners willing to take risks and share rewards.[52] There is a growing consensus that in an era of vendor-managed inventory, it may take the development of a strategic alliance between distributors, suppliers, and hospitals to improve hospital and system performance. The hospital gains additional benefits as the supplier takes on the costs of warehousing and excess merchandise.[53] Suppliers gain efficiency by having a stronger handle on use and an expected demand for goods.

Perhaps it is important to recognize that distributors are increasingly becoming knowledge management companies: allowing progressive managers to monitor their compliance with contracts and better manage standardization, understand use, engage financial modeling, and categorize materials. If they are able to continue along this line, they may become knowledge-creating companies.[54] Sophisticated distributor informatics provide systems with charts pertaining to top product categories (such as wound sutures, woven and nonwoven goods, adhesives, bandages, dressings and sponges, and surgical instruments). They also provide systems with data pertaining to purchase price and manufacturer contract information.

As progressive hospitals and systems seek to improve their own performance, they are clearly reevaluating an environment where their pursuit of strategic direction and strategic alliances is linked to the changing roles played by purchasing partners. Distributor organizations are separate from GPOs in the U.S. health care system. Without doubt, the presence of GPO contracts (Chapter Four) helps signal to suppliers that there will be a demand for their products and provides hospitals and systems with a potentially reduced range of items for accomplishing their goals. Hospitals also purchase GPO contracted products, as discussed in Study 1, through non-GPO sources, choosing to deal directly with a supplier and frequently purchasing goods that are not in a GPO contract from the lists of supplies offered by distributors.[55] In addition, hundreds of new products come onto the marketplace annually, many never securing a place in a GPO contract catalogue of goods. For this reason too, a significant amount of purchasing continues to be carried out directly with suppliers, and transactions with distributors are for a very large range of products. Distributors also may have their own label brands that compete with the products offered by GPO contracts. Thus, the nexus of purchasing partners is clearly not fully aligned, and it is not clear that the environment, where hospitals and systems are still considering the possibility of taking on inventory and distribution functions, will consistently lead to strategic alliances to strengthen the system. There is no question that inventory and distribution issues are complex issues that require carefully strategic consideration. The complexity described in this chapter, however, must be considered in relationship to a sector of the economy that has not yet given careful consideration to where order and supply errors occur and how such errors affect system performance, even in the presence of enhanced information technology.

CHAPTER SIX
_____

ORGANIZATIONAL DESIGN FOR HOSPITAL AND HEALTH CARE SYSTEM SUPPLY CHAINS
_____

This chapter assesses the extent to which organizational design and environment can be structured to facilitate excellence in hospital and hospital supply chain performance. The idea of the managers as architects of the organizational design is, of course, not new in the field of management. In the early 1960s Alfred Chandler provided strong evidence that an organization's strategy is a strong determinant of its structure.[1] The ASU/CHMR study found that progressive supply chain managers are able to articulate a strategy for their efforts. They understood that there are a variety of strategic alternatives related to their use of purchasing partners as well as their investment strategies for supplies. They also understand that the supply strategy must be a strategic fit for their organization's culture, and in achieving this level of fit, they must account for the various differences within the hospital and the system. In somewhat different terms, supply managers in progressive organizations see themselves as orchestrators of the supply function and seek structures to facilitate their success.

Supply chain departments can be thought of as boundary organizations that must manage both the internal organization of the hospital and the various upstream trading partners that are necessary to achieve supply chain management and strategy goals. Organizational design for a supply chain must thus be responsive to the dilemmas of a boundary organization that interacts with the very different environments of its internal and external customers.[2] The health care supply function must be designed to link with external suppliers and markets to deliver value to the company and to operationally link clinicians and other internal customers to "provide internal functions with external supply market intelligence and actionable opportunities."[3]

The ASU/CHMR study revealed that progressive hospitals and hospital systems are characterized by their diversity in organizational design, giving credence to the observation that contingency management is a key skill for health sector value chain.[4] While supply chain function centralization is touted in several systems as the key to high levels of savings and standardization on both clinical and commodity items, a number of decentralized systems attribute their success in cost reduction to being able to work at the local level. Peter Drucker wrote "that there is no one right or universal design but that each enterprise needs to design around the key activities appropriate to its mission and its strategies."[5] Hospitals and health care organizations are characterized by very different missions and strategies. They differ by market conditions, access to financial and human resources, financial structure (for example, investor owned versus nonprofit), regulatory environment, and geographical location. Mastery of understanding an organization's environment is one key to success. Study 3, an analysis of a large metropolitan hospital, describes the design characteristics of a hospital system following a merger. It clearly reveals the extent to which a hybrid form of organization is necessary in a system where members have very different missions and competencies.

Organizational Environment

Organizational environment is defined as the sum total of the elements that exist outside the boundary of the organization and have the potential to affect all or part of the organization. It has been suggested that ten factors (Exhibit 6.1) can influence the organization and the system. For the hospital supply chain, environment includes the legal and regulatory structure that affects both the hospital and the supply and distribution channels upstream from the point of delivery. What capital-level items can be purchased by a hospital continues, in many states, to be regulated

EXHIBIT 6.1.   ORGANIZATIONAL ENVIRONMENT FACTORS.

Industry dynamics	Economic conditions
Raw materials	Government regulations
Human resources	Sociocultural factors
Financial resources	Technology
Market conditions	International conditions

by the existence of certificate of need laws. The external environment, which also determines standards relating to infection rates and the shielding of employees from dangerous materials, affects the purchasing of goods and services.

The supply chain includes both the internal and external environment within the system. For instance, the market conditions of the physicians may affect the physicians' willingness to be supportive of hospital cost-containment and quality enhancement efforts. Environmental conditions may also include sociocultural factors, such as a hospital's linkage to a religious order with a strong commitment to bring health care to the poor.

These environmental conditions should be considered along several dimensions. The simple-complex dimension in Figure 6.1 refers to the degree of heterogeneity in an organization's operations. Hospitals and hospital systems generally operate in a complex environment with a large number of technologies and that is a focal point for cultural and value changes. At the departmental or specialty level, hospital environment is actually heterogeneous. It spans the range from simple to complex. A hospital laundry, for example, is a fairly simple environment, while a surgical floor is complex in its technologies, mix of staff, and range of services. The environments of such different organizations demand different strategies, as well as different structures. The hospital also has a complex mix of human resources and interfaces. Hospitals by their very nature serve a number of diverse customers, unlike most other industries.

System complexity also pertains to the mix of hospitals and other delivery units within the system. There are systems that are highly dispersed nationally,

FIGURE 6.1. ENVIRONMENTAL COMPLEXITY.

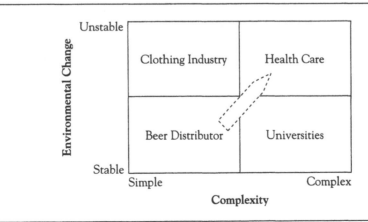

such as the Mayo Clinic, which has major operating units in Rochester, Minnesota, Scottsdale, Arizona, and Jacksonville, Florida, and HCA, with hospitals in over half the states and abroad. While centralization of the purchasing function characterizes the Mayo Clinic from a system-level perspective, its geographically remote operating units in Arizona and Jacksonville have substantial locally based supply chain management functions and different designs to meet the strategic goals of the different units. This kind of centralization is very different from the centralization that characterizes the supply chain function at HCA, which is increasingly built around a national materials formulary. It is also quite different from centralization at BJC HealthCare, which serves thirteen hospitals relatively near St. Louis, where a similar distribution model can be applied to the system's hospitals or the even smaller system detailed in Study 3. Centralization seems to mean different things to different systems.

The stable-unstable dimension refers to the extent to which elements in the environment are dynamic. An environmental domain is stable if it remains the same over a significant period of time. Hospitals are somewhat unstable because governmental regulations, reimbursements (economic or financial conditions), and technology are constantly changing. In addition, overall demand may be predictable (number of admissions), but the exact type of care is somewhat less predictable from day to day. Figure 6.1 demonstrates how the stable-unstable and the simple-complex dimensions generate the concept of uncertainty, that is, that decision makers do not have sufficient information about environmental factors and have difficulty predicting external changes. Uncertainty increases the risk of failure for organizational responses and makes it difficult to compute costs and probabilities associated with decision alternatives.

A good example of the difficulty that hospitals have planning in an unstable environment is associated with the decade-long controversy associated with the development of specialty heart and orthopedic surgical hospitals. Harvard University professor Regina Herzlinger has argued that such hospitals (or "focused factories") have the opportunity to become centers of clinical as well as administrative excellence (see Case 6.1 for policy background).[6] Even in the face of cyclical government-enforced moratoriums restricting the building of such hospitals, it remains uncertain that the environment will tolerate a set of new clinical efforts that are perceived to infringe on financially profitable units of comprehensive medical centers. For those who would design specialty hospitals or contemplate expansion of traditional hospital services, this is an uncertain environment. For those who would manufacture products for such services, anticipating the demand for capital items and materials for cardiac and orthopedic services is very difficult. Hospitals are complex. In such an environment, where supply management and strategy decision makers face a large degree of uncertainty, organizational design and strategy must be sufficiently flexible to facilitate the meeting of goals.

◆ ◆ ◆

Case 6.1 Specialty Hospitals

The Medicare Prescription Drug, Improvement, and Modernization Act of 2003 included an 18-month moratorium on the development of new physician- and investor-owned surgical facilities. These facilities, generally known as specialty hospitals, typically focus on a few areas of surgical practice such as heart surgery or orthopedic surgery.

Specialty hospitals offer high-quality health care in a setting outside of the traditional general hospital, care that often is delivered at lower cost. But specialty hospitals have drawn intense criticism from the general hospitals they compete with, who successfully lobbied Congress to include a moratorium on construction of new specialty hospitals in the Medicare Prescription Drug, Improvement and Modernization Act of 2003.

When the moratorium expired in June 2005, the Centers for Medicare and Medicaid Services refocused its efforts on ensuring that payments to such hospitals would not disadvantage general hospitals. The continued concern with such hospitals is grounded in a number of issues, which are discussed below.

Self-Referral

One major concern expressed by the American Hospital Association (AHA), which represents general hospitals and health care networks, is that because specialty hospitals are typically owned by doctors, there is an incentive for doctors to refer patients to a specialty hospital in order to generate profits, regardless of what is in the best interest of patients.

Two different studies conducted in 2003 by the Government Accountability Office (GAO) found a substantial majority (70%) of physicians with admitting privileges at specialty hospitals had no financial interest in the hospital. Of those physicians who had a financial interest, most owned 6 percent or less of the hospital.

Greg Scanlon, a health policy expert at the Galen Institute in Washington, D.C., expresses doubt about the charge that doctors improperly direct patients to clinics in which they have an ownership stake. Scanlon writes, "Given the scandalous track record of hospitals in patient safety and quality, it is entirely possible that physicians invest in facilities in order to assure better quality, and naturally refer their patients to facilities in which they have some influence over the quality of the care provided."

Limited Service

Another criticism leveled by the AHA is that specialty hospitals "do not have emergency departments."

The GAO research confirmed this. While 92 percent of general hospitals have emergency departments, fewer than half—45 percent—of specialty hospitals have emergency departments.

Health care experts, however, say this charge misses the point of specialization. "These hospitals are more efficient exactly because of specialization. They deliver the highest standard of quality care since they are not expected to be all things to all people by offering everything from an ER to a maternity ward," says Conrad Meier, senior fellow in health care for The Heartland Institute. "This is like a supermarket trying to shut down a drugstore because it doesn't sell fresh meat and produce, but it's ok for the supermarket to sell prescription drugs."

Many specialty hospitals, including MedCath, a chain of 13 specialty hospitals focusing on cardiac care, do have emergency departments. Those departments are open 24 hours a day, are staffed by physicians, and have an average of seven beds each. MedCath's emergency departments treated more than 60,000 patients over the past year, nearly two-thirds of them for non-cardiac-related conditions.

In a letter to Congress dated October 12, 2004, MedCath CEO John Casey and CFO James Harris point out that even large general hospitals typically don't offer every possible type of medical care, such as trauma or burn care. They note, "by focusing on cardiovascular disease and creating a center of excellence . . . MedCath hospitals have been able to improve the quality of care, reduce the average length of stay of our patients, save Medicare money, and achieve a high level of patient satisfaction."

Cherry-Picking

Critics say doctors at specialty hospitals refer healthier, more profitable patients to their own facilities while sending less healthy, more expensive patients to general hospitals. Because they do not operate emergency rooms, critics charge, specialty hospitals get a better mix of patients and serve fewer Medicaid and uninsured patients.

Caroline Steinberg, vice president of policy at the AHA, said, "Preliminary data from MedPAC . . . shows that cardiac surgery has greater profit margins compared to other types of surgery, and if you adjust for the severity of patient illness, orthopedic and general surgery also show greater profit margins, up to 15 percent more profit."

The American Surgical Hospital Association (ASHA), a trade group for specialty hospitals, strongly disputes those charges. They say their members provide services to Medicaid and uninsured patients. They also note the nonprofit status of most general hospitals allows them to better absorb the costs associated with lower-paying Medicaid and uninsured patients, compared to a hospital that must pay taxes on revenue.

Research by the Lewin Group also contradicts the charge that specialty hospitals are treating only the healthiest, most profitable patients. In a study of MedCath's 13 hospitals, Lewin researchers found Medicare cardiac patients treated by Med-Cath had a Case Mix Index (a measure of patient severity and case complexity) 20 percent higher than their counterparts at general hospitals, indicating MedCath facilities were generally treating patients less healthy than those of competing hospitals.

It is not difficult to understand why doctors might refer their most difficult cases to specialty hospitals, where they feel the most confident about being able to offer the best care to these patients. Linda Gorman, who follows health care policy for the Colorado-based Independence Institute, noted, "specialty hospitals may provide an alternative for doctors who are dissatisfied with the quality of care, efficiency, and bureaucracy of general hospitals."

Medical outcomes for cardiac patients at MedCath hospitals would seem to support that idea. Although MedCath patients generally enter the hospital sicker than average, they have shorter stays, lower mortality, and fewer complications when compared to patients at general hospitals in their peer group.

Draining Resources

Critics also charge that by focusing on procedures that attract higher reimbursement rates from insurance companies and government programs like Medicare, specialty hospitals drain away from general hospitals revenues that would otherwise be used to subsidize medical treatments reimbursed at less than cost. Cardiac, orthopedic, and general surgery are among the procedures with the highest reimbursement rates compared to cost, according to the AHA.

ASHA notes, however, that a survey of its 71 members shows they provide services in six different specialties on average, not just the three high-reimbursement specialties noted by AHA. Only five ASHA members are single-specialty hospitals.

Scanlon also notes specialty hospitals can hardly be blamed if general hospitals accept reimbursement from insurers and the government at less than cost for some procedures. He questions whether such internal cross-subsidies are appropriate. "Is it really fair or rational to have maternity or cardiac patients singled out to pay for the costs of a trauma center?" he asks. "If trauma centers are a valued community service, shouldn't the whole community subsidize the costs?"

Laws, Tougher Regulation Sought

Citing these complaints and others against specialty hospitals, the AHA, Federation of American Hospitals, state affiliates, member hospitals, and allies are fighting to stop the growth of specialty hospitals. They are seeking tougher and more widespread Certificate of Need (CON) laws, lobbying to make permanent the Medicare reform law's moratorium, and denying admitting privileges to doctors involved with specialty hospitals.

CON laws require that the construction or expansion of any medical facility be approved by government officials. Health policy experts say efforts to expand and strengthen CON laws are nothing more than using the government to stifle competition. "Certificate of Need and other anti-competitive regulations inhibit innovation and protect the market position of existing players," charges Scanlon.

A July 2004 report from the Federal Trade Commission and Department of Justice confirms Scanlon's criticism, finding that CON laws "are not successful in containing health care costs, and . . . pose serious anticompetitive risks. . . . Market incumbents can too easily use CON procedures to forestall competitors from entering the incumbents market."

Resistance to Innovation

Specialty hospitals are what many health policy observers term a "disruptive innovation," delivering health care in a new way that disturbs the status quo and reduces the market share of previously dominant players. A *Harvard Business Review* article in 2000, titled "Will Disruptive Innovations Cure Health Care?" notes, "health care may be the most entrenched, change-averse industry in the United States."

Specialty hospitals undoubtedly represent a change that threatens to disrupt the market dominance enjoyed by many general hospitals. By offering medical facilities that specialize in a few specific procedures, specialty hospitals can improve the quality of care while also reducing price through competition. It should come as little surprise that the dominant players, general hospitals, are fighting back and pointing out what they perceive as the negative consequences of upsetting the status quo.

Source: Parnell, S. "Specialty Hospitals." *Health Care News,* Dec. 1, 2004.

◆ ◆ ◆

Organizational strategy is a plan for interacting with the environment to achieve goals. Goals define where the organization wants to go, and strategies define how it will get there. For example, the goal might be to achieve 5 percent net income, while the strategy might be to reduce materials costs, improve operational efficiency, and improve employee productivity. Strategies can include any number of tactics to achieve the goal. Michael Porter developed a popular method for categorizing organizational strategies.[7] Each of the strategies (Table 6.1) attempts to maximize the organization's strengths in order to develop a competitive advantage within its environment, and in order to accomplish this goal, different organizational designs are required.

TABLE 6.1.   ORGANIZATIONAL STRATEGIES.

Strategy	Tactic
Low-cost leadership: Increase market share by increasing low-cost compared to competitors. Hospital example: Community hospital that competes by being the lower-cost, higher-quality alternative.	Tight cost control Process engineering skills across departments Intense supervision of employees, including professional staff Frequent and detailed control reports Intense efforts to reduce costs of product and service delivery
Differentiation: Attempt to distinguish products or services from others in the industry. Hospital example: A hospital that promotes its specialty, such as oncology.	Strong marketing emphasis Attempt to develop unique capabilities Purchase of high-quality capital equipment and development of unique specialties Emphasize research
Focus: Concentrate on a specific regional market or buyer group. Hospital example: A system focuses on obtaining dominant market share in a focused geographical region.	Combine the above tactics but focus on a unique market Attempt to promote one specialty over the others

Organizational Design and Structure

Before proceeding with this discussion, it is important to differentiate between organizational design and structure. The design is the overall look of the organization, including its formalization (the extent to which expectations regarding the means and end of work are specified and written), the centrality of authority and decision making, the complexity or number of distinctively different job titles or occupational groupings, and the number of distinctly different units or departments in an organization.[8] As depicted in Figure 6.2, organizational design emanates from dynamic strategic management, which takes into account an organization's culture, goal and work arrangements.

Organizational structure includes such items as:

- Division of work: Enhances the individual's proficiency in performing his or her work and thus improves the efficiency and effectiveness with which the work can be performed
- Departmentation: The grouping of work and workers into manageable units or departments

FIGURE 6.2. STRATEGIC CHOICE.

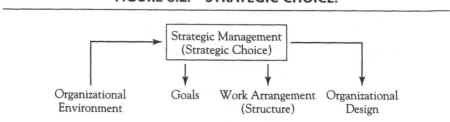

- Authority and responsibility relationships: Assigning individuals the responsibility and authority for the completion of work
- Span of control: Grouping workers according to the number of subordinates reporting directly to a manager
- Coordination: Assembling and synchronizing work to function harmoniously in attaining organizing objectives[9]

The appropriate structure flows from the goals, and the organizational design is required to implement the strategy in an efficient and effective manner.[10] The structural design of a supply chain requires:

- An "extra" design of the structure that is an interface with the outside world of suppliers and markets ("extra" here means focusing outside the company).
- The "inter" design, or the structure that is an interface with internal units, sites, and projects. ("Inter" here means interdepartmental across the company.)
- The "intra" design, or structure inside the company that translates, coordinates, and integrates the extra- and inter-designs. ("Intra" here means within the supply organization.)[11]

The ASU/CHMR research project was initiated around determining the best organizational design for the supply function. Early in the research, it became apparent that a hybrid approach, drawing on aspects of both centralization and decentralization, characterizes the most progressive systems. A review of the classic literature on organizational design indicates that both centralized and decentralized structures have advantages and disadvantages within supply chain management (Table 6.2). Both are characterized by facets of formalization and complexity. Managers contemplating design features will also see that trade-offs exist with each of the dimensions of organizational design—for instance:

- With centralization, it may be easier to develop a larger spend volume by coordinating across hospitals, BUT individualized specialized needs within a hospital may be lost.

TABLE 6.2. ADVANTAGES AND DISADVANTAGES OF CENTRALIZATION.

Advantages	Disadvantages
CENTRALIZATION	
Greater specialization of buying process: may specialize on a certain type of commodity, capital equipment, or physical preference items	Less ability to use generalized job skills across supply commodities or functions; greater propensity to become bored with job
Consolidation of supply requirements, resulting in greater buying clout	May overlook specialized needs in different hospitals
Bundling of suppliers so that fewer are required; improved administration of suppliers	Smaller and unique suppliers required for specialized services may be overlooked
Primary decision makers physically close to each other	May lose physical contact with users in different hospitals
Ability to develop critical mass of expertise in one location (economies of scale)	Critical mass may become psychologically isolated from users
Strong focus on strategy	Less focus on individual needs within the hospital
Improved control and universal policies and procedures	Individualized needs lost to universal control as a result of universal policies and procedures
Lower administrative cost of purchasing	Higher visibility of administrative costs of purchasing
DECENTRALIZATION	
Easier coordination with hospital users	More difficult to coordinate with other business units
Faster response to local needs	Become accustomed to responding on an ad hoc basis, with little planning
Effective use of local sources	Focus on local sources without using coordinated sources without using other units
Autonomy of local unit and pride in local efforts	Lack of commitment to entire system's objectives
Simple reporting lines	Poor coordination with the system
General job skills	Functional complex specialization more difficult
Better understanding of local cost structure	Poor understanding of total cost across the system

- As jobs become more complex, a greater level of specialization may develop, BUT flexibility is lost as personnel do not know how to quickly adapt to a local supply needs.
- Formalization may allow for a consistent way of recording and controlling costs, BUT the understanding of costs within a hospital unit may be difficult to understand.
- Local reporting lines of authority and responsibility make it easier to relate to local internal and external customers, BUT it is difficult to take advantage of leveraged buying across the hospitals.

Assessment of an organization's strategy should flow from the organization's assessment of its environment and its goals and the necessary trade-offs to ensure success.[12] A primary reason for these trade-offs is that most systems seldom have the same organizational environment and the same goals and strategies across system members. An example provides clarification for this statement. Consider a large system that has several large community hospitals, a small suburban community hospital that specializes in oncology, and another hospital that focuses on children, and still another with a large cardiac care center. In addition, the system has an assisted care center and a community outpatient clinic. Each of these facilities operates in a distinctively different community and clinical environment. Even the two large community hospitals have slightly different markets due to differing sociocultural factors within their regions. In addition, each hospital has different technology and financial environments. These are very complex systems.[13] Because of the different environments, each hospital has a different strategy for meeting these goals. One of the community hospitals, in a lower socioeconomic region, gains strategic advantage by attempting to be the low-cost provider within the community. Meanwhile, the other community hospital attempts to differentiate itself through customer satisfaction. It puts a lot of emphasis on promotional campaigns designed to develop an image of providing patient convenience and comfort in addition to quality care. The cardiac care and oncology centers focus on providing specialized treatment.

The different strategies should theoretically lead to different organizational designs, but a dilemma exists: How is it possible to have a separate organizational design for each unit within the system and a consistent design for the system as a whole? Charles H. Fine has advanced the concept of clockspeed to understand the rates of evolution in different industries.[14] He refers to the extraordinarily rapid clockspeed of the entertainment industry, the somewhat slower clockspeed of the semiconductor industry, and the even slower clockspeed of the aircraft industry. Each of these industries, given the changes within its environment, has a very different organizational design and very different structures and strategies associated with their supply chains. Fine suggests four keys to understanding supply chain architecture: (1) geographical proximity (physician distance), (2) organizational proximity (the relationships between customers and suppliers and their alignment of incentives and processes), (3) cultural proximity (commonality of language, business mores, and ethical standards), and (4) electronic proximity (the extent to which parties are connected through technology).[15]

Fine's classification of industries on the basis of such analysis brings together the aspects of clockspeed associated with products and technology, processes, and organizations. Taking a patient's ailment as the focal point for a health care product, Fine sees the architecture of the health care industry (except for emergency care) as dispersed, modular, and slow in both time and space.[16] But there are many different ways to look at health care. The hospital industry, while still having a large number of "general plants" in the form of hospitals, is increasingly characterized by outpatient clinics, relationships with contracting partners for services, and increased use of technology for communication. When the hospital becomes the focal point, with its various functions and services relating to the need for supply (both services and products), there is a very different view of the health industry. Perhaps what is most remarkable about the hospital is the various clockspeeds associated with different departments, products, and relationships. The clockspeed on an internal medicine or psychiatry ward may be very slow, with the introduction of few new, dislocating technologies. This is very different from the clockspeed in cardiac surgery, where new products, processes, and expectations continually challenge both the organization and the individual players. The supply function engaged in sourcing and contracting for food catering for patients, employees, and visitors has a very different clockspeed from the supply function engaged in sourcing and contracting for capital equipment on an enterprise systemwide basis.

In many ways, the introduction of new technologies changes the clockspeed of many different aspects of the hospital. A desktop specimen analyzer, for example, may allow a physician to diagnose and treat a patient in the same visit. This may lead to the dissolution of the relationship between the hospital and an outside laboratory that formerly did the test. It may also necessitate the availability of materials for a just-in-time intervention that is now possible as the result of the new information. The ripple of such an innovation can change many different things. What were once very modular patient encounters, requiring several visits to many different specialists, are now tight, integral procedures that require available products, expertise, and a highly coordinated organizational structure and effort.

The dilemma of the health sector supply chain is the very different clockspeeds and changing clockspeeds of units across the hospital and in ambulatory care. Because of this dilemma and the trade-offs already noted, it may be that the perfect fit is difficult to achieve. The centralized, complex, formalized organization does not fit all situations. However, the opposite of this—the decentralized, informal, or simple organization—does not fit all situations either. As a result, a hybrid form of organizational design is often more appropriate. In a hybrid organization, activities, responsibilities, and accountabilities are shared between operating units and the corporate office. Some activities are centralized at the system level, while others are decentralized to individual hospital units and even subunits within the hospital. For some situations, there may be extensive policies and procedures, and in others, individual flexibility is fostered. Some aspects of the supply chain structure may be complex, with many levels of hierarchy and rigid reporting relationships. Other parts of the organization may be flat, with loose reporting relationships. Consistent with research in other industries, the progressive hospitals and systems scrutinized for the ACU/CHMR study reveal that a hybrid organizational design is the most effective.[17]

Hybrid Organizational Design

Hybrid organizational design comprises a combination of centralized and decentralized, formal and informal, and complex and simple features. A hybrid design is an open system that does not seal itself off or exclude other possibilities. It may be said to be a loose-tight fit, with loose formalizations in some aspects of the organization and tight procedural controls in other parts. A number of progressive systems, for example, have tight, centralized control for use of a GPO for commodity items but loose control for physician preference items.

A hybrid system has the capacity to continuously adapt to its environment by combining organizational design elements with agility across parts of the system.[18] Combining elements is difficult because it means that ambiguous parameters may exist when considering control, responsibility, and accountability. A hybrid organizational design also requires communication and coordination where roles are not always clear. Perhaps what is most important is that the management of the supply design cannot be relegated to the hospital's tacticians; "rather it must be part and parcel of the organization's key strategic thinking."[19] Fine advises, however, that to accomplish design, "you need to have a clear image of what our supply chain design looks like, who is doing what for whom, and where the "clockspeed bottle-necks" are occurring."[20] Progressive hospital supply managers monitor the different hospital environments by employing clinical resource specialists to act in linking pin roles between supply chain department or other operational units.

Requirements of an Effective Hybrid Organizational Design

Information derived from the ASU/CHMR case studies as well as the current research literature, indicates that important attributes are necessary to have an effective hybrid organizational design in health care. These include an open systems approach in which there is flexibility in roles and responsibilities, clarity of goals, and high levels of employee communication and coordination.

Open Systems Approach. This approach requires a combination of external focus, operational flexibility, and interaction. The entire organization is seen as interacting systems open to the inputs and outputs of each other. This interaction requires that employees understand the importance of interaction and mutual dependency.

In an open system, the goals and outcomes of one unit are dependent on the goals of another unit. They are exclusive of each other. In operational terms, this means a physician, a quality control manager, and a supply manager depend on each other to meet their individual and organizational goals. In contrast, in a closed system, the supply manager may meet his or her goals by reducing the purchase price for an item such as a stent, but it may ultimately affect quality or physician satisfaction. The supply manager works to maximize his or her own goals without regard for others in the organization.

The open system in heath care is related to chaos theory. This theoretical approach states that employees live in a complex world full of randomness and uncertainty. This is true for complex health care environments, which are characterized by surprise, rapid change, and confusion. As a result, managers cannot measure, predict, or control in traditional ways the unfolding drama inside or outside the organization.[21] The open, hybrid organization recognizes this randomness and disorder and attempts to adapt to the chaos rather than completely change.[22]

Flexible Roles, Responsibilities, Authority, and Clarity of Goals. A supply chain executive in an ASU/CHMR progressive organization pointed to the importance of flexibility, agility, responsibility, and clarity of goals: "In the past, we defined ourselves by who we reported to. This is no longer the case. Now the important thing is to meet your individual, organizational, and project goals." This individual was expressing the importance of goals rather than just keeping the supervisor happy. In a rigid, closed, bureaucratic organization, often it is more difficult to meet systemwide markets than it is to align behaviors toward organizational goals. In an open system, goals dominate, and roles and responsibility must remain flexible in order to remain consistent with organizational culture.

Agility in reporting is an important attribute of progressive health care organizations. In one of the ASU/CHMR systems, the supply manager reported to the facilities manager when the hospital was refurbishing the birthing center. But on the next project in which the hospital was reconfiguring the storage areas and receiving docks, the facility manager reported to the supply chain manager. Responsibilities were reversed from one project to another. In one progressive ASU/CHMR study organization, it is clear that such a reporting scheme can lead to confusion among employees.

Some of the confusion associated with such reporting is expressed by a nurse who worked on standardization projects but reported to the supply management group: "Who I report to is not important, and those who think that it is will have trouble in this system." She went on to say, "When someone starts to ask me about my 'credentials' I know that they don't *get it*. And not everyone does at this point!"

Employee Communication and Coordination Skills. Greater communication skills are required in an open system than in a closed system because it is necessary to be able to influence others without line authority. In traditional bureaucratic organizations, influence is based on rules and procedures in addition to hierarchy of authority. In the hybrid system, authority is more likely to be based on technical knowledge, motivational abilities, and charismatic leadership. A senior manager who earned a master's degree before entering the workforce provided an interesting and humorous comment during one of the ASU/CHMR interviews: "I was fortunate to be well educated and join the workforce at a relatively high level back in the 1970s. It was great because people would listen to me. But now I realize they only listened to me because of my position. Now I have to convince them that what I am saying has merit. That is not always easy!! It has probably forced me to be a much better communicator."

Communication and coordination are vital for both vertical and horizontal linkages. As one supply executive of a large system commented, "Sometimes I wonder what keeps this place together. Not long ago, I realized that it was the communication that keeps us stuck together—the glue that keep the ship together, and sometimes it seems pretty wobbly!"

Characteristics of Effective Teams in Hybrid Organizations

The use of multidisciplinary teams made up of a wide spectrum of professionals is vital in a hybrid organization and has already been discussed to some degree in Chapter Three in the discussion of value analysis teams (VATs). VATs and other team efforts are generally characterized by the heterogeneity of membership and are cross functional. Such teams, which are important for both horizontal and vertical coordination and implementation of strategy, require careful design around several factors:[23]

- Team composition. The correct members must be included. For instance, a standardization committee on orthopedic implants without key users such as an orthopedic surgeon would have limited effectiveness.
- Team skills. The team members must have sufficient team skills. In several of the case studies, many of the participants had difficulty separating individual perspectives and the team goal. This is a particularly intense issue in health care because many of the key decision makers have had limited team-building training experience. Of course, the success of the cross-functional teams could be largely identified as superior team and leadership skills of everyone involved.
- Team incentives. This characteristic is highly related to the other two. The correct incentives must be in place for both individual and team contributions and for clinical and business contributors. This is not an easy task, but it is an essential one.

Strategic Questions for Organizational Design

The following strategic questions are designed to provide guidance in determining an appropriate organizational design for the supply function. It has already been stated that the hybrid approach is generally the most effective; however, it is necessary to determine the extent of centralization, complexity, and formality required.

- *What are the primary environmental factors that affect the supply chain organizational design?* A supply chain concurrently operates within two environments: (1) the internal clinical and business customers that it serves and (2) the external health care customers, political groups, governmental regulators, and financial markets. The relative importance and power of these environments must be determined. In some situations, it may not be possible to offset strong traditions of a particular internal group such as nursing or to counter the influence of physicians who have allegiances in multiple hospitals. An external group member, such as a major donor, may have an inordinate level of influence on organizational decision making. In other situations, it may be necessary to attempt to overcome these strong political barriers, which may stand in the way of an effective design. But a fair assessment cannot be made until the political environment is assessed.

Another crucial environmental factor is the market forces associated with the health sector, which can have an impact on both external relationships and internal dynamics. For instance, physicians who have high market demand, bringing a great number of admissions to a hospital, may have a different impact on supply decisions from physicians with low demand.

• *How do the goals and strategies of the system and each unit within the system affect the supply function?* It is within the context of mission that organizational design can make the greatest contribution to the system's goals and strategy. While the importance of linking the supply chain organizational design to the strategy cannot be overstated, only the most progressive hospitals and systems are characterized by written documents that link supply chain strategy and design to broader system strategy and design.

In the absence of clearly stated goals and mission, it is quite possible that confusion exists between the contending targets, such as low-cost and differentiation strategies. When strategies are developed to meet multiple goals concurrently, the organization is attempting to achieve "satisficing" goals rather than a maximum level of performance with a single goal.

The best way to satisfy goals is to thoroughly understand the goals and strategies of each hospital or unit within the system, which leads to the next question.

• *What are the goals and strategies of each unit within the system, and how can they be integrated?* Integration of strategies is extremely difficult, but supply management may be able to maximize integration opportunities much better than other functions. For instance, this may be accomplished through centralization of GPO and distribution policies while decentralizing implementation procedures.

• *What are the current structural elements of (1) division of work, (2) departmentalization, (3) authority and responsibility, (4) span of control, and (5) coordination? Also, what are the current organizational design dimensions of (1) formalization, (2) centralization, and (3) complexity?* In order for an organization to answer these questions, it may require a thorough mapping process throughout the system. The map that results from process analysis should provide an indication of the level to which the supply chain is supporting the organization's mission. It is particularly important to consider the difference between units and the interorganizational processes within the system. The result may indicate how the integration of goals could be better supported through supply chain design.

This process mapping may also indicate where communication linkages are deficient. For instance, it may be found that supply waste is occurring because one unit does not understand how excess supplies can be transported to another unit. Or it may be that one unit has lower GPO compliance because it is not aware of standardization processes that occurred in another unit.

FIGURE 6.3.   DIVISION OF WORK, AUTHORITY, AND RESPONSIBILITY.

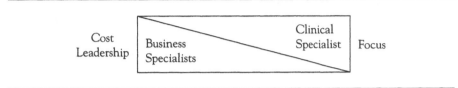

- *What is the appropriate division of work along with authority and responsibility between the supply management processes and the clinical process?* This could be restated as, "What is the role of the clinical staff within the supply process? Should the clinical staff be part of the supply process, or should they be separated?"

Figure 6.3 can assist with the answer to this question. On one end of the continuum is the cost leadership strategy. To meet the objective of this strategy, professionals are required with a strong background in cost analysis, strategic sourcing, and logistics management. These are highly specialized experts who have a lot of authority and responsibility within the supply process. But in a focus strategy, the supply specializations should be shared to a greater extent with the clinical staff.

In neither case does total authority and responsibility rest with one party. It is divided between the clinical and supply staff. Also, the division may vary within one hospital or throughout the system for different commodities and physician preference items. A hybrid organizational design is required in order to account for these differences.

Summary and Conclusion

Following Drucker's contention that organizational design begins with building blocks, this discussion has reviewed these building blocks within the context of environmental issues and strategy. Based on the current literature and the results of the case studies, a hybrid organizational design is recommended for most hospital supply chain situations. Because of the environmental complexity, differences in strategies may exist from one unit to another within a system. The idea of a hospital as an organization with units affected by a variety of clockspeeds further supports the need for a hybrid system with an open, flexible approach to organizational design.

It is noteworthy that hospitals, while characterized by different clockspeeds across departments, are also characterized by having units that are at very different stages in their life cycles and thus require different kinds of management.[24] One hospital participating in the ASU/CHMR project described the difficulties of managing an outpatient center that had very rapid turnover of patients and a demand pattern for materials that was quite different from in-patient units carrying out similar procedures. Another ASU/CHMR study site hospital, for example, had recently acquired a robotic surgical system that resulted in fewer complications, a shorter length of stay, and reduced complications. The technology was described as changing the demand for the surgical suites and staff.

Hospitals are a curious combination of continually growing and aging departments, processes, procedures, and technologies. New kinds of laboratories emerge to meet new technologies, and processes are outsourced due to changing time demands by patients and providers. No one supply design or strategy will fit all of a hospital's units.

The progressive supply manager must be prepared to assess not only the best strategy and consequent design for the overall supply function, but the strategy and design necessary to meet the demands of a variety of internal and external customers. In each case, the supply manager will find it necessary to determine the centralization, formalization, and complexity that is required within each unit.

CHAPTER SEVEN

LEVELS OF DEVELOPMENT FOR THE HEALTH CARE SUPPLY CHAIN

The ASU/CHMR study reveals that hospitals and systems vary considerably in their inclination, ability, and approach to controlling their supply chain. Over the course of the study, it became clear that progressive systems, committed to the control of the supply chain and cost reduction, have undergone a maturation process to adapt to the variety of pressures in their environments and the different clockspeeds that characterize their products and processes. This chapter describes the features of hospital and hospital system supply chain management characteristics observed in the course of the ASU/CHMR study. Management consultants have recognized that the foundation for understanding any organization is an assessment of the organization's level of development in its various business processes. On the basis of such analysis, they are able to make recommendations to improve strategic fit and advance the firm's ability to engage its environment at a more mature level. While tools to assist in such efforts have been designed for other industries,[1] no tool has been adopted by hospitals and systems to assess their current level of supply chain management sophistication.

Each level in the supply maturation process is characterized by different strategies associated with internally managing in the hospital (for example, inventory control mechanisms, distribution schemes, and engagement of clinicians) and externally with the system's purchasing partners. The idea of levels or maturation also implies an active process, with the possibility of change over time. Following the organizational life cycle idea,[2] some organizations exist at an infancy or emergent level, experiencing rapid periods of growth and adjustments in their supply chains to meet the contingencies of everyday practice.

As hospitals and systems become mature, they are able to put into place processes and procedures to reduce the burden of everyday management. Objectives include managing external partners, preventing suppliers from bringing unauthorized materials into the hospital, and internal decision making relating to physician product use.

Hospitals, hospital departments, and processes are characterized by very different structures, strategies, and clockspeeds pertaining to processes and organization. Strategies also differ across a system. One of the larger systems scrutinized is characterized by a value analysis team that was praised for its efforts to reduce the number of orthopedic implant manufacturers in one of its hospitals. In another hospital in the same system, the value analysis team has purposively worked not to reduce the number of suppliers but to standardize on price, thus having a ceiling or cap on how much it would pay for defined implantable items. The same manager heralded both efforts as great successes. Two different strategies in one system! In a third hospital, the system has not achieved cooperation from its two competing orthopedic groups and could not engage in standardization on either products or prices. Those that recognize this diversity and aspire to achieve excellence in their performance will require mature but agile supply chains to meet the challenges of the industry.

Figure 7.1 identifies the levels of development that the ASU/CHMR study uncovered for hospitals and hospital system supply chain management. While the ASU/CHMR study goal was not to classify the systems studied on the basis of

FIGURE 7.1.   LEVELS OF DEVELOPMENT.

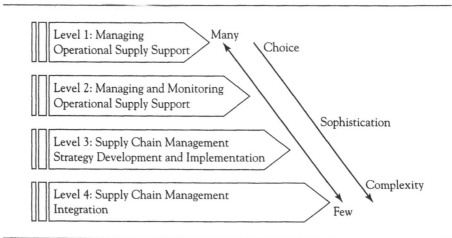

their hospital and system network integration, many of the attributes of progressive practice supply chain hospitals mirror the attributes of well-developed integrated delivery networks,[3] including the presence of highly committed and integrated physician groups and multiple sites with a wide range of services.[4] Yet progressive supply chain practices are not always part of larger, highly integrated systems. Single hospitals and small systems seem to be able to come together to establish progressive supply chains. Furthermore, some large systems, characterized by high levels of integration of administration, governance, payer alignment, and complexity of components, are not observed as progressive supply chain systems. Thus, one of the features of this chapter is a more extensive discussion of integration as an organizational design feature. As Burns and Pauley point out, "There are diseconomies from overcentralization of hospital systems and a need to blend both centralized and decentralized forms of management in such systems."[5] As suggested in Chapter Six, progressive systems recognize and are able to achieve such blends in both their design and other areas of their structure and operations.

Figure 7.1 challenges the reader to think about the various factors affecting health supply chain maturation and to begin to articulate, from experience, the factors that affect success. While it is possible to characterize hospitals and systems along a continuum or in terms of the developmental levels, a number of the supply chain management characteristics present in very mature organizations are also present in organizations that might be judged as being rather nonprogressive. At the same time, very progressive organizations frequently are characterized by some practices that one would not associate with organizational best practices. In a number of instances, large systems are characterized by hospitals that are all very progressive in their supply chain strategy and management. Some progressive systems, however, are uneven in the extent to which system hospitals and departments progressively engage their supply environment. These contradictions constitute a significant challenge for the supply chain executive.

Levels of supply chain development are best thought of as ideal types that are understood by the extent to which they reflect a strategic fit between a hospital and a system's environmental situation in relationship to its unique competencies.[6] A level of development constitutes a well-crafted strategic fit when it is successful in aligning the goals of the hospital and the system with the opportunities they encounter in their marketplace.[7] Achieving strategic fit is especially important in the health sector, where organizational cultures are very strong and clinician engagement is central to the production of successful outcomes.

The strategic fit between a hospital or system's level of development and its unique situation extends to how it manages and encounters its purchasing partners, including GPOs and distributors. When purchasing partners do not allow the organization to achieve its goals or to purchase within the framework of its culture, the hospital or system may attempt to change its existing purchasing partner's strategy or will seek different partners. An organization's purchasing strategy therefore represents its best attempt at resolution of this tension at a given period of time.[8]

Chapters Four and Five explored the idea of strategic fit for hospital relationships, respectively, with GPOs and distributors. In that context, strategic fit relates to the demand for products and the responsiveness of the supply chain to provide needed goods, in a cost-effective and timely manner, to hospitals and systems.[9] As hospital and system supply chain maturity is discussed in this chapter, a more macro and dynamic view of strategic fit is implied. This view takes into account the broad spectrum of issues associated not just with purchasing partners (such as GPOs or distributors) but with managing the variety of internal customers, processes, and designs of the organization itself.

The generic model of dynamic strategic fit identified by Northwestern University professor Edward Zajac and his colleagues, introduced in Chapter One, provides guidance for looking at how health care delivery organizations should approach their decisions regarding improved organizational performance (Figure 7.2).[10] Figure 1.2 identified the presence of a "system of exchange" as a

FIGURE 7.2.   STRATEGIC FIT FOR HOSPITALS AND HOSPITAL SYSTEMS.

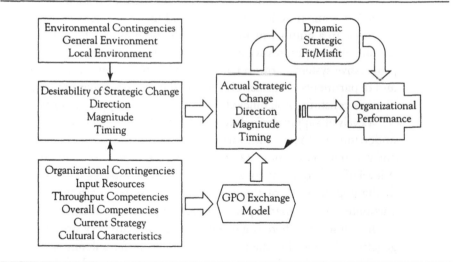

Source: Adapted from Zajac, E., Kraatz, M., and Bresser, R. "Modeling the Dynamics of Strategic Fit: A Normative Approach to Strategic Change." *Strategic Management Journal,* 2000, 21(4), 429–455.

key factor in the a hospital or system's ability to secure needed goods or services in the marketplace in which it exists. Figure 7.2 replaces the box labeled "system of exchange" with a box labeled "GPO" model. This reflects the observation that a system or hospital that lacks the organizational competency or inclination to gain the collaboration of its medical staff may find itself unable to be an active participant in a purchasing organization that demands compliance in using a limited number of products. Decisions must be made on the level of change required for improved performance, and decisions regarding organizational change will be successful only if there is ample consideration of organizational competencies and commitments.

Finally, adjusting organizational strategies is not a one-time decision. For some decisions, such as engaging the medical staff for increased collaboration, timing may be very important. In February 2005, just prior to the completion of this book, the federal government announced that it would reinterpret on a case-by-case basis laws regarding hospitals sharing savings with physicians (Study 4). Some systems report that this now provides them with a new set of incentives to align physicians with the organization's goals and advance the system's ability to reduce costs for physician preference items. A system that has had difficulty in achieving collaboration with medical staff may find that changes in the legal climate will facilitate their ability to move to a more advanced level of supply chain management development. Because changes in legal opinion regarding gain sharing are variable over time, there must be continuous vigilance by hospitals and systems toward their strategic decision-making process.[11]

Strategic Fit in Health Care Supply Management

Hospitals and hospital systems are differentiated by their organizational cultures, competencies, and aspirations. They are heterogeneous on the basis of levels of competition for patients, geographical dispersion, expectations by key stakeholders, medical staff organization and structure, focus (academic versus teaching), and power to influence their environment. Furthermore, they differ by their recognition of the centrality of supply, sophistication of purchasing executives, and the potential value of information technology.

As hospitals and systems develop strategies to solve clinical and business challenges and advance their missions, they must consider how their decisions and resulting practices combine to ensure strategic fit in managing its supply chain. A hospital with comprehensive surgical services in cardiology and orthopedics, for example, will have very different opportunities to negotiate directly for extensive supplier services and price concessions than a hospital with limited services in these areas. To the extent that volume can be leveraged to achieve better prices, hospitals may use contracting and purchasing options in different ways.[12]

Levels of Development and the Question of Integration

Overall hospital and system maturity is associated with the organization's level of horizontal and vertical integration. Horizontal integration occurs when two or more separate firms, producing either the same service or services that are close substitutes, join to become either a single firm or a strong interorganizational alliance.[13] Howard Zuckerman and Arnold Kaluzny describe alliances as being either service, opportunistic, or stakeholder focused; each requires different ways of thinking about organizations.[14] They require skillful management and an understanding of what each party hopes to achieve. Truly integrated supply chain partnerships are very complex, involving interrelationships of shared activities, processes, interests, objectives, and competitive information.[15] The principal drivers behind these horizontal linkages are potential economies of scale and a desire to increase market share.

Consistent with the discussion of organizational design for supply chain in Chapter Six, horizontal integration should involve consolidation of many duplicated resources among the organizations with the goals of increasing efficiency and taking advantage of economies of scale. The achievement of improved organizational performance through horizontal integration on operations is not clear. While there is continued debate regarding the extent to which mergers save hospitals money,[16] research by Dranove and Shanley[17] and Spang and her colleagues[18] concludes that hospital mergers do not result in lower production costs. The results of hospital consolidation require further study to assess implications for patient care and competition;[19] nevertheless, in one of the progressive systems in the ASU/CHMR study, there were significant cost savings associated with the reduction of supply chain personnel costs as a result of mergers, the centralization of the supply function, and the reduction of costs associated with standardization on items across the system.

Vertical integration refers to the bringing together of two more firms whose products or services are inputs to, or outputs from, the production of one another's services. Two reasons generally exist for vertical integration: to lower transaction costs between the units by substituting and exchanging within the organizations and to reduce average production costs by sharing common inputs (such as physicians and nurses) across related production processes. Extensive research has verified the benefits of vertical integration in a number of settings, including reduced transaction costs and collaborative savings associated with mutual problem solving.[20] Such integration can streamline products into lines of services and new business for a hospital or system. In many instances, more informal alliances, or "virtual integration," can achieve the advantages of firms coming under common ownership.

While the extent to which horizontal or vertical integration specifically affects supply chain operations, however, remains unexplored. It may be speculated that the extent of impact is related to the level of the integration.[21] A good articulation of the characteristics of integration, which follow quite closely with the ASU/CHMR features of progressive supply chains, is found in four stages of integration as developed by NCI.[22]

Supply Chain Functional Problems and Prerequisites

Four principal problems, or functional prerequisites, must be solved and achieved by all hospitals or systems in order to carry out every day functions: (1) strategic sourcing and product selection, (2) contracting strategy, (3) managing with the GPO, and (4) inventory and distribution.[23] While these have been discussed individually as important aspects of supply chain management in the preceding chapters, it is their orchestration at the hospital or system level that will determine the performance of the overall supply chain.

Strategic sourcing and product selection, as discussed in Chapter Two, is the process that identifies the need for the product, describes the product's attributes, identifies the potential suppliers, and evaluates them in combination with their products. This process involves the selection of the final supplier and product and the negotiation of price in the absence of a GPO. This process generally includes, as discussed in Chapter Three, the use of product selection teams such as value analysis teams (VAT). The supplier management plan may also be included in this strategic sourcing process.

After the product is selected, it is necessary to determine the best approach for contracting with the supplier. The question lies in whether this should be done independently (Chapter Three) or in collaboration with other organizations. This frequently depends on the nature of the product and whether it is a local, national, or international market. For instance, cleaning services may be a local market that would require contracting of local providers, so it would not be functional to use a national purchasing partner. However, if it was a system contracting for the cleaning of thirty different hospitals across five different states, a national service may be possible. Meanwhile, an international market is applicable to a product that has limited suppliers in the United States and abroad. Contracting strategies may also involve the employment of technologies such as reverse auctions to facilitate a more open and competitive marketplace. It is necessary to have a contracting strategy to determine the best approach for each of these items.

The third process is managing with the GPO (Chapter Four). On average, approximately 70 percent of the goods that a hospital purchases is through a GPO. It is for this reason that we have inserted the idea of the GPO model into Figure 7.2. It is vital, as we suggested in Chapter Four, that systems and hospitals select a compatible GPO from the variety of models that are grounded in some combination of alliance, price, moral, and communal characteristics.[24] In short, the GPO should be compatible with the overall supply chain strategy. This may be an arm's-length relationship that strictly focuses on price, or it may be a strategic development and collaborative relationship. GPOs may also facilitate independent purchasing for members by assisting with reverse auctions or advocating regional purchasing.

Whether contracting through a GPO or independently, distribution and inventory are necessary (Chapter Five). Distribution includes movement of the materials from the manufacturer to the end user in the hospital. Therefore, it includes transportation of materials to the hospital dock, material handling within the facility, and management of the item at the point of use. Most hospitals and systems use third-party distributors such as Cardinal or Owens and Minor to varying degrees and only in rare cases carry out these tasks completely independent of third-party providers.

Risk, as discussed in Chapter One, is also associated with each of the supply chain processes, thus requiring careful analysis and management. Strategy risk occurs when an inappropriate strategy is used for a good or service. For instance, a GPO may be used when it would be more appropriate to contract independently, or vice versa. The second type of risk is market risk. This occurs because the market may fluctuate rapidly without the knowledge of the supply chain professional. As a result, an inappropriate price may be paid for a commodity, the incorrect good or service may be acquired, or inferior goods may be purchased, resulting in inferior service. Demand risk, the third type of risk, develops because of fluctuating demands. Demand changes may mean that too much or too little of a commodity is available. The final risk, implementation risk, results when the appropriate strategy is attempted, but it is implemented incorrectly, resulting in high prices, poor clinical outcomes, or inferior customer service.

Successfully solving the four principal problems reduces the risk of organizational failure by ensuring that the appropriate products are selected, contracted for, and made available at an appropriate price.

Levels of Development

The ASU/CHMR study scrutinized the ways that hospitals and systems attempt to solve the four functional prerequisite problems associated with ensuring an effective supply chain through cost and value analysis, employment of information technology, and collaboration and integration. This section characterizes how progressive systems simultaneously work to solve the functional prerequisites for supply chain management. The characterization is completed with the recognition that issues such as marketplace dynamics associated with managed care and system integration,[25] differences in a hospital and system's definitions for success,[26] and system, geographical, and hospital diversity[27] will affect both supply management and strategy.

Level 1: Managing Operational Supply Support

Level 1 organizations are characterized by:

- Commodity-level focus
- Reactivity
- Emphasis on purchasing fundamentals
- Price metrics
- Unintegrated information systems
- No recognition that different units operate at different clockspeeds

At level 1, purchasing operations are managed at the departmental level, and few or no formal written strategies exist for working with GPOs, suppliers, distributors, or physicians. Furthermore, little collaboration exists among these entities. A total cost perspective is not used, and information systems are not integrated across functions. Although some strategic approaches may be used, they are not formally developed and articulated. Value analysis or product standardization is conducted on an ad hoc rather than a systematic basis. Benchmarking on prices and processes is limited to departmental-level activities. No attention is given to the various types of supply risk.

This level of development is likely to characterize freestanding hospitals or geographically dispersed systems. Both vertical and horizontal integration are low. Supply management receives little or no attention from the organization's top-level executives, and supply management employees have little formalized management or supply chain education. The supply process has extremely limited visibility within the organization.

Level 2: Managing and Monitoring Operational Supply Support

Level 2 organizations are characterized by:

- Purchasing strategies that dominate supply management thinking
- Integration that rarely exists beyond a unit

- Limited visibility of spend data
- Material management orientation (tactical)
- Price and limited cost metrics
- Minor recognition of the differences of unit clockspeeds

Level 2 is characterized by a facility-wide supply focus rather than just a departmental or commodity focus. The key concepts are the internal and external attention to supply management, as basic collaboration exists with the GPO and distributor. Both vertical and horizontal integration are beginning to emerge. Formal written strategies may exist, but they may not be thorough or related to systemwide corporate objectives. A price orientation exists rather than a total cost of ownership perspective. Formal VATs are in place, but they may have limited key physician input, and compliance remains weak. Traditional supply chain transactional metrics (for example, number of fulfilled orders or stock-out rates) may be shared with various executive levels, but they are not tightly integrated with corporate metrics.

Level 3: Supply Chain Management Strategy Development and Implementation

Level 3 organizations are characterized by:

- Unit-level, process focus
- Integration across the unit
- Total integration with suppliers, a sharing of vision and goals
- Integration with the corporate vision on resource use
- Global and strategic vision
- Total cost and strategy metrics
- Recognition of important clockspeed differences across units with managerial strategy developed for unique units

At this third level of development, the emphasis is on strategy. At the previous two levels, strategies may have been used, but at this level, the strategies are thoroughly developed and articulated among key constituencies throughout the hospital or hospital system. The strategies include thorough collaboration with GPOs, distributors, and key stakeholders within the system or hospital. Strategy effectiveness may be determined by total cost measures.

At this level, information systems are likely integrated across units; however, they are not robust. Also, extensive use of electronic purchasing (e-procurement) is beginning to emerge, but it is not fully implemented. Strategy implementation is still not at the optimal level due to information management limitations as a result of their ability to engage in collaboration and information systems that have a major impact on integration across the system.

Level 4: Supply Chain Value Integration

Level 4 hospitals and systems are characterized by:

- System-level, strategic, and value enhancement focus
- Proactive efforts to obtain competitive advantage
- Systemwide policy formation
- Integrated supply strategies with corporate strategy
- Integration of systems
- Physicians sharing the vision of the supply chain management team
- Long-term value metrics; value driven
- Clockspeed awareness that drives both strategy and tactics and leads to decision making at advanced levels

Strategy and implementation span the entire supply chain at this advanced level of supply chain development. The GPOs, distributors, and suppliers have a high level of collaboration with the individual units within the system, but the strategic relationships are generally developed at the centralized corporate level. Transaction, administrative, and product analysis takes a total cost perspective. VATs are highly structured, with key clinicians taking an active role in decision-making processes. Compliance is high throughout the system. At this level, a centralized information system is in place that provides real-time demand information.

The primary factor that differentiates this level from the others is that value is thoroughly analyzed in relationship to the system's overall mission and objectives. When considering value, supply risk is considered in relationship to clinical outcomes.

Advancing the Supply Chain Development Process

It is valuable to think of the four developmental levels in life cycle terms of organizational infancy, growth, stabilization, and maturity. However, developmental levels are not necessarily good or bad or indicative of an appropriate strategy. Rather, they are descriptive of supply function at a given time. The appropriate supply chain developmental level depends on the organization's history, environment, capacity, and aspirations. Each organization will vary, and the processes within the system will vary as well. But regardless of the current level of development, it is important to continue to advance in strategy and tactics in order to develop and maintain a competitive advantage and achieve strategic fit between the organization and its environment.

Solving the Principal Problems of Supply Management

Three principal tools or competencies are observed to be employed by managers in progressive systems to solve the challenges associated with each of the functional prerequisites:

1. Price and total cost analysis
2. Employment of information technology and e-commerce
3. Proactive efforts to manage collaboration and appropriate levels of integration

Although these tools and competencies are useful in solving the major functional prerequisites, they are employed differently, depending on an organization's structure, strategy, and level of sophistication. In addition, each of the prerequisites requires a number of unique managerial competencies and tools. Tables 7.1, 7.2, and 7.3 consider each set of management tools and competencies for each level of development (left-hand column) and how the competencies help to meet the functional prerequisite (top row) problems.

Cost and Value Analysis

Cost and value analysis at the most elementary level is viewed from an expenditure perspective (Table 7.1). How much must be spent to get something accomplished? While product price is frequently the focus,[28] at a more sophisticated level total cost analysis utilization takes a long-term perspective in order to understand all related cost and price issues. Also, cost is considered within the context of value, which may include aspects of safety and clinical outcomes. Total cost of ownership is defined as the sum of all expenses and costs associated with the purchase and use of equipment, materials, and services. To use a total cost approach, a firm must define and measure a purchased item's major cost components.[29] In writing about total cost of ownership (TCO), Ellram has pointed out that there "is no one standard 'model' or algorithm for understanding TCO across different types of buys, even within an organization." While unique models are required for major purchases, organizations are able to use "the same or very similar models for all purchases of production capital, or all low-value items."[30]

TABLE 7.1. COST ANALYSIS AND LEVEL OF DEVELOPMENT.

Levels	Problem 1: Strategic Sourcing and Product Selection	Problem 2: Contracting Strategy	Problem 3: Managing with the GPO	Problem 4: Distribution and Inventory
Level 4: Supply chain value integration	Integrates total cost, including clinical outcomes, when making product selection decisions	Compares the impact of value and total cost when comparing options	Develops a total cost model in conjunction with the GPO. Uses extensive VAT in conjunction with the GPO for value analysis	Sophisticated metrics and understanding of the overall value of buffer stock and a stock-out
Level 3: Supply chain management strategy development and implementation	Considers cost and quality in decision making in addition to price	Has a clear understanding of total spend and how the total cost will be affected by various contracting options	Begins to use cost and value analysis in evaluating the services provided by the GPO	Has appropriate metrics for different types of inventory items
Level 2: Managing and monitoring internal and external supply management	Historical price trends are analyzed	Price is the driving force in whether to use a GPO or other contracting approach	Attempts to reduce price by using GPO and is only beginning to consider total cost of services	Beginning to develop cost metrics for inventory levels
Level 1: Managing operational supply support	Considers only price; does not know total spend	Uses either the GPO or other alternatives because that is the way it has traditionally been done	Considers only the prices offered by the GPO	Does not understand the cost of carrying materials

Table 7.1 reveals the range of applications of cost analysis across the problems that hospitals and systems must solve in managing the supply chain. The most progressive systems use high-level cost of ownership and value analysis processes to solve each of the four management problems. In attempting to solve the problem of strategic sourcing, the progressive systems integrate total cost, including clinical outcome costs, when making product selection decisions. The information is carried into the contracting process to assess GPO opportunities and to make insourcing and outsourcing decisions. The analysis also provides metrics to understand volume-related purchasing and risks associated with stock outs. This approach contrasts dramatically with level 1 hospitals and systems that consider only price and have virtually no strategy for using cost of ownership data to assess the value associated the opportunities the hospital or system can command in the marketplace or the relative added value brought by the relationship with a GPO. Level 1 organizations take a very nonanalytical approach to assessing the costs associated with warehousing, distribution, inventory, and strategic options associated with outsourcing distribution functions. These organizations are likely to make mistakes in their assessment of opportunities in the environment.

Information Technology and E-Commerce

Information technology and e-commerce continue to grow in importance because there is a need to coordinate supply chain activities across many locations, assume an organizational rather than a functional perspective, and take on complex and strategic responsibilities. Internet-based systems that integrate processes within and between are recognized as critical to success.[31] In hospitals and systems in the United States, information management ranges from a simple spreadsheet at the most elementary level to total enterprise resource planning systems (ERPs). Supply chain management is also augmented by related transaction systems support from information management companies (such as Neoforma and Global Health Exchange) and by reverse auction technology provide by both GPOs and other technology vendors. Progressive systems report that ERP systems, while having had success in the area of general financial management, human resource management, and standard financial areas, fail to meet the needs for managing the core supply functions and linking these functions to the financial and clinical performance of the organization. Providing reports on use of materials, materials cost, and materials performance to support strategic initiatives with physicians is reported by even the most progressive systems as beyond the capability of their systems and the systems of their purchasing partners.

Table 7.2 reveals the range of applications of information management that hospitals and systems must solve in managing the supply chain. To address

TABLE 7.2. INFORMATION TECHNOLOGY AND LEVEL OF DEVELOPMENT.

Levels	Problem 1: Strategic Sourcing and Product Selection	Problem 2: Contracting Strategy	Problem 3: Managing with the GPO	Problem 4: Distribution and Inventory
Level 4: Supply chain value integration[a]	VAT has total access to market information and internal spend data	Includes commodities and a wide range of clinical preference items	Accurate compliance data provided on a real-time basis by the GPO and other IT partners	Distributor and system work together to provide accurate information and excellence in logistics, stock management, and other areas
Level 3: Supply chain management strategy development and implementation	VAT has access to extensive market information and internal spend data	Includes data on most commodities and limited clinical preference items	Systematic information on costs of different products	The distributor and system work together to provide accurate information and high levels of logistics, stock management, and other areas
Level 2: Managing and monitoring internal and external supply management	Limited internal VAT activity; high reliance on clinician preference	Limited use of internal or GPO VAT data in product selection at commodity or clinical preference item levels	Systematic information on product pricing used only to make majority of decisions	Compare availability across units
Level 1: Managing operational supply support	No internal VAT activity; market price information available	Little use of internal or GPO VAT in product selection at commodity or clinical preference item levels	Limited systematic information on product pricing compliance data	Spreadsheet analysis of availability

[a]Each of the primary processes uses a systemwide integrated data-based decision support system.

the problem of sourcing, the most progressive systems customize information from multiple sources in order to provide data for VATs and to assess their materials spend. This information then is carried over into contracting decisions.

Information on commodity item spend and performance is easier to obtain from GPOs and suppliers. This information provides the rationale for aggressively pursuing contracting decisions for commodity items. Information for these progressive systems has high payoffs. They are able to monitor their compliance with their own contracts and potential GPO contract opportunities. They are also able to engage in the most advanced inventory practices on the basis of understanding product demand and supply channels. Such information may be gathered through a hospital or system's own information system or outsourced to a third-party vendor that can provide such services and frequently benchmark the hospital or system in relation to the broader market.

The level 4 information technology demands and capabilities are in stark contrast to level 1 organizations, which have no internal or external (such as GPO-sponsored) VATs or standardization efforts to engage their medical staff. Level 1 hospitals and systems do not carefully monitor the value that various contract types bring to their bottom line and toward the improvement of care. There is a continued employment of information and information strategies to advance the hospital or system.

Collaboration and Integration

Collaboration and integration is defined as the process by which two or more parties adopt a high level of purposeful cooperation. This is not just the issue of whether a system is an integrated delivery system; it is whether the system expresses behaviors in which partners can find incentives and reciprocate through collaboration. This is the territory of customer, supplier, and purchasing partner relationship management. The relationships, when mature, are bilateral; both parties have the power to shape its nature and future direction. As demonstrated in Table 7.3, mutual commitment to the future and a balanced power relationship are essential to the process. Collaborative relationships are not devoid of conflict and must include mechanisms for managing conflict.[32] Developing trust in such relationships is a key to reducing transaction costs.[33]

Level 4 hospitals and systems work closely with physicians to develop formal and informal standardization processes. These systems recognize the value that both cosmopolitan and local physicians can bring to the management of resources. The level 4 capabilities are in stark contrast to level 1 organizations, which have no informal or formal plans in place to actively manage medical staff or engage suppliers.

TABLE 7.3.   COLLABORATION, INTEGRATION, AND LEVELS OF DEVELOPMENT.

Levels	Problem 1: Strategic Sourcing and Product Selection	Problem 2: Contracting Strategy	Problem 3: Managing with the GPO	Problem 4: Distribution and Inventory
Level 4: Supply chain value integration	Policy on physicians' role	Policy on collaboration with GPO	A supplier management strategy for continuous improvement	Policy on the role of independent distributor
Level 3: Supply chain management strategy development and implementation	Implementing VAT policy			Work with local market opportunities
Level 2: Managing and monitoring internal and external supply management	Managing VAT			Working with distributor for fulfillment
Level 1: Managing operational supply support	Ad hoc physicians' role			Independent materials handling

Strategic Fit and Levels of Development in Progressive Systems

The purpose of this discussion is to assist managers in understanding the current level of development of their supply chain management processes. Consistent with the focus on contingency management throughout this book, the appropriate strategies and tactics will vary from one system or hospital to another depending on how the levels across the four processes vary and the development of the three factors of total cost, information systems, and collaboration.

Regardless of the current level, making the transition from one level of development to the next frequently requires a systematic change effort. Unfortunately, many managers may believe that one or two tactical adjustments are all that is necessary to achieve a more sophisticated supply chain management effort. This is generally an incorrect approach. Tactical adjustments may be effective in moving an organization from level 1 to the beginning of level 2 because the various processes are basic. Sustained progress requires a more complex and continuous effort.

To move beyond level 1, an adaptive and flexible organizational culture is an essential driver for a systematic change. If the culture is not congruent with the advancement of the supply chain, little movement will occur. The reason that the culture is important is that it is the underlying values, assumptions, beliefs, and thought processes within the hospital or system.[34] Hospitals and systems typically have cultures that are very different from business enterprises because they provide services that are unique in society and are humanitarian in nature.[35] The tensions between the culture of business and the culture of professions represent a profound difference between health sector organizations and nonhealth counterparts. A cultural conflict also may exist between the business aspect of supply chain management and the humanitarian focus of the health care provider in general.

While a patient-centered or humanitarian perspective from the supply chain managers may exist, for most of systems involved in the ASU/CHMR study, cost containment was an interesting mix of superordinate and subordinate supply chain goals. Several systems clearly articulated a goal that recognized and managed supply chain to the advantage of the "physician as expert." At the same time, there was a growing recognition that even the culture of professionalism is undergoing change. This was probably best articulated by managers who advocated working closely with cosmopolitan physicians and building, within this group, an even stronger recognition of the positive aspects of effective supply management. This conflict is understandable, for culture is the historically developed sense of the institution's legacy—what it is, what it stands for, and what it represents for the people who work within the institution and the community it serves.[36] The hospital stands for humanitarian delivery of health care rather than cost containment.

The balance between a cost-efficient and a patient-focused and responsive health delivery culture is not easy. But it is vital for senior executives to develop and maintain this balance as they develop an overarching goal that meets the many competing and differing values within the hospital or health care delivery system.[37] A few enlightened executives observed in this study were able to articulate strategies to develop the balance between patient-centered and cost cultures. One of the ways that this is accomplished is that the executives have strong and tangible ways of expressing the visions to the executive group and to others. In some instances, they clearly stated, and presented tangible evidence, that the supply chain could have a direct impact on clinical outcomes, improved safety, and the ability of the system, through savings, to serve the community better. In addition, progressive executives clearly form strategies for change efforts designed to advance the level of the supply chain processes to contribute to the hospital's performance. Both written and spoken messages support and provide detailed change management programs.

It is important to turn vision into reality through consistent behaviors. First, the support must be present for hiring well-qualified people. This requires the appropriate funding so that highly qualified, experienced people can be hired for critical positions. To quote one director of supply chain in a large system, "We are almost afraid to hire well-qualified people at their market salary because we know that they would be the first to be laid off when the board wanted to reduce salary levels." The appropriate culture for transition to a higher level of development was not present in this system. Compare that to another system where the vice president stated, "We were told that it was critical to get the best. When the CEO set the goals for our supply management group, he made it very clear that we should pay above the going market rate for experienced health care supply chain professionals to ensure that we could hire the best. But in addition to giving us the green light to hire the best, he made it very clear that he wanted results that would hit the bottom line."

The second symptom of the appropriate culture is the organizational structure and where supply chain management is placed within it. At level 1 and level 2 organizations in which little visible evidence exists that much movement will be made, the supply chain effort is buried in the basement both figuratively and literally. In one case, the top supply management professional had the title of materials manager. His office was in the basement next to a warehouse, and the hall outside his office was cluttered with storage boxes. The image was that of a tactical support service for acquiring and moving materials with no strategic vision. He reported to the director of facility operations. Although this hospital was a unit within an integrated delivery network, the system was only a loose federation that had no central supply function.

Compare this to another hospital in which the top supply manager had the title of director of supply chain management. She had two direct reporting relationships: one was to the CFO of the hospital facility and the other to the vice president of supply chain management for the system. The vice president for the system reported directly to the system CEO. Her office was in the same general area of the corporate officers. The supply chain efforts in this case had a much greater visibility and cultural importance as a result of its organizational position.

Summary and Conclusion

In the dynamics of the twenty-first century, hospital and hospital system supply chain processes have increased their influence on other functions of the hospital, a result of greater professional skills and visibility within the organization. There is great interest in addressing progressive practices in order to confront the four problems all hospital and system supply chains face: strategic sourcing, contracting, managing with GPOs, and inventory and distribution. In this environment, there is also greater recognition of the need to develop a managerial tool box for problem solving. Tools associated with cost management, information management, and collaboration are recognized as the key to improved performance.

To move ahead in supply chain management will require investments in people and technology. In particular, total cost modeling requires sophisticated professionals who understand both the financial aspects of the hospital and the limitations brought about by clinical processes. Expensive and agile technology will be necessary for information management and collaboration needs. This is especially true in an organization characterized by units with many different clockspeeds and processes.

To advance supply chain practice, a preliminary understanding of the levels of development for supply chain processes can be a valuable tool. By identifying a system's placement within one of the four levels, it is possible to benchmark an organization and determine strategies for improvement. An analysis of the three management factors within the different levels provides specific opportunities. It is important to point out that not all hospitals or systems are expected to reach the same level of maturity in the management of their supply chain. Some will find themselves as a system (or part of a system) to be too geographically isolated and unable to take advantage of environmental factors that contribute to integration. Others will be poorly managed or make a conscious decision to achieve goals that are not focused on the management of the supply chain.

An example is provided by the analysis of risk. A total cost of ownership model should reveal the potential for supply risk. No doubt exists that risk is an important consideration throughout the health system.[38] However, this research revealed that risk management was considered only in systems at level 4 of development. Other hospitals or systems should be able to use the analysis presented here to determine the type of initiatives they should use to develop risk analysis and management systems. In addition to total cost, collaboration and information systems can assist supply chain managers understand their supply risk levels.

This chapter has been designed to provide the supply manager and strategist with the ability to take both a cross-cutting view of the supply function as it now exists in a hospital or system as well as a longitudinal view, assessing where the hospital or system has been and where it is capable of moving. It is a perspective that is consistent with the continuous quality improvement movement in U.S. health care. What is curious is that quality improvement most frequently is applied to clinical outcomes, not the outcomes of organizations and their processes. It is also not a perspective that has seen improvement in materials as leading to improvement in outcomes, safety, and overall organizational performance. In the most progressive systems, this is changing. Progressive systems question the strategic fit of their purchasing function with the overall strategies of the organization and work to determine how to improve its quality by analyzing its current level of development and determining how to advance to the next level.

CHAPTER EIGHT

BUILDING SUPPLY CHAIN LEADERSHIP AND RESOURCES FOR THE FUTURE

Supply chain leadership and management in progressive systems is orchestrated by individuals empowered by management to ensure that the supply chain function operates at a level that brings value to the hospital and system. Although they are charged to secure the best products, for the best price, at the appropriate location, their performance is assessed by their contributions to the organization's strategic goals. In many instances, these goals are related to cost savings. However, other goals, such as ensuring technological excellence, improving safety and outcomes, contributing to the organization's commitment to environmental protection, or ensuring high levels of physician satisfaction are also seen as principal ways that they bring value to the hospital or system. Ohio Health describes its goals for its medical resources management as (1) maximizing organizational performance by reducing processes to reduce clinical variation, (2) developing the business by facilitating the evaluation and introduction of new technology, and (3) focusing on and expanding the delivery system by supporting programs to meet financial goals for continued investment in facilities. These goals are beyond just the transactional aspects of materials management.

Senior supply chain leaders are skilled at positioning the supply function to influence the organization's mission regarding safety, patient outcomes, and acceptance of new technologies. A significant aspect of their job is to work diligently to ensure that the strategies they devise fit the organization's design and culture.

Making and managing insourcing and outsourcing decisions regarding supply functions are key aspects of these senior-level positions.

Progressive systems are also characterized by a group of clinical resource specialists or service line specialists who work with clinicians to assist in the selection and use of materials. These individuals, who frequently had very successful careers in nursing and pharmacy, are recruited on the basis of their ability to work with clinical staff. In larger systems, clinical resource specialists may report directly to a corporate director of clinical resource management who occupies a position between the vice president and various clinical resource specialists. In some instances, the clinical resource specialists represent fairly narrow service lines (such as cardiology), whereas others may have responsibility for working with a wide range of specialists. Regardless of their positioning, these individuals occupy the linking-pin roles that support successful value analysis teams and the implementation of supply strategy within the hospital. Together, supply chain management executives and those in operations work to reduce a hospital or system's exposure to risk (Chapter Two) including strategy, market, demand, and implementation risk.[1] Progressive supply chain leaders effectively categorize risk, create risk supply assessment tools, and include risk in supplier selection and evaluation.[2] As suggested throughout the book, risk reduction and other key supply challenges are fulfilled through performing the three supply chain macro processes of customer relationship management (CRM), internal supply management (ISM), and supplier relationship management (SRM),[3] as well as key issues pertaining to purchasing partner management (PPM).

This chapter takes an in-depth look at the human resource skills and support functions that are needed as health care facilities work to advance along the health care supply chain management continuum. In addition, it assesses the extent to which information technology can provide the solutions for health care managers.

Supply Chain Management and Leadership

In progressive systems, the leadership role of supply chain managers is evolving into an expanded role that includes a perspective of the entire health care supply chain. Table 1.1, which was developed as a result of a set of focus groups with supply chain managers at HCA, demonstrates how this fundamental shift in thinking is occurring. The materials manager of the 1990s was transaction focused, with relatively little interest in orchestrating the overall materials management processes. In somewhat different terms, Table 1.1 revealed a vision of the modern supply chain manager position as a career in which the manager works to align the supply chain operations with the overall goals and strategy of the organization.

It is a career in the sense that it must evolve over time, in a succession of positions, to prepare the individual to satisfy a wide variety of strategic constituent needs and demands.

As the supply chain management focus transcends the more transactional materials management focus, individuals are approaching their jobs with a new set of lenses (Chapter One), allowing them to act strategically on behalf of a variety of stakeholders and the organization. Given the diversity of the hospital environment, it is not surprising that the work of supply chain managers is played out along service lines that in many ways constitute organizational silos that are differentiated on the basis of their clockspeed, level mix of commodity and physician preference items, and complexity of processes.[4] Yet in the most progressive systems, executive-level supply chain management has a focus across the organization in a role that resembles other officer-level functions. This complexity suggests a need to balance, in staffing, the operational aspects of the supply function with the more strategic levels.

A better understanding of the strategic supply chain role is achieved through a comparison of the ASU/CHMR progressive respondent roles and capabilities in relation to their counterparts in both finance and informatics (Table 8.1). The supply chain strategic role is, without question, a cross-cutting role that requires the CFO's skills as an "architect of change"[5] in combination with the CIO's newly found power to lead and infuse materials that can transform how the business of the hospital is done.[6] Just as it is no longer sufficient for the CIO's role to focus on keeping the company's data centers up and running or the CFO to ensure the

TABLE 8.1. FUNCTIONAL AREA OFFICER ATTRIBUTES.

Attribute	Chief Financial Officer	Chief Information Officer	Chief Supply Officer
Value-based management	X	X	X
Activity-based management	X		X
Risk management	X	X	X
Streamlining	X	X	X
Shared services	X	X	X
Systems		X	X
Change management	X	X	X
Leadership	X	X	X
Transformational visioning	X	X	X

Sources: Pricewaterhouse Coopers. *Financial and Cost Management Team, CFO: Architect of the Corporation's Future.* New York: Wiley, 1997. Deloitte and Touche. *CIO 2.0: The Changing Role of the Chief Information Officer.* New York: Deloitte Development, 2004. http://www.deloitte.com/dtt/article/0,1002,sid percent253D26551percent2526cidpercent253D65595,00.html.

accurate recording of transactions, it is no longer good enough for the materials manager to sustain a uniquely transactional role. The supply chain strategic management role brings together both the inward- and outward-looking aspects of the role that drives the modern chief financial officer, chief information officer, and chief supply officer to be a service partner, business partner, strategic partner, and entrepreneur.[7]

As one looks across the hospital or system (the horizontal view), supply makes everyday performance possible by ensuring that the components for patient care and the business function are close at hand. Doing this efficiently and effectively has and will always be the minimum requirements for performance. Efficient transactions do matter! It is, however, at the vertical level where the new supply chain function truly brings value to the system in its role as orchestrator of change. By managing risk, organizing value analysis and technology evaluation teams, and understanding the life cycle returns of product investments,[8] the supply chain function is a key to the hospital as an engine of clinical excellence and improved efficiency. Carrying out this function is achieved through a clear understanding of the variety of individual actors within the supply chain as well as these actors within the context of a network.

Supply Chain Management as Network Management

Perhaps what differentiates the progressive chief supply officer (CSO) from his or her counterparts in finance and information management is the continuous focus on managing networks of strategic stakeholders. Issues of trust in the supplier/buyer/customer/end-user relations, for example, are complicated by the presence of diverse internal, external, political, and clinical interests. These complexities call for concerted efforts by managers to strategically align suppliers and buyers with the organization's goals and abilities. Johnsen and others identify three core components of networks: resource tying, activity linking, and actor bonding.[9] Discussions with managers at the ASU/CHMR research sites reveal that these factors require a great deal of hands-on management to coordinate efforts between parties, develop risk and benefit sharing, and regulate conflict resolutions.[10]

Harland and Knight identify six key roles required to proactively manage networks:[11]

> *Network structuring agent.* Monitors and influences the competitiveness of supply markets. Acts to protect critical suppliers from the detrimental consequences of fragmented purchasing. Restructures supply routes to work directly with manufacturers rather than wholesalers.

Coordinator. Acts to manage both ongoing and completed projects with network partners.

Advisor. Provides advice on supply policy and strategy matters to internal network partners.

Information broker. Collects, analyzes, and disseminates information to network partners in order to better manage the interests of the relationship as well as focus on key issues and performance metrics.

Relationship broker. Facilitates inter-network communication and negotiation as well as encourages change to deal with specific performance-related issues.

Innovation sponsor. Promotes and facilitates product and process innovation.

These roles demand skills that create and help establish a sense of trust and collaboration among the various parties involved with the network, which include clinicians, GPOs, distributors, and manufacturers.

Information systems enable both sides of the relationship to benefit. On a more subtle level, managing relationships involves the use of information: how to gather it and how to use it. With the establishment of measurable metrics and the use of information technology data, supply chain managers will not just be able to view their own progress, but will establish responsibilities and accountability for all members of the supply chain. For example, by working with suppliers to implement long-term solutions, both parties can benefit from captured efficiencies such as reductions in the number of orders or order mistakes. A smoothly functioning network relies on members acting together to produce the greatest benefit for everyone involved.

To capture the greatest amount of efficiency and value from supply chains, health care organizations must put into place a system that involves creating a full integration of network resources.[12] This process combines an understanding of supply chain management techniques with the organizational concepts of policy, strategy, management, and operations.[13] These efforts need to be coordinated across departmental lines, while supporting the service line differences within the hospital and at the same time ensuring that a silo mentality does not prohibit the organization from achieving its larger systemwide goals.

Health care systems are still having troubles developing the processes necessary to capture the advantages of an integrated system.[14] Today's hospital system or integrated delivery network (IDN) can consist of acute care hospitals, outpatient clinics, physician practices, surgery centers, long-term care facilities, health plans, and a variety of community and social services that span across cities or even states. Helping to bring these various interests and abilities together can be a daunting task, but therein lies the greatest potential to capture the real benefits of an integrated network through standardization, stock-keeping units and contracts reduction, committed purchasing programs, benchmarking, and integration of information technology systems.

Network Leadership

Network leadership involves a manager's ability to motivate his or her team. This includes establishing a solid base of structured responsibilities, accountability, expectations, and goals. Strong leadership requires the development of a strategic plan that provides a clear vision for the direction of the division as well as the processes that need to be followed.[15] While flexibility and adaptability are certainly necessary in today's hybrid organizational designs, the ability to maintain a focus on the goals of the organization keeps tasks and projects from deteriorating into disorder.

Network Management Skills

Separate from leadership, managerial skills enable supply chain managers to monitor and direct the resources in their department. In the most progressive systems, this involves developing a set of metrics that are translated into markers for supply chain performance and useful for managing both upward to those to whom the supply chain executive reports (most frequently a chief financial officer) and laterally and downward to those in clinical specialist roles. There are a number of necessary skills.

Financial Management and Accounting. These skills allow one to deduce the implications of sourcing and contract decisions, the impact of noncontract spend, and the results of cost tracking and internal auditing. For reports and presentations, supply chain managers can extrapolate the costs of holding versus removing inventory or demonstrate the need for process changes revealed by activity-based costing. This allows the manager to develop a broader picture of the cost of doing business.

Computer and Information Technology. Knowledge in this field allows greater dialogue and use of enterprise resource planning (ERP) systems, unique supply chain management platforms, e-procurement, bar coding, universal product numbers, e-auctions, supply replenishment automation, automated report generation, and automated ordering and invoicing. These tools offer great opportunities for more effective cost management by using technology to reduce transaction costs associated with purchasing and engage in more effective inventory management.

Data-Driven Quantitative Analysis. Perhaps the top challenge facing a manager is knowing where and how to make value-added changes. A key to success in supply chain management is the development of metrics as they relate to effectiveness. This advances the concept that behavior needs to be driven by measurements and that there is real value in benchmarking.[16] While a uniform and agreed-on set of metrics to assess the supply chain has not yet been developed, information on the performance of the supply chain is increasingly available from GPOs and consulting firms. The Health Sector Supply Chain Research Consortium at ASU's W. P. Carey School is currently carrying out an assessment of such metrics to better understand their power for advancing supply chain performance. Data management has the power to provide managers with valuable tools in their decision-making processes that include statistical process knowledge, contract compliance and tracking, demand forecasting, process improvement, and study follow-up. For example, end-to-end product tracking allows users to track the progress of materials from delivery to disposal or return. For rental items, this provides a record of time spent in various locations for charge purposes, an assessment of turn-around times to evaluate process efficiencies, and accurate, active inventory records to evaluate future purchasing decisions. For disposables, this helps track inventory turnover and shelf storage time to provide more accurate information for ordering purposes.

Continuous Process Improvement. New materials and procedures are continually changing how medicine is practiced and make major demands on the resources of the hospital or health care delivery system. A new product such as drug-eluting stents, for example, has the potential to reduce the demand for open heart surgery. The introduction of robotics for the delivery of pharmaceuticals has important process implications for both pharmacy and nursing. The ability to analyze, design, implement, and monitor a process helps ensure progress toward an established goal. This procedure is often referred to as Plan-Do-Check-Act (PDCA Cycle) or the Deming Wheel. Supply chain manager training in process improvement becomes invaluable for change initiatives.[17] The supply chain manager should be a resource not only to the department but also to the entire organization as they contribute to change processes across a variety of settings.

Managing Internal, External, and Executive Networks

Managing the complexity of the hospital and hospital system supply function is related to the extensive number of internal and external network organizations and individuals that characterize the health sector value chain. While the following sections discuss these networks as though they are stable and identifiable, in reality it is sometimes difficult to distinguish between internal and external network issues. Community-based physician groups are external to the hospital in many ways. Yet when they have contracts that link their practice to the hospital or are employed by a hospital (for example, Mayo Clinic), they are truly part of an internal network. Supply partner relationships also are frequently structured to raise both internal and external network management issues. Distributor organizations that provide employees to carry out a full range of distribution functions within the hospital require management as part of a hospital's internal and external networks.

External Network Issues. Managing the external network requires customer relationship management (CRM), supplier relationship management (SRM), and purchasing partner management (PPM).[18] In even the most progressive systems participating in the ASU/CHMR study, these activities are hampered by the inability of information systems to provide timely and relevant data pertaining to internal and external purchasing partners.

The external network includes all of the players outside the organization with a directed interest in how the institution purchases, moves, uses, disposes of, and pays for materials. This includes (but is not limited to) GPOs, distributors, regulators, financial institutions, software providers, manufactures, third-party payers, and patients. Although supply chain managers may not directly interact with each of these groups, they do have to be aware of and proactively manage each of these relationships.[19] The degree of network management will depend on the facility's strengths, assets, needs, goals, and nature of its association with the other players in its network. The role of the supply chain manager essentially becomes "engaging in network management (that) would neither be controlling, nor merely coping within, the network. Controlling and coping can be seen as extreme positions on a spectrum of (the) actor's potential behavior within a network."[20] Ideally, in dealing with external networks, the supply manager must assume a role that has the characteristics of both a business and strategic partner.[21] This gives the supply chain manager great flexibility in choosing how to work with these partners and manage the relationships.

Internal Network Issues. In addition to elements outside the organization, the supply chain manager's role increasingly demands skills that facilitate the management of internal networks. The rapid rise of spend for items other than labor has increased the supply chain manager's span of influence.

Curiously, it is within the supply chain's environment that the worlds of health care, management, and medicine meet. To communicate effectively, supply chain managers must be able to speak both clinical and business languages. To this end, they need to understand the complexities of the clinical, cultural, and political issues that span these internal networks. Perhaps it is best to think of the outcomes of internal supply management in terms of success in services provided to key end users and influencing organizational performance through innovation in supply chain practice and technology.[22]

Executive and Clinical Network Issues. The executive officers and clinical leaders of an organization constitute a special internal network for supply chain management attention:

- Chief financial officer (CFO). Coordinating activities with this officer goes beyond simple evaluation of departmental budgets. In progressive systems, the CFO and supply chain manager work together to monitor and effectively manage facility expenditures through the development of performance metrics, such as spend per patient, spend per diagnosis-related group (DRG) or procedure, product transport costs, and contract and off-contract spend. These categories provide the groundwork for a facility's budgeting decisions, strategic planning initiatives, and evaluation of purchasing options. The work of these executives is frequently hampered by the lack of standardized metrics and, as suggested by leading executives in the industry, the absence of clear return-on-investment information on supply chain management technology.

- Chief operations officer (COO). Closely working with this position will help ensure that high-quality and timely services are delivered to the patient as well as to clinical and nonclinical staff. For example, decisions about staffing levels and unit stocking schedules directly affect when an operating room or dialysis center will be able to receive patients. In addition, coordination between the positions proves essential for the introduction of new product lines, communication of informational technology systems, and restructuring of departments or job roles. Many clinicians tend to exhibit resistance to new technology; therefore, the supply chain manager needs to be able to bridge this gap between clinical and business operations in order to ensure successful integration.

- Chief executive officer (CEO). Communication with the CEO should be directed toward ensuring that the time and effort of projects are worth the investment of resources. In working with the CEO, the supply chain manager is also working to address the concerns of the board of trustees, to whom the CEO is accountable. In addition to financial concerns, there are issues of the public perception of decisions, the added value of an initiative, outsourcing decisions, and, if the information is available, the final return on investment. In this working relationship, the supply chain manager must be able to speak to the business side of issues as well as demonstrate the benefits to the facility. For example, in making recommendations for change, the supply chain manager must be able to justify changes by addressing the CEO's clinical and operational concerns.

• Clinical leaders (chief medical officer, director of nursing). Clinical selection of materials is often seen as the biggest opportunity for savings in the health care supply chain.[23] As discussed in Chapter Three, progressive systems have established value analysis teams to evaluate clinical material decisions. These groups are given the responsibility for assessing the multitude of products available for use, making recommendations for use guidelines, and purchasing contracts based on efficacy and patient outcome optimization. The goal of these groups is not just to reduce choice or simply cut costs; it is to help clinicians make informed logical choices based on data. In order to contribute to these deliberations, the supply chain manager must be able to gain the trust of clinicians to participate and communicate with members not just on the basis of costs or efficiencies but in terms of quality and use.

Information Technology in Support of Transformation

It is argued that "information replaces inventory" in the modern supply chain. This line of reasoning, however, underestimates the importance of having the correct products available at the correct time. Information takes on a central feature in the supply chain to the extent that it:[24]

• Helps reduce variability in the supply chain.
• Helps suppliers make better forecasts, accounting for promotions and market changes.
• Enables the coordinating of manufacturing and distribution systems and strategies.
• Enables retailers to better serve their customers by offering tools for locating desired items.
• Enables retailers to react and adapt to supply problems more rapidly.
• Enables lead time reductions.

The transformation of hospital and hospital system supply chains from a transactional to a strategic perspective relies on information and organizational intelligence as key enablers of change. Even if supply managers understand the potential for a new role, enacting the role as described above requires the support of information technology.

In the ideal world, information technology allows managers to gain access to data, provide transparency to how their systems work, and target plans that move

the organization toward greater efficiency. However, while the idea of using technology as a competitive advantage has been around for several years, the health
care industry is lagging almost a decade behind other industries. There are several
issues contributing to the lack of technology in health care, ranging from complexity and cost management problems to the difficulty in changing processes.

With the growing complexity of hospital systems and integrated networks in
tandem with an increase in outsourcing services to group purchasing and distributor organizations, the health care industry is poised to break through the information technology barrier. At the same time, the design of many of the
enterprise resource planning systems, which fail to integrate financial, supply use,
and clinical data, is not meeting supply chain management needs. Value analysis
processes and value analysis team performance are hampered by the absence of
sound data linking materials to performance. In order to create activity-based
management that is functional, the database should contain the following
components:[25]

- Market, product, and customer informant
- Product profitability
- Product and price assessment
- Value analysis and cost reduction identification
- Business process and reengineering data
- Performance measures and benchmarking
- Resource planning and sourcing decisions
- New business and product evaluation and investment appraisal

Hospitals and systems have learned that the wide variety of systems and software implementations that they have accrued fail to support the core business of
the company. Such technologies frequently serve the back office (human resources
and payroll) and, more recently, aid in revenue recovery. However, they rarely
bring together the necessary data that allow an assessment of quality of care or
outcomes.

Some of the difficulties facing health care systems that wish to implement
large-scale changes are their own legacy systems. Legacy systems are so named because they were created specifically for an organization and are critical to the nor-
mal functioning of the company. Many of these systems were created using
software and technology that are now obsolete and have interfaces that are complicated and expensive. Another part of the reason for this complicated structure
is a lack of data and information standardization at the time these systems were
initiated. Due to the fact that these systems are deeply ingrained in the day-to-day
working processes of a hospital or system, they are often extremely difficult and

expensive to replace. In addition, because of the length of time these systems have been in place, they have become customized not only to the industry but also to a particular company; hence, legacy systems cannot just be removed in order to start over. Significant effort and planning have to go into the process of integrating legacy systems with newer ones, thus ingraining the legacy applications even further.

Looking to IT for Solutions

Information technology offers an array of data-gathering and analysis capabilities. However, in order to make the investment count, the health care organization has to know what it wants and which program will help to obtain these goals. Here are some products currently on the market and the capabilities that they possess.

Enterprise Resources Planning Systems. ERP systems have an impact on all the operations of a company. The system takes information from accounting, finance, supply chain, human resources, and customers and provides it to anyone who is able to use it. The advantages to systems like this are endless, with synchronized and up-to-date information available to everyone at the click of a button. ERP systems were developed from materials resources planning systems, which helped revolutionize the way managers could track inventory and manage their replenishment cycles in the 1970s. In the 1980s, manufacturing resources planning systems integrated other job functions such as shop floor management, distribution, and accounting. The next step was to integrate engineering, project management, finance, and human resources to form the current ERP systems.

There are significant risks to such implementations, though. ERP systems tend to be extremely expensive not only to purchase, but also to integrate, especially when legacy systems and applications exist. Implementations often require significant planning and business process modeling and change. The health care industry can benefit significantly from ERP systems but faces several challenges in purchasing them due to expense and lack of implementation knowledge. Progressive systems have mixed success in harnessing ERP systems to help manage the supply chain more effectively. Their greatest success appears to be in assessing overall purchasing patterns for specific materials. However, they appear to provide less value in answering questions related to product use, safety, efficacy, and outcomes.

E-Procurement Systems. E-procurement generally relates to providing business-to-business (B2B) services over the Internet. E-marketplaces propose to link buyers and sellers as efficiently as possible by "enticing many purchasing execs to shift their procurement into these venues."[26] A B2B process is any process that takes place between two companies and uses technology such as e-commerce as the facilitator. The technology can be as simple as information or transaction based, or it can be as complex as a shared ERP or e-procurement system. The basic use for B2B systems is the automation of previously manual functions and the removal of paper-based technology. Burns has written, "Hospitals and IDNs exhibit weak capability in several supply chain functions. These include logistics, procurement, utilization, pricing, and support for the materials management role."[27] While the six years since Burns has carried out his research have led to the development of more sophisticated B2B systems, a great number of transactions are still carried out manually in hospitals. There is a belief in progressive systems that electronic marketplaces continue to have a potential to link price purchasing, and clinical data in ways that have not yet been fully met.

With the growth of health care, B2B companies such as Global Health Exchange and Neoforma, which merged in 2005, are moving toward a more efficient electronic environment. What remains to be demonstrated is how savings achieved through reduced transaction costs will affect the broader performance of the health sector supply chain.

IT and Supply Chain in Hospitals

The systems described above can help play a large role in improving the supply chain of hospitals by affecting purchase, transaction, and administrative costs. E-procurement systems can help to significantly reduce purchase costs through the consolidation of supplier networks and creation of supplier partnerships. Transaction and administration costs can be reduced through the use of ERP systems, which provide an automated and paperless format for information to flow throughout an organization. Finally, market analysis can be conducted with significant success and accuracy using the data generated from these systems. With this in mind, there are several significant drivers for cost reduction and revenue improvement in the health care industry:

- A 1999 Ernst & Young study estimated that the potential savings through e-commerce in supply chain cost for hospitals could range between 13 and 27 percent. With the average IDN's operating expense at $1.5 billion, there is potential for huge savings.[28]
- The recently opened Indiana Heart Hospital, which has been built to be completely digital and virtually paperless, boasts a reduction in accounts receivable days to fewer than sixty, with an expectation to lower it to forty-five.[29] This success shows the possibility of faster revenue generation for hospitals.

- Administrative costs have grown 24 percent from 1999 to 2002 according to a report by Cap Gemini Ernst & Young.[30] A large number of these costs are from manual processes, associated with the supply chain, with potential for automation.
- Billing errors, insurance underpayments, denials, and self-pay bad debt account for 13 percent of lost revenue for hospitals.[31] Many errors in the supply chain are associated with the inability to order reconciliation and the ability to determine appropriate pricing.
- Only 25 percent of surgical services and materials managers acknowledge that their operating room computer systems automatically place orders to replenish supplies by procedure for each physician.[32]
- An interesting contrast between competitive industries such as the automotive industry and the health industry is the relative lack of emphasis on the inventory and distribution network. Yet it is these networks that can provide the greatest opportunity for cost management, and after process improvement, information technology has the potential to help derive the greatest value from cost management techniques.
- The Sachs Group's 1999 survey of customer satisfaction found a direct link between the information provided to customers by their HMO and their satisfaction.[33] Consultants have identified the provider's customer service as a customer service organization in which "the entire materials management team understands and is dedicated to fulfilling customer needs."[34] Yet few progressive systems appear to effectively use customer service relationship management technology (CRM) to assess how they are meeting the needs of their key customers.

Barriers and Concerns in IT Implementations

As the federal government continues to mandate new standards for information systems and the movement to electronic medical records,[35] the health sector is poised for major investments in this area. Yet hospitals have not seen information technology as an avenue to help them contend with cost growth, increasing malpractice insurance, poor decision making, and the shortage of nurses. In addition, physicians are frequently reluctant to consistently use these new technologies, which they frequently believe do not contribute to increased efficiency. While investment may be even greater in the next five years than the $34 billion projected by the Garner Group estimates,[36] it is not clear how these investments will, in a short period of time, change the landscape of health care supply chain technology.[37] Of even greater concern is the inability to assess how such investments will improve system performance. Perhaps the best news is that newer information applications are anticipated, by directors of progressive supply chain systems, to better meet the level of complexity associated with the health sector supply chain. This is facilitated by the increased standardization in applications such as bar coding and performance metrics between systems and departments.

Despite the reservations suggested, the health care industry is as excited today about information technology and its applications as the telecommunications industry was ten years ago. In its 2001 report, the Institute of Medicine "identified the use of technology as one of four main healthcare environmental structures or processes that must change for redesign of the healthcare delivery system to take place."[38] In recent years, there has been an increasing demand that both medicine and management become evidence based. Yet while a great deal is being written about the advances to be accrued from providing clinicians and managers with increased data, evidence regarding improved outcomes is not yet forthcoming.[39] It has been pointed out that there are few data to assess the effects of many leading management techniques and strategies.[40] In many ways, the failure to develop an evidence-based environment is significantly hampered by the inability of information systems to drill down to analytical levels that support such decision making. In the most progressive systems, profiling the contribution of materials to both clinical and cost outcomes is a key component to success, but the ability to assemble such data in ways that are meaningful to the medical staff is beyond the capabilities of supply chain management. The principal cause of this is the great fragmentation between clinical, management, and financial information systems.

Information technology itself cannot solve all of the problems associated with strategic management of the health care supply chain. The implementation, systems, and people that use the technology determine the ultimate value.

Summary and Conclusion

While the vast majority of hospitals and systems in the United States have not achieved the strategic levels for health care supply chain management described in Chapter Seven, progressive health care organizations are characterized by a new generation of managers who understand their organizations through a strategic lens, understand that their organizations are characterized by departments and services with variable clockspeeds, and are seeking support systems as they work to become part of a movement by which evidence-based management supports evidence-based medicine. One cannot work with clinicians on value analysis teams without comprehensive and credible data about product performance, outcomes, safety, and cost. The skills necessary to support such endeavors are a mix of managerial epidemiology and cost-benefit analysis supported by evidence based management and practice.

The ASU/CHMR study identified a continuous recognition by progressive systems for better-trained staff to mount the supply chain management process. Continued education through either a structured program or a professional organization is perhaps the most powerful means by which to increase the abilities of individual managers. For managers who have advanced through the organization, this becomes even more imperative as it is important to bring in outside ideas and information, which can then be adapted to a manager's own situation. Structured courses in supply chain management help provide an understanding of both concepts and tools by which modern supply chains are effectively managed. Perhaps one of the biggest failings of the current system is the lack of effort in encouraging educational development among managers and the entire materials management organization.[41] Without the dissemination of knowledge, a facility's ability to develop and implement sophisticated ideas is limited.

For their own benefit, supply chain managers must establish their own sense of professionalism and leadership capabilities.[42] If they want their contributions to be recognized and respected, they must be able to show them off. This involves active participation in the health care management process. Opportunities need to be taken to volunteer and be active in committees that expand their exposure to people within the organization. This allows the sharing of information about roles and job functions throughout the various departments. By making themselves known to other members of the organization, supply chain managers also open the opportunity to expand their internal network capabilities.

Professional organizations such as the Association for Healthcare Resource and Material Management and the Institute for Supply Management are playing an ever increasing role in research and knowledge dissemination in the industry. Through membership in such organizations, supply chain managers gain the opportunity to network with other professionals, participate in certification programs, and gather news on the latest advancements and research in the field. Other avenues for improving the skills and capabilities of hospital and hospital system purchasing executives include programs developed by purchasing partners as well as in-house programs. While these programs have not been systematically studied, there is a strong belief that exposure to these programs has assisted in refocusing the time and energy of purchasing employees on the strategic aspects of practice.

Effective management of the health sector supply chain presents an important opportunity for improved hospital and hospital system performance. Executive education programs with CEOs have revealed a growing interest in this area, as well as a recognition that the potential for supply chain is hampered by a lack of training and an inability to set goals pertaining to cost savings and risk reduction. These managers also recognize that they have often failed to understand that their organizations are characterized by very different process, product, and organization-level clockspeeds that require very different managerial strategies. Yet as new technologies, such as drug-eluting stents, threaten to change practice patterns and the demand for many hospital services, these executives recognize that not giving attention to the supply chain will only lead to increased losses in their organizations. The evidence is mounting that after the cost of labor, the cost of supplies as a percentage of any discharge can make the difference between a surplus or a loss on a case.

As suggested above, the Health Sector Supply Chain Research Consortium, with members from a wide variety of hospitals, systems, group purchasing organizations, and informatics companies identify return on investment and metrics as two of the most important problems requiring research. The health care supply chain may be a difficult process to manage, but this should not keep organizations from trying. The efficiencies and advantages gained by other industries as a result of their efforts show that even complex situations can be essentially understood and frameworks developed in order to provide better management. While the work to develop the frameworks for managing the health care supply chain continues, so do efforts to bring a greater degree of professionalism and knowledge. The first step along the road to building this vision involves understanding the skills and job responsibilities that are necessary. By raising expectations, the profession of health care supply chain managers will take greater roles in the future management of the health care system. In addition, as the organization moves along the continuum of functionality in how it manages its supply chain and resources, the supply chain manager is in an excellent position to be the champion of information technology initiatives and projects that build unity among the various segments of the organization's network.

STUDY 1: THE VALUE OF GROUP PURCHASING IN THE HEALTH CARE SUPPLY CHAIN

This study scrutinizes key writings and research on the cost of hospital contracting and the role of group purchasing organizations (GPOs).[1] A recent series of case studies conducted by Novation, the supply company of VHA and UHC, on the value of group purchasing will be used to determine the factors associated with contracting cost. At a time when regulations such as the Balanced Budget Amendment and pressures associated with managed care are reducing hospital margins and jeopardizing the viability of many hospitals, understanding how and where efficiencies will emerge is critical. With the proliferation of new pharmaceutical products and emerging technologies, increased in-patient acuity, and a sustained competitive environment, it is important that hospital management understand the potential for improving organizational effectiveness by advancing a strategic vision for the supply chain function.

Group purchasing is a principal strategy by which companies in many sectors, especially health services, have sought to achieve cost containment, improve the quality of goods purchased, and allow staff to focus their efforts on other activities.[2] A Health Industry Group Purchasing Association (HIGPA) report

This study was originally published and circulated as an industry white paper by Eugene Schneller, W. P. Carey School of Business, Arizona State University, in 2000. The research for this report was supported by Novation and the data collected in collaboration with B&D Consulting.

stated that goods and purchased services accounted for the second-largest dollar expenditure (55 percent labor and 45 percent nonlabor supplies, services, and capital equipment) in the hospital setting. Therefore, achieving a better understanding of the health care supply chain is key to the management of a health care delivery organization. It is noteworthy that 72 to 80 percent of every health care (acute care setting) supply dollar is acquired through group purchasing. The bottom-line rationale for group purchasing is to achieve (1) lower prices, (2) price protection, (3) improved quality control programs, (4) reduced contracting cost, and (5) monitoring market conditions. Estimates place the GPO market for hospitals and nursing homes at between $148 and $165 billion and growing to $257 and $287 billion per year by 2009.[3]

While the HIGPA report documents the many products and services that GPOs offer their members, it reveals that GPO members purchase a significant proportion of their goods through direct negotiations with suppliers. These observations add credence to the contention that today's most pressing supply chain issue, for suppliers[4] as well as for group purchasing organizations,[5] is contract compliance by members. Currently, there are no precise estimates of the cost savings generated by GPO contract compliance. The work reported in this case study makes a contribution to understanding the value of group purchasing by scrutinizing the costs of contracting with and without group purchasing.

In multihospital systems, the purchasing function continues to have the focus at the individual hospital level, with inconsistent approaches toward systemwide corporate purchasing and negotiation. In addition to contract portfolios, GPOs offer information sharing, clinical and operational benchmarking, and value analysis assistance that could strategically differentiate GPO members in their markets. Moving health care organizations to take advantage of these GPO products and services is dependent on rising above the belief that securing price savings for products is the sole or unique benefit of GPO participation.

Background on Group Purchasing

A 1996 survey of 131 group purchasing firms (principally nonhealth) carried out by the Center for Advanced Purchasing Studies (CAPS) at Arizona State University revealed an average GPO annual dollar saving of 13.43 percent with an impressive average return on investment of 767 percent.[6] The CAPS study also confirmed that executives identified price savings as the principal rationale for group purchasing. Data reported in *Business Week* and HIGPA reveal the substantial savings associated with health sector group purchasing.[7] It is estimated that group purchasing saved hospitals $12.8 to $19.2 billion or 10 to 15 percent of total purchasing costs.[8] The promise of group purchasing for achieving cost saving appears to meet GPO membership goals for price savings.[9]

Despite the fact that seven GPOs account for 85 percent of the U.S. hospital market, the substantial reconfiguration of the U.S. health care industry has raised issues about the future role of GPOs. Frequently cited by GPO executives as threatening to their industry is the rise of integrated delivery networks (IDNs), which, like their GPO counterparts, attempt to provide value by seeking to secure low prices for their facilities.[10] The breadth of these organizations has grown so substantially that almost three hundred IDNs are reported to have the scale necessary for group purchasing.

Almost half of the members of GPOs are also affiliated with or owned by an IDN.[11] It is not unusual for IDN executives to report they find it convenient to use the GPO quoted price as the ceiling from which they can enter into negotiations with suppliers or to reenter negotiations with other GPOs. While the purchasing activities of IDNs have been discussed as threatening to GPOs, this activity comes as no surprise to supply chain experts. A study of 450 CEOs and 159 purchasing and supply professionals concluded that because of the high dollar volume that could potentially be spent in these areas, "it will be crucial for purchasing and supply professionals to track the performance of suppliers."[12] One of the ways to track performance is by comparing the GPO performance to one's own network-associated purchasing power in the marketplace. A 1999 survey of hospital materials executives revealed almost unanimous (96 percent) commitment to using the GPO to reduce supply expenses and improve operating margins. The survey also reported that 68 percent would compare prices to GPO contracts to verify market and price competitiveness. It is interesting that respondents did not report that the outcomes of such comparative efforts led to substantial cost reductions, nor did they report the cost of engaging in such comparative activities. Rather, they report that product standardization and entering into GPO contracts were the most effective cost-reduction strategies.[13] Independent comparative shopping for best price continues to be a behavior to gain confidence in the value of GPO membership.

The Value of Group Purchasing Case Studies

Novation conducted the Value of Group Purchasing Case Studies to determine (1) the cost of hospital contracting, (2) the cost avoidance of using group purchasing contracts, (3) member expectations of group purchasing, and (4) operational performance measures of purchasing. This was accomplished by day-long on-site interviews at ten multihospital systems across the United States. The study sites represented fifty-five hospitals with varying levels of participation with group purchasing with more than $600 million combined annual purchases. Novation engaged B&D Healthcare Consulting and Services to conduct the interviews and data collection.

Departmental interviews were conducted with seven departments within each study site: pharmacy, cardiology, materials management, radiology, laboratory, surgical services, and food and nutrition. Respondents were questioned about their perceptions of GPO value; how their department, the hospital, and the broader system use the GPO; and on their own measures and benchmarking of procurement. They were also asked to provide information that detailed the costs and activities associated with their contracting costs with and without group purchasing. Senior management within the GPO was interviewed to assess their expectations for group purchasing.

Departmental Use of Group Purchasing Contracts

Robert Betz, executive director of HIGPA, contends that the most successful compliance programs allow GPO members the choice to use or not use contracts, as contracts fit their needs—but reminds them that there is added value for use contracts. Greg Firestone, president of National Contracts Inc., contends that contract compliance is an effective way for group purchasing to provide value to suppliers for their administrative fees and help drive costs out of the system.[14]

Table Study 1.1b indicates the range in group purchasing contract use by department across study sites. It should be noted that Pharmacy had the lowest gap variance from highest contract usage to lowest contract use. In general, it was observed that Pharmacy had the highest departmental contract participation across all study sites.

Contracting Costs

Entering into a GPO contract is not cost-free to a hospital department. Table Study 1.2 reveals the cost of self-contracting in dollars and hours per contract. The cost per contract was determined by taking the labor hours per contract multiplied by the annual salary of the staff involved in the contracting effort. The average cost avoidance with using group purchasing by department was also determined and showed an average cost avoidance per contract of $1,367.

Table Study 1.3 shows the activities involved in contracting, the average cost associated with such activity, and the cost avoidance of using group purchasing. It is difficult to judge whether the search for best price actually yields a better price and offsets the average cost avoidance of $1,367 per contract when using group purchasing.

(a)   TABLE STUDY 1.1.   GROUP PURCHASING CONTRACT USE.

	Study Site	Number of Facilities	APDs[a]	Annual GPO Purchases
1	Baptist Health, Little Rock, AR	8	264,502	$66,881,839
2	Baylor Healthcare System, Dallas, TX	7	894,927	142,916,367
3	Baptist Health System, San Antonio, TX	6	325,910	68,710,588
4	Medical University of South Carolina, Charleston, SC	1	155,095	24,012,922
5	Memorial Hermann Healthcare System, Houston, TX	12	786,739	177,749,413
6	Pinnacle Health System, Harrisburg, PA	7	232,023	50,981,982
7	Rush-Presbyterian St. Lukes, Chicago, IL	7	555,454	45,710,585
8	UCLA Healthcare, Los Angeles, CA	5	164,318	53,237,832
9	University Hospital, University of New Mexico, Albuquerque, NM	1	134,044	20,215,943
10	University Medical Center, Southern Nevada, Las Vegas, NV	1	169,281	19,672,635

(b)

Contracts	Study Site Highest Number of Contracts Used	Study Site Lowest Number of Contracts Used	Study Site Average Number of Contracts Used	
Pharmacy	192	138	167	87%
Medical	65	26	47	72
Surgical	63	17	41	65
Capital equipment	58	18	37	64
Anesthesia/respiratory	49	23	31	63
Radiology	33	10	16	48
Orthopedic	31	11	24	77
Laboratory	25	9	20	80
Facilities	25	2	7	28
Cardiology	23	10	17	74
Food and nutrition	19	2	6	32
Business products	17	1	10	57
TOTAL	600	267	423	71

[a]APDs = adjusted patient days.
Source: Value of Group Purchasing Case Studies.

Cost Avoidance with Group Purchasing

If group purchasing did not exist, it would cost a hospital $353,147 annually to perform the same function (Table Study 1.4). The annual cost avoidance per hospital with using group purchasing is $154,927. It is noteworthy that many hospitals are part of larger, multihospital systems, and the savings opportunities are

TABLE STUDY 1.2.   HOSPITAL COST OF CONTRACTING AND COST AVOIDANCE WITH GROUP PURCHASING.

Contracts	Hospital Cost of Self-Contracting per Contract	Hospital Cost Using GPO per Contract	Cost Avoidance with GPO per Contract	Hospital Time Self-Contracting (in hours) per Contract	Hospital Time with GPO (in hours)	Time Cost Avoidance with GPO (in hours)
Radiology	$5,707	$4,046	$1,661	188.2	126.7	61.5
Laboratory	3,325	2,070	1,255	135.8	85.4	50.4
Operating room	3,021	1,410	1,611	111.3	54.0	57.3
Pharmacy	2,429	1,324	1,105	89.2	46.5	42.7
Cardiology	2,287	1,193	1,094	90.6	46.5	44.1
Food and nutrition	1,927	451	1,476	71.0	17.8	53.2
Average contract cost	3,116	1,749	1,367	114.4	62.8	51.6

Source: Value of Group Purchasing Case Studies.

TABLE STUDY 1.3.   COST AVOIDANCE WITH GROUP PURCHASING PER CONTRACT.

Activity	Hospital Self-Contracting Cost	Hospital Contracting Cost with GPO	Cost Avoidance	
Determine product requirements	$265	$174	$91	34%
Determine product use	251	120	131	52
Department meetings user input	20	109	99	48
Access suppliers lists	68	20	40	59
Bid or request for proposal preparation	379	14	365	96
Send bid or request for proposal	40	2	38	95
Respond supplier questions	150	48	102	68
Analyze bid proposal	295	101	194	66
Conduct product evaluation	520	450	70	13
Decision product selection	180	143	37	21
Implementation contract	633	462	171	27
Record retention	25	16	9	36
Monitor contract compliance	70	65	5	7
Monitor market competitiveness	33	26	7	21
Total	3,116	1,749	1,367	44

Source: Value of Group Purchasing Case Studies.

**TABLE STUDY 1.4. HOSPITAL CONTRACTING COST AND COST
AVOIDANCE WITH GROUP PURCHASING.**

	Self-Contracting Costs per Hospital (340 contracts)	Cost Avoidance with Group Purchasing per Hospital	Self-Contracting Cost for Multi-hospital System (five hospitals, 1,700 contracts)	Cost Avoidance with Group Purchasing Multi-hospital System (five hospitals, 1,700 contracts)
Cost per contract	$3,116	$1,367	$15,580	$6,835
Total cost of contract (340× cost per contract)	1,059,440	464,780	5,297,200	2,323,750
Annual cost (average term: 3 years)	353,147	154,927	1,765,733	774,583

more significant for the broader health care system because purchasing has not
been consolidated to achieve economies of scale.

Member Expectations of Group Purchasing

In addition to understanding contracting cost avoidance, it was important to determine the member expectations of group purchasing (see Figure Study 1.1). Overwhelmingly, departmental-level management and senior executives reported "best
price for best product" as their principal expectation for group purchasing.

The second and third most frequent expectations were cost analysis and attaining leverage with suppliers. Senior management also expected to use GPO expertise
to optimize use of their resources and provide a benchmark for purchasing decisions.
In addition, executives thought GPOs helped drive standardization throughout the
system. These responses are consistent with the literature identifying the role that
GPOs play in assisting their members in achieving best prices.

Value of Group Purchasing Findings

Three distinct philosophies on contract utilization with group purchasing were
found among department managers interviewed:

1. Contracts were viewed as valuable and allow resources to concentrate on operational and clinical issues.

2. Group purchasing contracts were viewed individually based on perceived departmental value and savings based on cost of conversion to alternative products.
3. Contracts were considered starting points for the health care organization's own negotiation.

It is critical to recall that participants frequently use group purchasing to monitor price. Interviews revealed that most respondents did not have an understanding of the cost of contracting and did not routinely study their own costs associated with purchasing; thus, their ability to truly understand the actual cost of a contract and goods purchased was limited.

The findings below do not include cooperative returns, manufacturers incentives, and resources which provide additional value to members.

Pharmacy Model

Perhaps the most striking observation between departments pertained to pharmacy—in respect to both the number of contracts used and their

FIGURE STUDY 1.1.   EXPECTATIONS FOR GROUP PURCHASING.

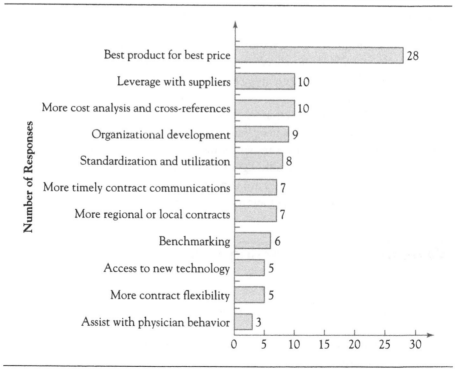

**TABLE STUDY 1.5.   REASONS THAT PHARMACY DEPARTMENTS HAVE
HIGH GPO CONTRACT COMPLIANCE.**

Reasons for Compliance	Reasons Pharmacists Believe They Comply with Contracts	Reasons Other Departments Believe Pharmacists Comply with Contracts
Engaging in search for better price is not good use of clinician's time	47%	23%
Pharmacist expertise with standardization and formularies	21	23
Pharmacists believe GPO price is advantageous	16	15
Other	16	16
Don't know	—	23
Total	100	100

confidence in group purchasing. Pharmacy departments reported they did not see contract negotiation as optimizing the use of their resources. Table Study 1.5 identifies reasons pharmacists support group purchasing as well as the reasons their counterparts outside pharmacy attribute to pharmacy compliance. Both pharmacists and their nonpharmacist counterparts attribute pharmacy contract compliance to the pharmacist's expertise in standardization and belief in group purchasing price advantage. Pharmacists were more likely than the nonpharmacists to believe that engaging in contracting is not a good use of clinician time.

Measuring Outcomes of Purchasing Practices

The Value of Group Purchasing Study was also conducted to determine if performance measures such as benchmarking were used to measure purchasing outcomes. Carr and Smeltzer have pointed out that benchmarking as a process involves comparisons: "the assumption that an organization will improve its own performance if it copies an organization that exhibits the best performance, product, or process."[15] Their research has found a positive relationship between benchmarking and firms' performance.[16] They also found positive relationships between benchmarking and engaging in strategic purchasing in small and large firms.

FIGURE STUDY 1.2.   TOTAL SUPPLY EXPENSE PER ADJUSTED DISCHARGE (WEIGHTED PER CASE MIX INDEX) VERSUS GPO PARTICIPATION.

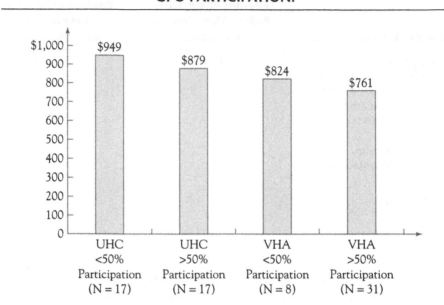

In 1997, University HealthSystem Consortium (UHC) and VHA collaborated on a Purchasing Process Benchmarking Survey with forty-six UHC hospitals and forty-one VHA hospitals. Figure Study 1.2 indicates a lower total supply expense per adjusted discharge with the organizations that had a higher use of group purchasing. Organizations with more than 50 percent contract participation with group purchasing were compared to organizations that used less than 50 percent contract participation. Data presented excluded pharmacy and dietary products.

Conclusions from the survey suggested benchmarking and improvement efforts should be targeted to supply-related expenses:

1. Creation of an organizational cost management focus
2. Establishment of performance measures and the provision of feedback
3. Creation of end user accountability for supply cost management
4. Increasing involvement of key physicians
5. Implementation of incentives and gain-sharing programs to increase results
6. Identification of acceptable products and the control of information on new ones

EXHIBIT STUDY 1.1.   INDICATORS OF PERFORMANCE.

Demographics
- Case mix index (hospital and medicare)
- Total hospital supply costs
- Total hospital purchased services cost

Materials Management
- Materials management "influenced" supply cost ratio
- Materials management "influenced" supply cost per $1 of labor
- Materials management hourly rate

Organizational
- Total hospital supply cost/adjusted discharge
- Total hospital supply cost/operating expenses

Department Specific
- Total hospital surgical service supply cost per procedure
- Total cath lab supply cost per procedure
- Laundry and linen pounds per adjusted patient-days

7. Increasing the use of group purchasing
8. Concentrating on areas with the largest opportunities for improvement
9. Using key suppliers as partners in the cost management initiative

In a separate study, the VHA West Coast developed a Materials Management Report Card and Data Collection Tool to support performance improvement and benchmarking. What is significant about this tool is its concentration on materials management beyond line item price.[17]

Participants in this project recognize that benchmarking indicators provide an important basis for managing realistic expectations for improvement. The report recommends that organizations come together to (1) conduct self-audit of performance against each category means and best performance, (2) contact better-performing organizations to discuss processes and procedures that contribute to their success, (3) share results with participating organizations, and (4) apply findings as baseline for improvement efforts (see Exhibit Study 1.1).

Advocating Compliance

Manufacturers and suppliers recognize that both GPO and IDNs cannot always secure commitment from their membership on specific items. GPOs must assist in the development of an environment in which unit price is not the only measure of their value. Furthermore, IDNs must develop system integration to deliver compliance.

GPOs and IDNs will find new competition for their business as new technologies and agencies of exchange concentrate buyers to reduce expense and transaction costs. Advocating compliance requires that GPOs become customer-centric. Today's end user is a pharmacist, physician, nurse, or administrative employee of a department who gathers information from a variety of modalities. These strategic constituents frequently have very different understandings of the factors associated with the various products involved in the delivery of health services. Physicians, for example, frequently report that those who advocate GPO commitment undervalue the positive aspects of intensive involvement with manufacturers and their representatives. Reflecting on the health care industry, Hurwich and Lanigan have argued that "the emerging business model for health purchasing in the 21st century is the "connection company" that relates to various customers (patient, physician, administrator) not simply as a supply need, disease, or condition, but holistically as a complex amalgam of wants and needs.[18] Pressures on GPOs will continue to mount, and new opportunities will emerge as health care leadership comes to grips with the implications of the shift from measures associated with discharges to measures that reflect costs and outcomes associated with episodes of care. Purchasing success will require tools and strategies that track and meet the needs of the customer/patient over a longer period of time and in multiple settings, including the home.

Compliance requires executive commitment. A recent survey of CEOs reveals that procurement organizations should provide strategic advantage and revenue enhancement. Interviews with executives suggest that health care organization administrators have not yet embraced this position for the purchasing function. Failure to articulate a vision for the value attached to purchasing leads to managerial decisions "by default." Kearney's recent attention to this issue concludes that creating advantage revolves around "building a mindset that procurement counts."[19] Strategies associated with this include the development of joint product development teams between suppliers and hospitals that "move beyond sharing information to sharing ideas, collaborating on how and where products or components are made, or how services might be redefined for mutual advantage." GPOs emphasize "total supply chain management," the overall process by which products are ordered, delivered, inventoried, paid for, used, and disposed of.[20]

GPO compliance requires facilitation and linkage of clinician supplier relationships. Clinicians have established strong relationships with suppliers that manufacture a wide variety of products such as prostheses and pacemakers. Without an institutionally shared vision for purchasing and standardization, efficiencies will not evolve in the clinical arena. Clinical leadership that embraces a vision of improved patient outcomes as a result of standardization will lead to the ultimate success. Schneller has argued that health sector executives must become skilled in selecting physician collaborators who have a strong appreciation for resource use and collaboration: "While healthcare delivery organizations may be able to tolerate some percentage of physicians who have little appreciation for ongoing change processes, failure to develop 35 to 40 percent of the medical staff who will be strong collaborators in both resource management and corporate development will be a prescription for organizational failure."[21]

GPO success will be dependent on the ability to harness an integrated business and clinical perspective to improve organizational performance. By achieving an organizational focus, GPOs can shape the environment in which their members become accountable for optimal resource use by achieving integration across departments, establishing and enforcing performance measures, and ensuring that incentives are in place to achieve system-level efficiencies. In this context, structural changes will be necessary in both the membership organization and the GPO that includes building new ties to the supplier community. Schneller has written that health care executives frequently feel uncomfortable in an environment that necessitates advanced business skills in supply management and information technology.[22] Executive education in total health care supply chain management will be necessary to establish an environment where leadership has the vision to move the purchasing team from a focus on the "product" as the center of attention toward systemwide purchasing initiatives that incorporate many of the components of market strategy.

As health care organizations downsize, employees must seek ways to work smarter, allotting their time on those activities that truly make a difference in both cost and patient outcome. Understanding where compliance makes a difference, as recognized in pharmacy, is an important step that health care organizations must take in the near future. In a customer-focused organization, where customers actually promote change, purchasing leaders will be required to give extensive time to the various constituencies with which they interact on a day-to-day basis. To avoid cost increases, this will require redirecting time away from everyday purchasing activities toward satisfying customer needs.

This is an era of enormous change for the entire field of supply chain management. Purchasing for health care organizations has always been an extraordinarily complex process of struggling to meet the needs of management, key business stakeholders, clinician partner preferences, and patients. To date, the enormous push to achieve standardization and manage for improved outcomes has achieved only modest success.

Across the health care industry, there are numerous forces attempting to employ new technologies and business models to impose a new discipline on the organizations and professionals that come together to make up health care. In "E-Commerce Coming to Health Care Industry," the *Wall Street Journal* depicts purchasing in the typical hospital as an antiquated process in which multiple customers independently access suppliers, distributors, and hospitals, with the GPO being only one of a number of customers.[23] The new supply chain is different by virtue of providing an online market in which a wide variety of customers, hospital departments, physician offices, and even GPOs access an online market—a virtual new exchange system. Our analysis suggests that while e-commerce and business-to-business models will have a striking influence on how health care manages its supply chain, the role of knowledgeable exchange agents, especially GPOs, will become even more important. In such an environment, achieving a level of discipline in the supply chain may even be more complex than in the past. Group purchasing organizations have been the centerpiece for reducing the burdens associated with effective supply chain management. Strategies that advocate full use of group purchasing have the potential to shape improved efficiencies and effectiveness in the changing health care industry.

Discussion

A wide range of contract use characterizes the multihospital systems scrutinized in the Value of Group Purchasing Case Studies. With few exceptions, GPO members are not willing to take as a matter of faith that membership automatically leads to their principal expectation: lowest possible price. Rather, these organizations test the marketplace for achieving lower prices for goods and engage in contracting behavior that, while costly, is believed to help achieve organizational goals. And to the extent that each of the sites studied is not tightly integrated into collective systems for purchasing, there appears to be substantial intramember variance in GPO contract use. Further study will be necessary to determine just how such intrasystem compliance affects overall system cost and success.

The HIGPA report argues that GPOs present an opportunity for membership choice and flexibility. This contention is tempered, however, by the observation that in "their capacity as brokers and facilitators, GPOs walk a fine line, balancing their members' desire for flexibility and freedom to suit their needs with suppliers' desire for standardization and increased market share."[24] The case studies reported here reveal that the tension between flexibility and standardization is not systematically managed across the hospitals and systems studied. Pharmacy departments recognize the value of compliance with contracts and have institutionalized mechanisms for achieving standardization. Leadership is not consistent in other areas, with few models being advanced to achieve effective supply chain management. Yet the savings associated with contract compliance, as demonstrated in this case study, are profound in terms of both time and cost avoidance.

The growing body of literature on clinical outcomes is rapidly becoming baseline knowledge for clinical and insurance decision making. This now has the potential to serve as the intellectual capital to drive standardization and, subsequently, purchasing behavior. As this progresses, the purchasing profiles of clinical departments should begin to look a great deal more like pharmacy departments, with data on outcomes strongly informing purchasing decisions. Sarpong's research on pharmacists engaged pharmacy and therapeutics (P&T) committees revealed that the vast majority of respondents had received training or continuing education in either pharmacoeconomics or outcomes research in the past two years.[25] Progress in applying such information outside pharmacy may be accelerated by developing a series of continuing education experiences in clinical economics and decision making for managers in clinical departments and their allied physician leaders.

Maltz and Ellram have identified the duality associated with purchasing within complex organizations. On the one hand, purchasing involves locating and screening suppliers, structuring and requesting proposals, negotiating final agreements, and monitoring ongoing relationship.[26] At the same time, purchasing professionals also need to develop clear sets of expectations regarding outcomes and performance objectives associated with the supply management function while recognizing that many specific decisions regarding purchasing may take place throughout the organization. Within this context, they suggest that "someone in the organization must always oversee and monitor the purchase of outside goods and services, analyze options, select suppliers, and monitor ongoing performance."[27] Giving continued attention to the activities of the GPO to which one belongs is an obvious aspect of doing good business and recognizes that the purchasing function cannot be totally outsourced. The Value of Group Purchasing Study, however, did not reveal organizational recognition or management of the complexity of purchasing or specify how modern tools for supply chain management are best employed to improve organizational effectiveness.

Conclusions

Disciplined models for achieving compliance with GPO contracts cannot emerge without executive commitment to excellence in purchasing, a recognition of the legitimacy of clinician-supplier relationships, developing an integrated business and clinical organizational focus, ensuring the employment of advanced business skills in supply chain management and information technology, and advancing an organizational focus in which everyone works smarter to optimize resources for the task at hand. Such a model for compliance retains fidelity to price as a principal goal for the GPO but ensures that the GPO activities will have an ongoing fit with the organizations they serve.

STUDY 2: CLINICIAN, SUPPLIER, AND BUYER WORKING AS ONE TO IMPROVE PATIENT OUTCOMES

Plymouth Hospitals NHS Trust provides general hospital services to a local population of 430,000 in Plymouth, West Devon, South Hams, and East Cornwall, England. Derriford Hospital also provides a number of specialist hospital services to more than 1.6 million people in Devon and Cornwall and in some cases to bordering areas of Dorset and Somerset. The main specialist or tertiary services provided are:

- Cardiothoracic surgery and cardiology
- Neurosurgery and neurology
- Renal transplant surgery
- Some specialist cancer treatments
- Plastic surgery and burns

The Trust's vision for the next five years is to be recognized as a leading center of excellence for a wide range of general hospital services and complex specialist services for people living within the Southwest Peninsula, a geographical area covering Devon and Cornwall providing health care to a population of over 1.6 million people. The Trust has established an agenda to work with its health partners to ensure that services are planned and delivered around the needs of the patient.

This study was written by Ian B. Shepherd in March 2003.

Of the Trust's specialist services, the South West Cardiothoracic Centre represented the biggest commercial challenge given its growth potential and the opportunity to influence significant expenditure.

The Cardiothoracic Centre opened late in 1997, treating 274 patients as finished consultant episodes (FCEs). Since then, the center has increased the number of patients treated each year, reaching 2,105 FCEs during 2001. More patients have been able to benefit from coronary artery bypass grafts and other heart operations. In addition, the center is leading the introduction of a new day case technique for performing coronary angioplasty and stenting on patients with heart disease. The standard approach is to gain access to the coronary artery from the groin (femoral artery), which involved an overnight stay for the patient. The new procedure involves introducing a tube through the wrist (radial artery), a procedure known as transradial intervention. The risk of bleeding is reduced, patients can regain movement earlier, and they can often go home the same day, helping to reduce waiting times for other patients. "The first patient sat up and read a newspaper within thirty minutes of the procedure and he was discharged without complication in less than four hours," says Joe Motwani, consultant cardiologist. "I now use this route of access in over 90 percent of patients, and we are using the procedure more extensively than any other center in the UK."

In the most recent survey, November 2003/04, the center was rated as the top hospital in the UK on its combined results for all heart operations, according to the Society of Cardiac Surgeons. The mortality rate for the period April 1998 to March 2000 was the lowest, at just 2.3 percent. This compares with a national average of 4.0 percent.

In the last year we have implanted 430 pacemakers for bradycardia indications (new implant rate about 700 per million). The center prescribes using the British Pacing and Electrophysiological Group guidelines. Many patients have additional arrhythmia, particularly atrial fibrillation, and we have actively developed a program of using new devices with anti-atrial fibrillation therapy.

As part of our collaboration with our suppliers, we have had a productive research program and are about to publish a study into onset mechanisms of atrial fibrillation and flutter after coronary bypass graft surgery. For this, the center used an advanced dual chamber pacemaker with excellent Holter functions. In addition, we are now pacing for heart failure with biventricular pacing systems.

Dr. Andrew Marshall and Dr. Guy Haywood, consultant cardiologists, both participated in the Multi Site Stimulation in Cardiomyopathy (MUSTIC) trial, making Plymouth one of the seventeen European centers at the forefront of this clinical development. Figure Study 2.1 shows that expenditure has been brought in line with budget while treating more patients.

FIGURE STUDY 2.1.   BUDGET, EXPENDITURE, AND PATIENT ACTIVITY, CARDIOTHORACIC CENTER (IN POUNDS STERLING).

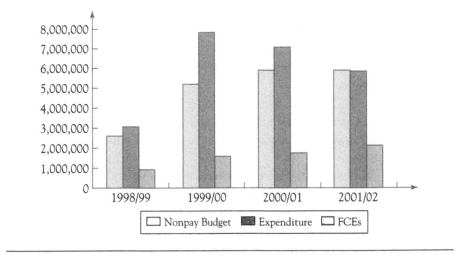

The Perennial Challenge

The perennial challenge facing most Trusts is to treat more patients sooner while improving clinical outcomes, within a finite budget. Increasingly, the vast array of products required to meet this demand are subjected to dynamic market forces where the introduction of innovative devices attracts premium prices. Commercial aims to meet this challenge were to:

- Widen purchasing influence over core expenditures with increased commitment to contracts
- Improve supply chain operational efficiency
- Reduce our supplier base
- Rationalize catalogue line items
- Manage the introduction of new technologies
- Reduce inventory value and associated replenishment costs
- Ensure 100 percent stock availability
- Generate annual savings of at least £800,000

In consideration of these primary aims, we set ourselves the overall goal of treating 10 to 15 percent more patients within the existing budget. Subsequently, the

Trust's purchasing and logistics strategy was developed as a by-product of taking this approach.

Purchasing Strategy

In support of realizing our aims, the Trust Board endorsed our vision and mission statements as:

Vision: Development and management of an integrated supply chain optimising total costs of acquisition, possession and use

Mission: To provide all customers with the timely delivery of the right quality and quantity of products and services at the lowest overall cost

Recognizing that we did not have the skills or resources available to influence all of the Trust's nonpay expenditure, our initial focus was to meet the needs of the South West Cardiothoracic Centre. Demand for treatment of coronary heart disease was growing at an annual rate in excess of 30 percent, and the center's budget would need to increase to approximately 10 percent of the Trust's annual revenue to meet this need. Furthermore, following a Pareto analysis of expenditure, just 180 key products and eight of the Trust's top twenty suppliers accounted for 60 percent of the Cardiothoracic Centre's budget.

Figure Study 2.2 represents an analysis of the Trust's supplier portfolio. It links expenditure of each operating division within a corporate entity by aggregating sales values. These revised and validated data were then used to identify the Trust's top 50 suppliers. However, compiling this list highlighted that 150 suppliers represented 79 percent of expenditure and 10 percent of transactional volume. At the other end of the spectrum, 1,500 suppliers represented 10 percent of expenditure and 70 percent of transactional volume. In developing objectives in pursuit of partnership relationships, it was essential to determine our starting point and understand the relative strategic significance of existing and prospective suppliers. Our objective was to develop partnerships with a number of category A suppliers, ensuring sales growth, while consolidating transactional activity and significantly reducing the number of category D suppliers.

The added advantage of pursuing a different approach with the Cardiothoracic Centre was that suppliers in this market were few and therefore potentially more manageable, and in most cases, suppliers were able to meet the majority of the Trust's demand for key categories of products from within their corporate

FIGURE STUDY 2.2.   ANALYSIS OF THE TRUST'S
SUPPLIER PORTFOLIO.

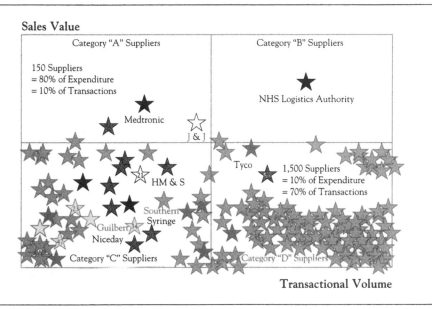

portfolios. In addition, niche suppliers were already known to the Trust, and we had a good understanding of their potential for growth.

Our overriding strategic aim was to test and develop the concept of partnership working from both the clinical and commercial perspectives. Our criteria for appointing suppliers to this program were:

- Year-on-year commitment to improve clinical outcomes
- Sound research and development track record with innovative product improvement programs for the future
- Robust communication and information links
- Willingness to share information on costs
- Commitment to training, education, and development of clinical and managerial staff
- Consistent high-quality customer service
- Process efficiency and cost containment in working toward e-business solutions
- Shared risk and benefits associated with market growth

Figure Study 2.3 is a summary of how one of our key supplier's strategic focus influences patient outcomes, maximizing the use of new technologies and therapies

FIGURE STUDY 2.3.   INFLUENCE OF STRATEGIC FOCUS ON PATIENT OUTCOMES.

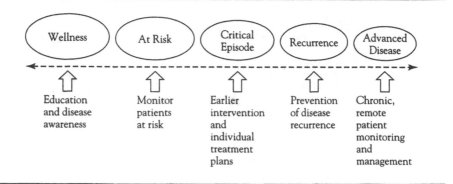

as the enabler. By working together with our clinical colleagues and suppliers, we hoped to influence and improve the quality of life for patients with coronary heart disease and reduce the overall cost of each finished consultant episode.

Market Analysis and Segmentation

Continuous monitoring of market dynamics is essential for products that have continued growth or have yet to reach maturity. Given that new entrants are launched at premium prices and in a competitive market, mature products are priced to protect or increase market share. Figure Study 2.4 shows the dynamic nature of the cardiothoracic market. This serves to illustrate the point that new product launches or additional features to existing products, dependent on their positioning within the life cycle, are often priced at premium rates. The challenge for the buyer is to work with clinical staff to determine whether these new devices provide differentiated clinical outcomes and therefore represent value for money.

We are currently working on two business cases to determine the benefits of drug-eluting stents and cardiac resynchronization therapies. If these are proven to be cost-effective, we will then have the added challenge of convincing commissioners of health care and budget holders, of the need to change their outlook by focusing holistically on budget provision, to meet these new treatment regimes.

By working more closely with our clinical colleagues, we not only gained a better understanding of their needs but also used this opportunity to improve our knowledge of the products and suppliers within the cardiovascular market. Examples of the level of detail we believed was required in understanding product

FIGURE STUDY 2.4.   PRODUCT LIFE CYCLE.

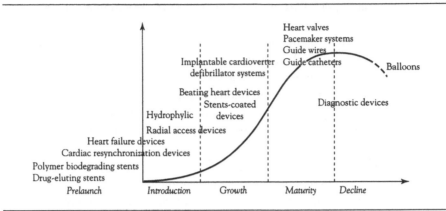

FIGURE STUDY 2.5.   MARKET DYNAMICS.

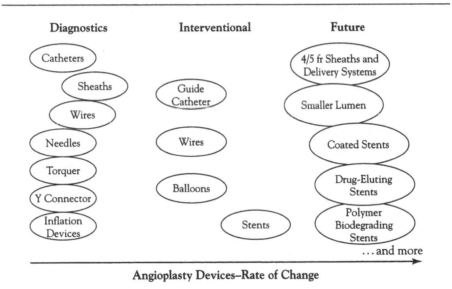

use and the stability and growth in demand for products is demonstrated in Figures Study 2.4 and 2.5.

The interesting dynamic here is that clinical staff are pioneering transradial intervention. This change in clinical practice uses niche products where technological advancements are producing smaller lumen sizes in the hope that this will improve patient outcomes. Products are increasingly being coated with hydrophilic agents to improve speed of access and reduce the risk of infection. As the market develops, these products should see sustained growth, and this commercial opportunity is not lost in our relationships with niche suppliers. The challenge we have set them is to provide product improvements with pricing to match established equivalent items.

At the opposite end of the spectrum, we have a decreasing need for balloon catheters given that interventional cardiologists are continuing to increasingly use direct stenting to reduce overall procedure costs. Managing market share and leveraging these commercial opportunities for maximum benefit is not possible without accurate, up-to-date information. In recognizing this need, we have implemented plans to continually develop our information systems and the sharing of data to support commercial negotiations.

To avoid monitoring other than the significant differentiated clinical or cost benefits, we have, for example, built into our contract for pacemaker systems the clinical option to select next-generation products at contract prices. Taking this approach enables us to efficiently manage the introduction of new therapies, such as atrial fibrillation with Medtronic's Prevent AF device.

Having gained an understanding of market dynamics, including the increasing trend for supplier mergers and acquisitions, we established an approach to further segment the market by risk in terms of awarding contracts on the basis of single, dual, or multisource commitments. Duration of contract term was an added consideration given our desire to reduce administrative costs and develop longer-term commitments based on partnership relationships.

Following this detailed analysis of market conditions, we awarded a number of contracts. First, we awarded a seven-year single-source contract for the supply of generic commodity items (cardiology diagnostic devices). Items in this category would not be influenced by technological change (stable market). Given strong competition in the NHS market, this represented minimal risk. Price would be easily managed by benchmarking and cost analysis, with performance reviewed annually.

Second, we awarded a twelve-month contract for the supply of catheter-mounted stents, given that this was considered to be a highly volatile market in terms of falling prices, growth in demand, and technological advancement. There was a prior agreement with clinical colleagues that as the market matured, we would increasingly commit larger volumes to a primary supplier and ultimately move to a dual-source contract. This has recently been honored with the award of contracts for a three-year commitment. The added complication in managing this market in the future is around the introduction of premium-priced drug-eluting and coated stents.

Figure Study 2.6 shows the considerable change in demand for stents, with future growth anticipated at 30 percent annually. The added dynamic in managing

FIGURE STUDY 2.6. CONTRACT VERSUS ACTUAL PROCEDURE VOLUMES FOR STENTS, MARCH 2002.

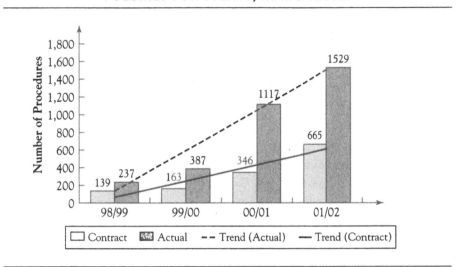

products in this category of expenditure is the variance in clinical preference as to whether to predilate vessels with a balloon or to direct-stent the lesion.

Sustained monitoring and annual negotiation have seen unit prices fall from £800 to £250 per bare metal stent.

Third, we awarded a five-year multisource contract for the supply of mechanical and tissue heart valves. The overriding dynamic in this contract was that products are in a stable market, but there was a desire within the center to undertake a comprehensive, randomized research project. This was agreed as part of the procurement process with the award of contracts, including the provision of significant research funding coterminous with contract expiration. It was believed that by taking this approach, we would develop increasingly closer relationships with our core suppliers.

Finally, we awarded a two-year dual-source contract for pacemaker systems. The primary supplier had previously acquired the secondary supplier, and risk was considered to be minimal given that separate research and development platforms and manufacturing processes were retained. Following successful completion of the initial term, the option to extend the contract period by a further three to five years was recently granted.

In taking this approach, we have significantly reduced the number of primary suppliers serving the Cardiothoracic Centre, and further rationalization is to continue given sustained performance monitoring leading to partnership status. However, in recognizing this change, there was still a need to provide access to new and innovative enhancements to products. Evaluations of items in this category were conducted within a maximum 10 percent of total sales value. This flexibility in the evaluation of products was easily accommodated given the growth in demand for interventional angioplasty and cardiac rhythm management therapies.

The Procurement Process

The procurement process was not unlike any other invitation to tender except for real emphasis on:

- Clinical outcomes and growth in demand for specific treatment regimes
- Commitment for the long term with mutual benefits
- Product quality and reliability of performance in use
- After-sales support services
- Added-value services (for example, training, education, and research)
- Performance management
- Information sharing
- Reducing costs and of course price

However, the key differentiator from the traditional approach was that the lead consultant from each clinical specialty signed the invitation to tender, participated in pretender negotiations, and cosigned the contract award schedule. The purpose of this was to clearly demonstrate to the market that we were serious about aggregating and consolidating our requirements and would support this through absolute commitment to contract volumes.

The sample contract schedule in Figure Study 2.7 serves to emphasize that the commitment stated at the beginning of the purchasing process is reflected in the contract award. All parties have signed the schedule in recognition of each other's obligations.

Postcontract performance reviews have further demonstrated our sustained commitment to contract volumes and growth. For pacemaker systems, 99.9 percent of volume is shared with two manufacturers. Figure Study 2.8 is an example of this approach as applied to monitoring the commitment given to our preferred supplier of surgeons' gloves. The figure clearly demonstrates commitment to primary supplier B, as changes introduced in October 1998 have resulted in sustained erosion in the use of alternative suppliers products.

Instead of inviting tenders for each category of expenditure, a notice was published in the *Official Journal of European Communities* inviting tenders for devices to meet the Cardiothoracic Centre's entire need. We believe that this approach to aggregating expenditure is unique within public sector procurement, and it is interesting to note that this approach was well received by participating suppliers, due in part to its significant reduction in tender administration costs.

FIGURE STUDY 2.7. CONTRACT SCHEDULE FOR PLYMOUTH HOSPITALS, NHS TRUST.

CONTRACT FOR: IMPLANTABLE PACEMAKER SYSTEMS	BUYER: IAN B SHEPHERD MCIPS SUPPLIER CONTACT: STEWART WOOD LEAD CLINICIAN: ANDREW MARSHALL	DATE OF ISSUE: 5th May 1999 DATE LAST REVISED: 31st March 2001 SUPPLIER CATEGORY: 'A'
CONTRACTOR: MEDTRONIC LTD SUITE ONE SHERBOURNE HOUSE CROXLEY BUSINESS CENTRE WATFORD HERTS WD1 8YE TEL: 01923 212213 FAX: 01923 241004 MOBILE: 0802 160935 EMAIL: stewart.wood@medtronic.com	TERMS OF CONTRACT: NHS Standard Terms and Conditions of Contract apply, with formal annual review to take place in April each year. In addition, quarterly review meetings will be held in July, October and January each year, throughout the contract term. TYPE OF CONTRACT Alliance agreement as the primary supplier for the single and dual sourcing of products at reference. Preferred supplier status.	REFERENCE NO: 98/S247-169988/EN CONTRACT NUMBER: IBS/001/A/T/PAD PERIOD OF CONTRACT: 1st April 1999 to 31st March 2001, with options to extend to 31st March 2004 and 31st March 2006. 36 month maximum price agreement. ACCOUNT MANAGEMENT: Pacing product specialist - Stephen Allen (Medtronic) - David Todd (Vitatron) Technical Support - David Rowley (Medtronic) - David Todd (Vitatron)

This contract covers the terms and conditions relating to the supply of implantable pacemaker systems by Medtronic and Vitatron to the Trust and will form part of the overall 'Partnership Agreement' between Medtronic Corporation and Plymouth Hospitals NHS Trust.

APPROVED BY:

DR ANDREW MARSHALL
Consultant Cardiologist

01 March 2001

APPROVED BY:

IAN B SHEPHERD MCIPS
Head of Procurement and Logistics

01 March 2001

APPROVED BY:

GEOFF MORRIS
Country Manager, UK &Ireland
Medtronic Limited

01 March 2001

APPROVED BY

GARY SLACK
Country Manager Vitatron Ltd

01 March 2001

FIGURE STUDY 2.8. PRODUCT USE COMPARISON.

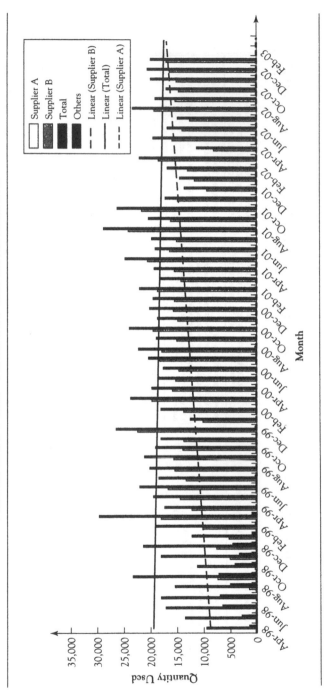

The core product categories representing 80 percent of expenditure included in the invitation to tender were:

- Pacemaker systems
- Implantable cardioverter defibrillator systems
- Heart valves (mechanical and tissue)
- Coronary artery bypass graft (procedure packs)
- Coronary stents
- Diagnostic cardiology devices
- Interventional cardiology devices
- Perfusion devices for bypass surgery
- Electrophysiology devices

Key items used within these core product categories are summarized in Table Study 2.1.

The price comparator in Table Study 2.1 shows that effective price management has been sustained throughout the contract term. The cumulative total saving as a result of this approach currently stands at £1.4 million.

TABLE STUDY 2.1.   PRICE COMPARATOR FOR CARDIOTHORACIC CORE PRODUCTS.

	1997/98	1998/99	1999/00	2000/01	2001/02
Coronary stents	£800	£700	£427	£350	£315
Pacemaker systems (average price)	2,370	1,800	1,570	1,450	1,400
Implantable cardioverter defibrillator systems (average price)	22,000	18,500	14,500	13,000	12,000
Heart valves (mechanical)	1,930	1,650	1,405	1,405	1,350
Heart valves (tissue)	1,700	1,650	1,350	1,350	1,300
Angioplasty balloons	275	200	140	125	100
Blood cardioplaegia	54	49	47	45	45
Guide catheters	60	50	35	32	25
Guide wires (average price)	80	60	49	42	39
Thoracic cannulae		8.48	6.00	5.83	5.83
CABG procedure pack (increased components)		218.08	218.08	175.38	175.38
Angiography pack (increased components)			64.20	34.23	32.50

Invitation to tender prequalifying criteria determined a short list of suppliers from whom tenders were invited. Our next step was to invite all interested parties to a supplier briefing, where clinical colleagues and I presented our expectations in terms of improving clinical outcomes and reducing costs. Consistency of approach in communicating with each prospective supplier was ensured as a lead clinician for each clinical specialty was assigned to speak on behalf of his peers.

The process and benefits of developing relationships with clinical colleagues are illustrated by the innovative purchasing solution developed for the supply of pacemaker systems. Having gained senior management support of the concept to commit absolute volumes to longer-term contracts, in the hope that this would leverage lower prices, a series of meetings were held with clinical colleagues to confirm their needs and explore options of how best to structure invitation to tender documentation and determine the contract award criteria. Andrew Marshall, a consultant cardiologist, was very receptive to the concept of a longer-term commitment but wished to ensure his team received the appropriate level of training and education required to keep them at the forefront of pacing technology. His primary concerns were to improve clinical outcomes, have freedom of choice in selecting a therapy to treat patient need, and to share risk should there be an unfortunate future occurrence of a manufacturer's product being recalled.

Invitation to tender documentation made reference to these primary concerns and specifically forewarned prospective suppliers that addressing these key elements would feature in our pretender negotiations. During these meetings, suppliers were asked to demonstrate their track record and, subject to nondisclosure agreement, advise us of their upcoming product launches and future research and development plans. An essential feature of their response to this criterion was how they demonstrated their corporate philosophy in terms of ability to work in partnership. It is worth noting that price was not a factor at this stage.

Subsequent pretender negotiations ensured that there was no ambiguity about the clinical and commercial expectations of the Trust. During these meetings, it was reiterated that we would honor absolute commitment to current and projected future contract volumes.

Following analysis of tenders received, Andrew Marshall and I, together with representatives of senior management and the finance department, invited a short list of suppliers to formally present their tender submission. This aided clarification of technical aspects of product detail and ensured parity of approach for commercial comparisons. Because of the ongoing openness among all parties, it was relatively straightforward to select our preferred partners.

Engaging suppliers early in the process met a primary objective of the Trust's purchasing strategy regarding developing partnership relationships. Parity of approach ensured open discussion on how suppliers could play a part in this process. Indeed, they were invited to comment on draft documents prior to their inclusion within the invitation to tender. I am sure this approach enabled prospective suppliers to focus on meeting our needs, within their tender submission, by highlighting key differentiators that would impact on clinical outcomes and cost.

Benefits

Taking this innovative approach yielded a number of benefits.

Clinical Benefits

The benefit for clinical staff and patients is the ability to access leading-edge therapies with device selection based on the need of each patient. Price is no longer a consideration given the introduction of average pricing, within a capped budget.

Continued training and development ensures that clinical staff have access to supplier networks with a high level of technical support. This is supported by sustained provision of genuine added value.

We now have the opportunity to work with market-leading suppliers on the introduction of new technologies with whom there is potential to conduct clinical studies and research. One example is to evaluate the potential of devices that may be upgraded by software downloads as a patient's disease progresses. The benefit for the patient is that no further invasive treatment is required.

British Pacing and Electrophysiology Guidelines are adhered to in prescribing the mode and type of device suitable for each patient. However, the unknown is whether future patient demand would be skewed toward the higher-cost, more complex modes. By adopting an average price for all therapies, the supplier shares the risk associated with unknown patient demand, as all patients' needs are met from a finite budget. Annual reconciliation of the account, if skewed to less complex modes, would result in a rebate to the Trust if the total value of sales, at unit prices, is less than the total expenditure based on the agreed average price per pacemaker system.

Figure Study 2.9 illustrates actual activity during the past two years. The adoption of average pricing with risk transfer, compared to mode and lowest benchmark equivalent prices, has proved to be of benefit. However, the real significance of using this review model is the benchmarking intelligence it provides in negotiating revised prices for the coming year.

FIGURE STUDY 2.9. BENCHMARKING COST/BENEFIT ACTIVITY.

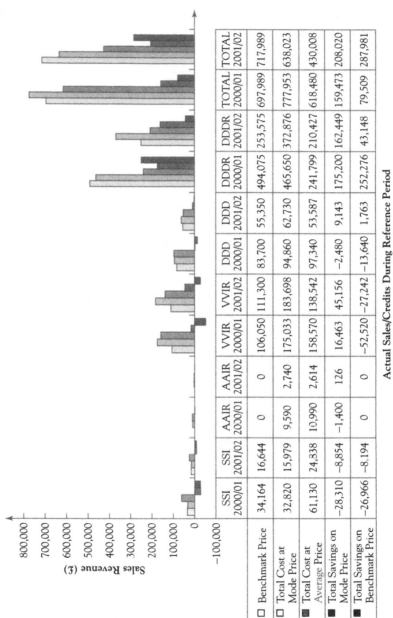

	SSI 2000/01	SSI 2001/02	AAIR 2020/01	AAIR 2001/02	VVIR 2000/01	VVIR 2001/02	DDD 2000/01	DDD 2001/02	DDDR 2000/01	DDDR 2001/02	TOTAL 2000/01	TOTAL 2001/02
Benchmark Price	34,164	16,644	0	0	106,050	111,300	83,700	55,350	494,075	253,575	697,989	717,989
Total Cost at Mode Price	32,820	15,979	9,590	2,740	175,033	183,698	94,860	62,730	465,650	372,876	777,953	638,023
Total Cost at Average Price	61,130	24,338	10,990	2,614	158,570	138,542	97,340	53,587	241,799	210,427	618,480	430,008
Total Savings on Mode Price	−28,310	−8,854	−1,400	126	16,463	45,156	−2,480	9,143	175,200	162,449	159,473	208,020
Total Savings on Benchmark Price	−26,966	−8,194	0	0	−52,520	−27,242	−13,640	1,763	252,276	43,148	79,509	287,981

Actual Sales/Credits During Reference Period

Sales Revenue (£)

800,000
700,000
600,000
500,000
400,000
300,000
200,000
100,000
0
−100,000

□ Benchmark Price
□ Total Cost at Mode Price
▨ Total Cost at Average Price
■ Total Savings on Mode Price
■ Total Savings on Benchmark Price

Supplier Benefits

Our primary suppliers have been successful in developing our relationship due to their:

- Aggressive pricing
- Service excellence
- Quality products
- Education and support infrastructure
- Mutual desire to work toward long-term goals
- Open and consistent communication
- Belief and realization that mutual commitment has been and will continue to be honored

Being able to demonstrate we are in it for the long term has meant that we have worked together in an environment where the supplier's business is not at risk, save acceptable performance. This has allowed all parties the ability to focus on continuous improvement and improved clinical outcomes and have a trusted partner with whom to pioneer new ideas and technologies. The development of our relationship is based on shared objectives and a mutual belief that we are playing on the same side. There are additional benefits for the supplier as well:

- Long-term absolute commitment
- Prompt payment and in some cases prepayment
- Reduced sales, marketing, and associated administrative costs
- Opportunities to test new ideas
- Ongoing education of how the NHS functions
- Better mutual support mechanisms

Buyer Benefits

In addition to preferential pricing in return for long-term commitment are these commercial benefits:

- All expenditure is visible; therefore, off-contract creep, if any, is kept to a minimum (during financial year 2001–2002 just £61,000 of the Centre's £6 million expenditure was not influenced by the purchasing department).
- Continued development of our product knowledge and understanding of market dynamics provides intelligence to be used in a nonthreatening way when reviewing the market, costs, and prices annually.

- Continuous improvement in transforming supply chain processes has led to improved efficiency in managing:
    Receipting and quality control
    Product catalogue data conversion
    Business protocols and policies
    New product introduction protocols
    Invoice matching and payment performance
    Compliance in the use of a standard (agreed) product range
    Inventory levels and associated acquisition costs
    E-commerce solutions

The most important benefit is the collective energy of clinician, industry, and buyer working together as a team to provide the best possible outcomes for patients at the lowest overall cost.

Continuous Improvement

The iterative process of ongoing performance monitoring has led to the development of the performance management schedule in Figure Study 2.10. In addition to assessment of supplier performance in completing Figure Study 2.10, we review service provision with customers in consideration of less objective criteria:

- Has sincere desire to serve customer needs
- Supplies all necessary information on demand

FIGURE STUDY 2.10.   SUPPLIER PERFORMANCE MONITORING.

Supplier Name:		Reviewed with:		Reviewed by:		
Date: Period of review: To		From:				
	100	90	80	60	40	20
Price: supplier's prices have:	Exceeded Expected Reduction	Been Reduced	Stayed Constant	Increased By < Inflation	Increased at Inflation	Increased By > Inflation
Delivery: % on time	100%	99%	> 98%	> 96%	> 94%	> 90%
% complete	100%	99%	> 98%	> 96%	> 94%	> 90%
% packaging damage	0.1%	0.2%	0.3%	0.4%	0.5%	0.6%
Invoicing: 0% matched zero tolerance	100%	99%	> 95%	> 99%	> 85%	> 80%

- Consistently provides agreed level of support to meet our business aims
- Willingly helps in emergencies
- Answers all communications within defined time
- Advises on progress or trouble
- Keeps promises
- Maintains good usable records in support of data exchange targets
- Reacts well to adverse incidents, criticisms, and rejections
- Proactively offers efficiency gains, service improvements, and cost reductions
- Has well-trained, courteous staff
- Able to make prompt decisions

The objectivity in assessing performance by using the criteria in Figure Study 2.10 has meant that complacency by either party is avoided. Indeed, the opposite applies: performance management has enabled the relationship to be increasingly more challenging than would have been the case without its introduction.

Beyond ensuring that the right products are available to meet clinical need at the lowest price, our performance review with suppliers has increasingly become focused on continuous improvement of supply chain processes—for example, the average invoice settlement period of Trusts throughout the NHS with our primary supplier is seventy days. This is at odds with the public sector payment policy (PSPP) of thirty days. In Plymouth we have done much to improve our payment performance with all suppliers, and this is reflected in Figure Study 2.11.

FIGURE STUDY 2.11.   UNIT OF PURCHASE PRICE INVOICE RATE VERSUS VARIANCE REPORT.

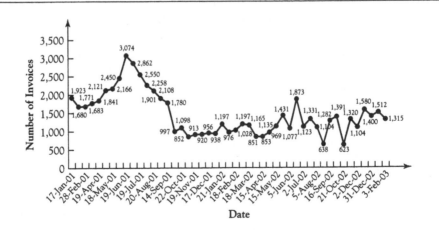

Figure Study 2.11 illustrates the transformation in payment performance from a position in 1999 where 60 percent of the Trust's invoices did not match purchase order unit prices first time within a tolerance of £10 or 2 percent whichever was the greater. Current performance stands at more than 90 percent of invoices first time-matched with zero tolerance. In early 2001, we believed we had performance under control but failed to recognize that process change was not embedded. However, we have learned from this and now have greater understanding of what is required to improve further.

Taking ownership of the entire process of purchase to payment has helped to build stronger relationships with our top fifty suppliers. Increasingly, we are able to pinpoint the root cause of errors that would result in significant upstream corrective action if they went undetected. Transformation of our payment performance has not been just about validating item catalogues and unit prices to enable an invoice match, but has had more to do with continuous improvement of core tasks and managing the whole process to drive greater efficiency throughout the supply chain. For example, if items are not correctly reconciled to match goods receipted as invoiced, in a timely manner, then poor payment performance could result. Our approach to improving management of this function has been the creation of a central goods receipting facility and if required, for technical purposes, the use of second-stage receipt processes as close to the point of use as is practicable. This proves a qualitative (technical) assurance, as opposed to a first-stage quantitative acceptance. Further improvements are in hand as we explore the use of manufacturers' bar codes to facilitate an end-to-end match of data, ultimately enabling point of receipt self-billing.

Our e-trading capability will increase e-commerce following the introduction of system-to-system data transfer using the Global Healthcare Exchange. GHX provides a fully integrated solution for business-to-business transactions. Information is converted to the standard GHXml language for transmission. The Trust's EROS catalogue is maintained by the suppliers via the Internet. Prices that we put on orders are automatically compared with those held by our suppliers in their price files, making error-free trading realizable for the first time in the NHS. Orders are raised in EROS itself, not in a browser, and are then forwarded directly to the supplier's order processing system; the system then sends an order acknowledgment back to the Trust confirming product availability and the date of delivery. Working in partnership with our suppliers and GHX, we will continue to develop these new technologies to improve and automate our transactional processes even further, as shown in Figure Study 2.12. This diagram shows the full extent of our processes. Every shaded activity can be eliminated or simplified significantly using GHX technology.

FIGURE STUDY 2.12. PURCHASING CYCLE.

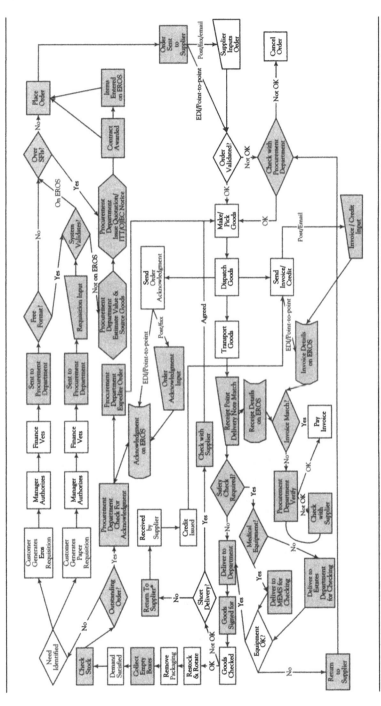

The ability to place orders directly into our supplier's systems within seconds and send and receive real-time information is just the start. GHX will be constantly adding to the functionality of its product, and features such as electronic invoicing will soon be available. Additional mutual benefits will accrue as we implement the next phase of our e-commerce strategy with our top twenty suppliers. This phase is to integrate the products required to meet predictable patient demand into our supplier's production forecasting. We hope that this approach to sharing data will lead to increased operational efficiency and reduced inventory and ensure 100 percent availability to match patient demand.

Lessons Learned

The iterative strategic approach adopted in managing aggregated revenue expenditure has without doubt proven to be a success. The benefits are significant; however, the experience in itself and application of lessons learned are of equal importance.

By refining our thinking, reviewing actions, and occasionally taking time out for a reality check, we have maintained our focus to enable sustained continuous improvement. This systematic appraisal of what is really going on, together with an eye on the future, has resulted in our ability to maintain influence over expenditures and ensure compliance in the use of specialized high-value core products.

Sustained use of Trust item catalogues is essential in controlling expenditure of generic commodity items. Our approach in managing these less contentious products was to adopt a policy of "commodity item best value denominator," defined as the evaluation of a lowest-price generic product and the next lowest and so on until a standard item is agreed by a representative customer group. Initially, this approach was applied to noncontentious commodity items and then extended to all other products residing within validated supplier catalogues, subject to clinical or end user specific evaluations. Not only has this approach enabled rationalization and standardization; it has also aided the promotion and compliance in use of a Trust-wide catalogue across clinical specialties.

Our key to success has been ongoing performance management. An example of where this has led to a practical operational improvement is the introduction of a policy for suppliers visiting the Trust to evaluate new products. Previously suppliers would cold-call or prebook time with clinical staff to use products and then submit their invoice for payment. In effect, this unmanaged approach was eroding preferred suppliers' market share, often at premium prices. Ongoing performance monitoring enabled identification of this off-contract activity. Given its significance, a revised policy has now established an agreed price, which is lower than the contract price. This price is applied with absolute parity to all visiting suppliers for a stated generic product such as a stent. Prices are reviewed annually in line with contract renewals. The major difference in taking this approach is that instead of the supplier just presenting an invoice, as was previously the case, the supplier is now required to submit its item catalogue to the purchasing department so that we may preload this prior to the good's being presented to clinical staff. Failure to adhere to this policy will result in the invoice being returned to the supplier, advising that retrospectively presenting an invoice is not acceptable and the goods used are considered to have been donated free of charge. Implementation and compliance with this policy were not possible without maintaining excellent working relationships with clinical staff and suppliers' sales representatives.

Sustained benefits realization has required tenacity, strong management, and effective communication to ensure our focus is not eroded. This has required dedicated resources with the skills and knowledge to lead the change. Commodity specialization to support ongoing development is an essential requirement in a dynamic market, such as the continued innovation in cardiac rhythm management. In addition to developing product knowledge, we have learned that success requires:

- Focusing on wants and needs to identify what clinicians and key stakeholders are really interested in and then developing an innovative solution to meet their needs, which also maximizes the commercial opportunity.
- Developing robust plans and sticking to them, ensuring change is embedded.
- Validating data and, if comparing this with information provided by the supplier, making sure we are looking at the same reference period. We were surprised at the magnitude of difference caused by not agreeing on the same cut-off date against which to compare data. Do not assume their data are any more accurate than your own.
- Benchmarking what you have achieved and then devising plans to leapfrog better performers.
- Being selfish about maintaining and further developing relationships. Resist the temptation to apply what you have learned elsewhere too soon, as this could erode or destroy the good work accomplished thus far. Relationships of the type described have taken longer to achieve than anticipated. We underestimated the skill shift and resources required by a factor of at least three.
- Recognizing that realizing the big prize takes longer than expected, but when it is reached, avoid complacency and strive for further improvements as they are achievable.

- Promoting your ability to add value, beyond price, by making life easier for your stakeholders. This helps build individual relationships and has ultimately broadened commitment, as awareness increases our role to genuinely add value.
- Celebrating your mistakes as well as your successes. By trying to make a difference and occasionally failing, we have learned much more about what is required to improve that which has not worked.
- Keeping it simple. We have explored numerous approaches to managing price and the application of discounts and rebates for growth. In the light of this experience, we now believe that the best approach is to keep it simple and apply validated prices to each line of a supplier-specific catalogue. The benefit is less administration to monitor and validate pricing and provides easy assimilation of data matching on presentation of invoices.
- Recognizing that rigid organizational structures restrict our collective ability to influence all expenditures within a corporate entity, although we have modified our organizational structure to embrace customer and supplier relationship management and associated category management. A virtual organization with the ability to augment established policies and essential practices with innovative business solutions is what we now aspire to.
- Challenging cherished values and the status quo with credibility and a well-thought-out plan. Otherwise, the likely result would be to alienate those stakeholders without whom change would be impossible. Finding common ground, on occasions through compromise, to build a platform for success has worked.

Partnership is not about cozy relationships or complacency. Our experience is that to deliver short-, medium-, and long-term benefits of the magnitude described here, all parties must have mutual commitment to continually challenge the current. Without the right relationships and a passion to make a difference, sustained improvement is not possible.

The Future

During the progressive development of our approach in managing cardiothoracic expenditure, we transferred the principles of our strategy and applied them to other key categories of products within the Trust. Parallel procurement initiatives have resulted in the realization of savings totaling £4.7 million during the past three and a half years. However, relationships in other market sectors are not as clearly defined and efficiently managed as in the cardiothoracic market, and to ensure sustained performance, improvement plans are in place so that we continue to develop our skills, knowledge, and experience and apply these to maximize our influence over expenditure and outcomes. To achieve this will require transformation of the existing purchasing and supply organizational structure and the continued development of the team to focus on new skills as commodity and customer relationship management increasingly become core competencies.

The recent appointment of a clinical nurse adviser to the purchasing team has already enhanced the department's capabilities. All staff, in addition to conducting traditional operational tasks, are increasingly taking on a new role as resource managers, monitoring product use and taking a holistic approach in understanding how products perform in use. Focused product management at an operational level, however, is just the start. As skills and knowledge increase, staff will proactively influence buying decisions in support of an overall strategic sourcing agenda. In some markets, change will be incremental; in others, a more radical and rapid transformation is likely. Figure Study 2.13 shows the resource impact of this change.

This new role was considered essential to sustain the development of commodity buyers in gaining an in-depth appreciation of medical products and their performance in use. Having someone on the team from a clinical background will also aid further rationalization and standardization of user-specific and Trust-wide catalogues. The ability to liaise with clinical colleagues from a position of knowledge and experience will enable focused product evaluation of new products and support determination of best value when evaluating variances in use from existing standard catalogue items. The ability to be more responsive to customer

FIGURE STUDY 2.13.   THE CHANGING ROLE OF PURCHASING AND SUPPLY.

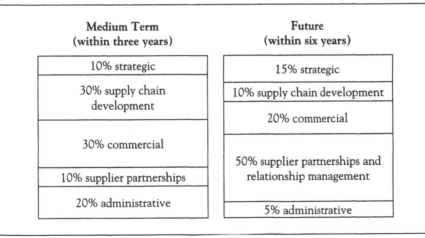

Medium Term (within three years)	Future (within six years)
10% strategic	15% strategic
30% supply chain development	10% supply chain development
	20% commercial
30% commercial	50% supplier partnerships and relationship management
10% supplier partnerships	
20% administrative	5% administrative

FIGURE STUDY 2.14.   POTENTIAL RESOURCE SHIFTS.

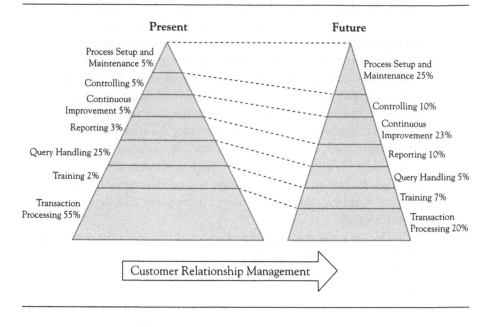

needs and to proactively support the introduction of new clinical legislation and policies is an additional significant advantage of this dynamic role.

As an enabler of our strategic direction, Figure Study 2.14 highlights the resource shift needed to develop our e-trading systems and supporting processes to enhance our performance management capability, freeing up operational time so that this may be more productively used.

Future changes toward modernizing the NHS and shifting the balance of power need to be better understood regarding the challenges and opportunities that this presents to the purchasing and supply profession. Our strategic focus in developing commodity and customer relationship management must embrace and support the development of clinical networks. This extended role will augment an even greater understanding of clinical need and associated economic drivers so that our influence of market dynamics provides further added-value benefits to a broader customer base. This holistic approach of meeting patient needs is to review the total cost of the clinical care pathway and explore the introduction of new therapies such as cardiac resynchronization and atrial fibrillation management for the life of the patient rather than comparing the price of a specific clinical intervention with current budget provision. We must engage commissioners of health care within the local economy to explore alternative funding arrangements and recognize that short-term levels of higher investment will reap medium- to long-term cost reduction benefits. Working together on evidenced-based outcomes supported by robust cost models is where purchasing in the future must demonstrate its ability to add real value. This collaborative activity is to be prioritized to match the effort with potential benefits.

In taking a more holistic view of the market by cutting across existing purchasing and supply operational boundaries, we must analyze current practices, support treatment regimes, and develop innovative solutions that provide efficient process redesign. In addition to having the right skills, knowledge, and experience available to meet this challenge, our future is also about recognizing the value of investing to save, for strategic advantage, rather than expending disproportionate time managing marginal price improvement.

We must establish a strong relationship with the clinical lead of the South West Cardiac network once established. It is anticipated that by becoming an active member of this network, we would be in a position to manage the extension or creation of new contracts on behalf of the wider health economy and influence the range of products used. Given that the number of locations where patients may be treated with interventional therapies is likely to increase, it is essential that we manage the logistics infrastructure to provide this service and ensure optimum inventory controls are applied.

Conclusion

The Cardiothoracic Centre has developed a reputation for clinical excellence, and it has expanded enormously to catch up with unmet demand. By working together, clinicians, suppliers, and the purchasing team have exceeded the initial aim of treating 10 to 15 percent more patients within the same budget. A saving of £1.2 million has been achieved, which represents 19 percent of existing expenditure. It has resulted in the Trust's ability to treat an additional four hundred heart disease patients who might otherwise have had to wait longer for their treatment. We must now extend our influence to all clinical activity by developing strategies to optimize product, services, and operational costs.

STUDY 3: METROPOLITAN HOSPITAL SYSTEM—A STUDY OF A HYBRID ORGANIZATIONAL DESIGN

Supply chain design should evolve from the environment and strategy in order to have the appropriate levels of formality, centralization, and complexity. Metropolitan Hospital System represents a case of a good theoretical fit because it matches the requirements of the environment and the goals and strategy of the system.[1]

Metropolitan Hospital System is a 720-bed hospital in one of the largest U.S. metropolitan areas. This hospital was in a relatively good financial position and had one of the strongest reputations in the area. In the late 1980s, another major community-based hospital with approximately 450 beds was facing financial issues and experiencing a great deal of turmoil on the governing board.

Initial merger discussions were initiated by two of the most prominent board members, who were well-respected businesspeople in the city. In retrospect, it seemed that merger discussions focused on political realities more than on transaction costs or potential economies. The overriding objective was to develop a strong public image by bringing together two hospitals that already had strong reputations in the community. A horizontal merger occurred that was publicized as a joining of equal institutions, and the names were joined with a hyphen to facilitate the image. Most of the community and many of the employees believed that it was a horizontal merger of equals, but top management and the board knew that the larger hospital had substantially greater power in the marketplace and a reputation as a superior institution.

According to their advertising campaigns, these two hospitals merged to generate increased market share or economies of scale. However, no extensive analysis was completed prior to the merger to determine the precise source of these economies of scale or scope that would hypothetically result. Also, only a few finance and accounting specialized postmerger task forces were charged with identifying merger efficiencies. Increased market share was a natural by-product of the merger, but economies of scale were not natural. This was largely a loose, horizontal merger of two parties with equal functional capabilities.

Shortly after these two institutions merged, the board of directors became more interested in other possibilities for both vertical and horizontal mergers. This was during the era in which mergers were seen as the way to resolve both cost and competitive pressures.[2] Within five years, Metropolitan Health System consisted of seven hospitals and several nursing homes and home care units. One of the hospitals focused on neurological disorders and another on oncology. In total, the system had approximately three thousand beds.

The system could be classified as a loosely knit confederation of hospitals in one geographical region. The system had one board of directors, but each hospital also had a board of trustees. In some of the hospitals, the board of trustees had a much stronger political and strategic power than in other hospitals. The chairman of each board of trustees was on the Metropolitan Health System board of directors.

Until the mid-1990s, the system was essentially decentralized. The strongest centralization was around the finance and accounting operations, with some limited centralization around public relations and advertising. Each hospital had its own materials management group, which also had purchasing and distribution responsibilities. The corporate director of materials management had two people reporting to him, and they served largely as a corporate internal consulting group. The hospital materials groups had no reporting relationship to the corporate office. The corporate staff assisted with writing procedures for standardization committees and worked on group purchasing organization (GPO) relationships and distribution activities. The decentralization was demonstrated by the fact that Metropolitan Health System did not have a universal GPO; rather, it had arrangements with three large GPOs. As one manager stated, "At that time we were like a loose confederation of countries with separate armies. And on occasion, a war broke out among ourselves!"

But in the mid-1990s everything changed. Typical of many other systems at the time, the board of directors began to question why the system was not realizing any clear economies of scale or scope from the merger.[3] The CEO retired, and after a lengthy search, a new CEO was appointed. The new CEO was not previously part of the system, so he had no allegiance to any particular hospital or unit. He had a varied health care background, including experience with one of the largest governmental health care providers in the United States and a government health care adviser role, and he had been a CEO of a fifteen-hundred-bed hospital.

The CEO had a future vision that was dramatically different from the existing one. One of the first actions he took was to get the board to support a Metropolitan Health System management vision that simply stated, "One System with One Vision." The vision was to be the low-cost, top-quality health care provider of choice within the market area. This may be considered a satisficing goal because it included cost leadership, differentiation, and focus strategies across the system. A satisficing goal "is a design decision that has been chosen to satisfy a specific non-functional requirement goal."[4] It is a goal that seeks a strategy that, given lack of knowledge and uncertainty, settles on what is good enough, if not best. The challenge was to integrate the diverse parts of the system into one whole that did not sacrifice the goals of a single unit.

Supply Chain Management Foundation

The corporate director of materials management took over as director of materials in one of the system's hospitals as the incumbent resigned. A new corporate vice president of supply chain management was established and filled. The new vice president had an extensive background in health administration at both a large, complex hospital and an integrated delivery network. His most recent position prior to joining Metropolitan Health System was as the director of supply management for two and a half years at a smaller system. He had a broad managerial perspective with experience relating to diverse groups.

A consulting firm was retained to conduct a high-level plan for the corporate supply management group. The vice president immediately saw, however, that this firm was focusing only on supply cost reduction and emphasized standardization, GPO compliance, and leverage of buy across the hospitals. The vice president believed that insufficient attention was given to the focus and differentiation strategies, so he decided not to continue with the firm.

At the same time, he was establishing a supply chain management steering committee with members from across the system. This was an extensive undertaking. He said that he had individual discussions with nearly one hundred people across the organization and around thirty group meetings just to determine who should be on the steering committee. The ostensible purpose was to discuss the purpose of a steering committee with a wide variety of constituents, but at the same time, he was attempting to find supply chain management champions throughout the organization.

The vice president also was analyzing the internal environment. He was especially interested in the financial and political environments of each hospital. It was also important for him to understand the depth of local management's commitment to the stated strategies of the system as well as the different hospitals. It was his position that the integration of strategies was important because of the differences across the system. For instance, the hospital with a neurological focus had been rated as one of the top fifty hospitals in the United States in this area. It did not compete as a low-cost provider as did one of the general community hospitals.

The goal was to keep the supply chain management steering committee to around fifteen to eighteen people so that everyone would have a voice. But the vice president knew that this would leave various groups unrepresented throughout the system. Therefore, at its first several meetings, the steering committee developed a subcommittee structure that would integrate all of the supply processes and systems across the system. Again, this was an enormous task, and a specialist in process analysis was hired. This individual had a background in industrial engineering with approximately four years of experience in health care. His charter was to map processes to determine which groups were interdependent and how they coordinated activities.

To bring the entire system together as one voice, the need for cross-functional teams became apparent. These teams were set up under the direction of the supply chain management steering committee. Furthermore, the committee endorsed the position that all members of a cross-functional team would complete training designed by the human resource group.

Supply Chain Management Plan and Organizational Design

As a result of these activities, a foundation had been established for integrating supply management across the organization. However, a specific organizational design had not been established. To quote a director of materials in one of the hospitals, "The organizational chart for supply chain management looked like a spider web spun by a spider who had gone without sleep. But it was effective." In other words, a complex, hybrid design was implemented.

The organizational design was reconfigured so that each unit (hospital) had a supply chain director who reported to both the CEO of that hospital and the corporate vice president of supply chain management. These individuals were on the corporate supply chain leadership team and sat in on the supply chain steering committee meetings. However, they were only ex officio members of the steering committee.

This reconfiguration was approved because the new vice president of supply chain management developed an elaborate explanation of a hybrid system. The term he used was *adaptive system*. He explained that it was critical that supply management was adaptive to both local and global environments, and this could be done only with a flexible system. It was important for the system to be able to adapt to the needs of the different hospitals while at the same time supporting the goals of the entire health system.

Each director was responsible for establishing supply chain goals and strategy that had to be approved by both the corporate vice president and the hospital chief executive officer. This ensured that the plan integrated with the goals of both the hospital system and the individual hospitals. And to ensure coordination among the units, the plan had to be reviewed and discussed by the leadership team.

The vice president of supply chain management declared that only one GPO and one distributor would be used throughout the system. This was a centralized, autocratic decision. The manner and extent to which each unit would use the GPO and distributor, however, was decentralized. Selection of a GPO and distributor required extensive coordination among the units.

The issue of GPO and distributor selection and use was a classic example of a hybrid system. Some decisions were centralized, while others were decentralized. Implementation was definitely decentralized. But even at the hospital unit level, some of the decisions regarding GPO use were centralized while others were decentralized. For instance, in one hospital, the use of orthopedic implants was centralized, while at another unit that had an especially strong focus on orthopedics, the use of implants could vary.

These differences were necessary because each unit had different goals and strategies for meeting the goals. It was anticipated that the hospital with the orthopedic focus strategy, characterized by specialists from many different groups, would have a larger proportion of physician preference items, while the hospitals with cost leadership strategy would attempt to use the GPO more in an effort to reduce the cost of commodity items. This differentiation in strategy was especially important because the orthopedic-focus strategy hospital was committed to providing differential treatment to the most renowned physicians, who brought extensive business to the hospitals. Those with cost leadership strategies had to be much more aggressive with their standardization and utilization efforts in order to reduce costs. Control was centralized in the cost leadership units and decentralized in the focus strategies. The political and financial environments drove the strategy, which in turn drove the organizational design.

Because of environmental and strategic differences, the hybrid form was also used for complexity and formalization. In the low-cost hospitals, standardization and utilization efforts resulted in highly formalized policies and procedures. To ensure that these procedures were implemented, more complex structures also were needed at the cost leadership hospitals. But the political environment and strategies were different at the focus strategy units. Here the authority and responsibility for supply selection and use were much more decentralized. As a result, the organizational design was much less formalized and complex.

Another way to view complexity is that at the corporate or systems level, there was a shallow hierarchy. Six people reported to the vice president. But the organizational design was much more complex at the low-cost hospital unit level with as many as twenty-five employees and three or even four hierarchical levels. This complexity was necessary because a high level of centralized control within the hospital was needed to meet the low-cost goals. Formalization (extensive policies and procedures) was extremely high for GPO use of commodity items but looser for physician preference items. In the hospitals with the focus strategy, more physician preference items were used so the extent that there was less formalization.

The corporate level was generally rather informal. Few policies and procedures drove the job activities, with the staff generally serving as advisers to the local units. They provided assistance with standardization and utilization efforts, GPO compliance, sourcing of specific items, and tracking of various metrics.

The organizational design throughout Metropolitan Health System varied from centralized to decentralized, formal to informal, highly complex to less complex. To understand the reasons for this hybrid design, it is valuable to return to the five elements of organizational structure: (1) division of work, (2) departmentation, (3) authority and responsibility, (4) span of control, and (5) coordination. For instance, division of work was different in one hospital than in another one. In addition, it is important to understand that environmental factors (see Exhibit 6.1 in Chapter Six) affect the strategic differences and opportunities for both hospitals and systems. It can be seen that the dramatic differences across the Metropolitan Health System meant that different design characteristics were needed. These differences make it much more difficult to manage because there is not one correct way of doing things. But the hybrid approach leads to greater effectiveness because the organizational design supports the strategy.

STUDY 4: OFFICE OF INSPECTOR GENERAL ADVISORY OPINION NO. 05–06, FEBRUARY 2005

Chapter Three addressed a role that value analysis teams (VATs) play in assessing products that attempt to achieve standardization to reduce costs and improve outcomes. VAT success relies substantially on the collaboration between supply chain and clinical leadership to act, without personal gain. In fact, the sharing of savings (gainsharing) between a hospital and its medical staff's efforts to limit items or services has been seen as illegal. In February 2005, the Office of the Inspector General (OIG) of the Department of Health and Human Services approved a number of gainsharing arrangements between hospitals and physicians. The provisions have profound implications for the management of materials by specifically targeting product use and standardization. This study provides the full text of OIG Opinion No. 05–06. Case analysis by both students and practitioners will lead to a better understanding of the variety of constraints that affect the management of the supply chain and provide the opportunity to assess the extent to which gainsharing can be an effective incentive to reduce cost while sustaining high-quality patient care.

We are writing in response to your request for an advisory opinion concerning a proposed arrangement in which a hospital will share with a group of cardiac surgeons a percentage of the hospital's cost savings arising from the surgeons'

We redact certain identifying information and certain potentially privileged, confidential, or proprietary information associated with the individual or entity, unless otherwise approved by the requestors.

implementation of a number of cost reduction measures in certain surgical procedures (the "Proposed Arrangement"). The cost savings will be measured based on the surgeons' use of specific supplies during designated cardiac surgery procedures. You have inquired whether the Proposed Arrangement would constitute grounds for sanctions arising under: (i) the civil monetary penalty for a hospital's payment to a physician to induce reductions or limitations of services to Medicare or Medicaid beneficiaries under the physician's direct care, sections 1128A(b)(1)-(2) of the Social Security Act (the "Act"); or (ii) the exclusion authority at section 1128(b)(7) of the Act or the civil monetary penalty provision at section 1128A(a)(7) of the Act, as those sections relate to the commission of acts described in section 1128B(b) of the Act, the anti-kickback statute.

You have certified that all of the information provided in your request, including all supplementary letters, is true and correct and constitutes a complete description of the relevant facts and agreements among the parties.

In issuing this opinion, we have relied solely on the facts and information presented to us. We have not undertaken an independent investigation of such information. This opinion is limited to the facts presented. If material facts have not been disclosed or have been misrepresented, this opinion is without force and effect.

Based on the information provided and the totality of the facts as described and certified in your request for an advisory opinion and supplemental submissions, we conclude that:

(i) the Proposed Arrangement would constitute an improper payment to induce reduction or limitation of services pursuant to sections 1128A(b)(1)-(2) of the Act, but that the Office of Inspector General ("OIG") would not impose sanctions on the requestors of this advisory opinion, [names redacted] (the "Requestors"), in connection with the Proposed Arrangement; and (ii) the Proposed Arrangement would potentially generate prohibited remuneration under the anti-kickback statute, if the requisite intent to induce or reward referrals of Federal health care program business were present, but that the OIG would not impose administrative sanctions on the Requestors under sections 1128(b)(7) or 1128A(a)(7) of the Act (as those sections relate to the commission of acts described in section 1128B(b) of the Act) in connection with the Proposed Arrangement.

This opinion may not be relied on by any persons other than the Requestors and is further qualified as set out in Part IV below and in 42 C.F.R. Part 1008.

I. Factual Background

A. Parties

The Hospital. [Name redacted] (the "Hospital") is an acute care hospital in [city and states redacted] that offers a broad range of inpatient and outpatient hospital services, including cardiac surgery services. The Hospital is a participating provider in the Medicare and Medicaid programs.

The Surgical Group. [Name redacted] (the "Surgical Group") is a professional association composed exclusively of cardiac surgeons who are licensed in [state redacted] and have active medical staff privileges at the Hospital.[1] The cardiac surgeons refer patients to the Hospital for inpatient and outpatient hospital services.

The Program Administrator. The Hospital has engaged [name redacted] (the "Program Administrator") to administer the Proposed Arrangement. The Program Administrator will collect data and analyze and manage the Proposed Arrangement.[2] The Hospital will pay the Program Administrator a monthly fixed fee certified by the Requestors to be fair market value in an arm's-length transaction for services to be provided by the Program Administrator under the Proposed Arrangement. The fee will not be tied in any way to cost savings or the Surgical Group's compensation under the Proposed Arrangement.

B. The Proposed Arrangement

Under the Proposed Arrangement, the Hospital will pay the Surgical Group a share of the first year cost savings directly attributable to specific changes in the Surgical Group's operating room practices, including standardization of certain cardiac devices. The Program Administrator conducted a study of the historic practices at the Hospital's cardiac surgery department and identified twenty-seven specific cost-savings opportunities. The results of the Program Administrator's study of the Surgical Group and the specific cost-savings opportunities are summarized in a "Practice Patterns Report."[3] The Hospital and the Surgical Group have reviewed the Practice Patterns Report for medical appropriateness and each has adopted its recommendations and conclusions.

In general, the Practice Patterns Report recommends that the Surgical Group change current operating room practices to curb inappropriate use or waste of medical supplies. The twenty-seven recommendations can be roughly grouped into four categories.

The first category consists of two recommendations that involve opening packaged items only as needed during a procedure. Most of these "open as needed" items are surgical tray or comparable supplies.

The second category, involving three recommendations, is similar and involves limiting the use of certain surgical supplies, such as gelfoam, surgicel, and vancomycin paste, to an as needed basis (hereafter, the "use as needed" recommendations). The Requestors have certified that the individual surgeon will make a patient-by-patient determination as to whether these items are clinically indicated and that the surgical supplies will still be readily available to the surgeons. The Requestors have further certified that any resulting limitations on the use of these products will not adversely affect patient care.

The third category, involving eleven recommendations, consists of the substitution, in whole or in part, of less costly items for items currently being used by the surgeons (hereafter, the "product substitution" recommendations). In this case, the substitutions involve types of items and services for which a product substitution will have no appreciable clinical significance (e.g., substituting disposable head supports, disposable k-thermia blankets, and instrument pouches). For example, currently a foam donut is used in each surgical case to support the patient's head. Under the Proposed Arrangement, surgeons would be asked to utilize a less expensive reusable head support that has similar characteristics to the surgeons' historic preference.

The final category, involving eleven recommendations, consists of product standardization of certain cardiac devices and supplies where medically appropriate. For this category, the Surgical Group would be required to work in conjunction with the Hospital to evaluate and clinically review vendors and products.[4] The Surgical Group would agree to use the selected products where medically appropriate, which may require additional training or changes in clinical practice.

The Proposed Arrangement contains several safeguards intended to protect against inappropriate reductions in services. With respect to the substitution recommendations, the Proposed Arrangement would utilize objective historical and clinical measures reasonably related to the practices and the patient population at the Hospital to establish a "floor" beyond which no savings would accrue to the Surgical Group. For example, surgicel is currently utilized on 28% of the cases specified under the Proposed Arrangement. According to the Program Administrator, national data indicate a best practice usage of 5% for surgicel. Thus, the Program Administrator has set a 5% floor for this recommendation. The Surgical Group will receive no share of any savings resulting from the reduction in use of surgicel beyond the 5% floor. With respect to the product substitution recommendations in the Proposed Arrangement, as the identified substitutions[5] will have no appreciable clinical significance, no floors are set.[6]

Importantly, with respect to the product standardization recommendations, the Requestors have certified that the individual surgeons will make a patient-by-patient determination of the most appropriate devices and supplies and the availability of the full range of these items will not be compromised by the product standardization. The Requestors have further certified that individual physicians will still have available the same selection of devices and supplies after implementation of the Proposed Arrangement as before and that the economies gained through the Proposed Arrangement will result from inherent clinical and fiscal value and not from restricting the availability of devices and supplies.

According to the Program Administrator, if implemented in accordance with the Practice Patterns Report's specifications, the twenty-seven recommendations would present substantial cost savings opportunities for the Hospital without adversely impacting the quality of patient care.

The Hospital will pay the Surgical Group 50% of the cost savings achieved by implementing the twenty-seven recommendations in the Practice Patterns Report for a period of one year. At the end of the year, cost savings will be calculated separately for each of the twenty-seven recommendations; this will preclude shifting of cost savings and ensure that savings generated by utilization beyond the set targets, as applicable, will not be credited to the Surgical Group. This payment will constitute the entire compensation paid to the Surgical Group for services performed under the contract memorializing the Proposed Arrangement between the Surgical Group and the Hospital. For purposes of calculating the payment to the Surgical Group, the cost savings will be calculated by subtracting the actual costs incurred for the items specified in the twenty-seven recommendations when used by surgeons in the Surgical Group during the specified surgical procedures (the "current year costs"[7]) from the historic costs for the same items when used during comparable surgical procedures in the base year (the "base year costs"[8]). The current year costs will be adjusted to account for any inappropriate reductions in use of items beyond the targets set in the Practice Patterns Report. The payment to the Surgical Group will be 50% of the difference between the adjusted current year costs and base year costs, if any.

The Hospital will make an aggregate payment to the Surgical Group, which distributes its profits to each of its members on a per capita basis. Payments to the Surgical Group will also be subject to the following limitations:

• If the volume of procedures payable by a Federal health care program in the current year exceeds the volume of like procedures payable by a Federal health care program performed in the base year, there will be no sharing of cost savings for the additional procedures.

- To minimize the surgeons' financial incentive to steer more costly patients to other hospitals, the case severity, ages, and payors of the patient population treated under the Proposed Arrangement will be monitored by a committee composed of representatives of the Requestors, using generally accepted standards. If there are significant changes from historical measures, the surgeon at issue will be terminated from participation in the Proposed Arrangement.
- The aggregate payment to the Surgical Group will not exceed 50% of the projected cost savings identified in the Practice Patterns Report.

The Hospital and the Surgical Group will document the activities and the payment methodology under the Proposed Arrangement and will make the documentation available to the Secretary of the United States Department of Health and Human Services, upon request. In addition, the Hospital and the Surgical Group will disclose the Proposed Arrangement to the patient, including the fact that the Surgical Group's compensation is based on a percentage of the Hospital's cost savings. The disclosure will be made to the patient before the patient is admitted to the Hospital for a procedure covered by the Proposed Arrangement; if pre-admission disclosure is impracticable (e.g., the patient is admitted for an unscheduled procedure or the need for the procedure is determined after admission), the disclosure will be made before the patient consents to the surgery. The disclosures will be in writing, and patients will have an opportunity, if desired, to review details of the Proposed Arrangement, including the specific cost savings measures applicable to the patient's surgery.

II. Legal Analysis

Arrangements like the Proposed Arrangement are designed to align incentives by offering physicians a portion of a hospital's cost savings in exchange for implementing cost saving strategies. Under the current reimbursement system, the burden of these costs falls on hospitals, not physicians. Payments to physicians based on cost savings may be intended to motivate them to reduce hospital costs associated with procedures performed by physicians at the hospitals.

Properly structured, arrangements that share cost savings can serve legitimate business and medical purposes. Specifically, properly structured arrangements may increase efficiency and reduce waste, thereby potentially increasing a hospital's profitability. However, such arrangements can potentially influence physician judgment to the detriment of patient care. Our concerns include, but are not limited to, the following: (i) stinting on patient care; (ii) "cherry picking" healthy patients and steering sicker (and more costly) patients to hospitals that do not offer such arrangements; (iii) payments in exchange for patient referrals; and (iv) unfair competition (a "race to the bottom") among hospitals offering cost savings programs to foster physician loyalty and to attract more referrals.

Hospital cost savings programs in general, and the Proposed Arrangement in particular, may implicate at least three Federal legal authorities: (i) the civil monetary penalty for reductions or limitations of direct patient care services provided to Federal health care program beneficiaries, sections 1128A(b)(1)-(2) of the Act; (ii) the anti-kickback statute, section 1128B(b) of the Act; and (iii) the physician self-referral law, section 1877 of the Act.[9] We address the first two of these authorities; section 1877 of the Act falls outside the scope of the OIG's advisory opinion authority. We express no opinion on the application of section 1877 of the Act to the Proposed Arrangement.

A. The Civil Monetary Penalty, Sections 1128A(b)(1)-(2) of the Act

Sections 1128A(b)(1)-(2) of the Act establish a civil monetary penalty ("CMP") against any hospital or critical access hospital that knowingly makes a payment directly or indirectly to a physician (and any physician that receives such a payment) as an inducement to reduce or limit items or services to Medicare or Medicaid beneficiaries under the physician's direct care. Hospitals that make (and physicians that receive) such payments are liable for CMPs of up to $2,000 per patient covered by the payments. See *id.* There is no requirement that the prohibited payment be tied to a specific patient or to a reduction in medically necessary care. The CMP applies only to reductions or limitations of items or services provided to Medicare and Medicaid fee-for-service beneficiaries.[10]

The CMP prohibits payments by hospitals to physicians that may induce physicians to reduce or limit items or services furnished to their Medicare and Medicaid patients. A threshold inquiry is whether the Proposed Arrangement will induce physicians to reduce or limit items or services. Given the specificity of the Proposed Arrangement, it is possible to review the proposed opportunities for savings individually and evaluate their potential impact on patient care.

Having reviewed the twenty-seven individual recommendations, we conclude that, except for the unopened surgical tray items and the product substitutions (discussed in more detail below), the recommendations implicate the CMP. Simply put, with respect to the recommendations regarding the "use as needed" surgical supplies and the product standardization, the Proposed Arrangement constitutes an inducement to reduce or limit the current medical practice at the Hospital. We recognize that the current medical practice may involve care that exceeds the requirements of medical necessity. However, whether the current medical practice reflects necessity or prudence is irrelevant for purposes of the CMP.

With respect to the recommendations regarding "open as needed" surgical tray items and product substitutions, we reach a different conclusion. To the extent that the sole delay in providing items or services is the insubstantial time it takes to open a package of supplies readily available in the operating room, we believe there will be no perceptible reduction or limitation in the provision of items or services to patients sufficient to trigger the CMP. With respect to the specific product substitution recommendations, the identified substitutions will have no appreciable clinical significance; therefore, we believe there will be no perceptible reduction or limitation in the provision of items or services to patients sufficient to trigger the CMP.

In sum, while the recommendations for the "open as needed" surgical tray items and the specific product substitutions do not run afoul of the CMP, we find that the CMP would apply to the remaining recommendations involving limitations on use of certain surgical supplies and product standardization. Notwithstanding, the Proposed Arrangement has several features that, in combination, provide sufficient safeguards so that we would not seek sanctions against the Requestors under sections 1128A(b)(1)-(2) of the Act.

First, the specific cost-saving actions and resulting savings are clearly and separately identified. The transparency of the Proposed Arrangement will allow for public scrutiny and individual physician accountability for any adverse effects of the Proposed Arrangement, including any difference in treatment among patients based on nonclinical indicators. The transparency of the incentives for specific actions and specific procedures will also facilitate accountability through the medical-legal professional liability system.

Second, the Requestors have proffered credible medical support for the position that implementation of the recommendations will not adversely affect patient care. The Proposed Arrangement will be periodically reviewed by the Requestors to confirm that the Proposed Arrangement is not having an adverse impact on clinical care.[11]

Third, the payments under the Proposed Arrangement are based on all surgeries regardless of the patients' insurance coverage, subject to the cap on payment for Federal health care program procedures. Moreover, the surgical procedures to which the Proposed Arrangement applies are not disproportionately performed on Federal health care program beneficiaries. Additionally, the cost savings are calculated on the Hospital's actual out-of-pocket acquisition costs, not an accounting convention.

Fourth, the Proposed Arrangement protects against inappropriate reductions in services by utilizing objective historical and clinical measures to establish baseline thresholds beyond which no savings accrue to the Surgical Group.

The Requestors have certified that these baseline measures are reasonably related to the Hospital's or comparable hospitals' practices and patient populations. These safeguards are action-specific and not simply based on isolated patient outcome data unrelated to the specific changes in operating room practices.

Fifth, the product standardization portion of the Proposed Arrangement further protects against inappropriate reductions in services by ensuring that individual physicians will still have available the same selection of cardiac devices after implementation of the Proposed Arrangement as before. The Proposed Arrangement is designed to produce savings through inherent clinical and fiscal value and not from restricting the availability of devices.

Sixth, the Hospital and the Surgical Group will provide written disclosures of their involvement in the Proposed Arrangement to patients whose care may be affected by the Proposed Arrangement and will provide patients an opportunity to review the cost savings recommendations prior to admission to the Hospital (or, where pre-admission consent is impracticable, prior to consenting to surgery). While we do not believe that, standing alone, such disclosures offer sufficient protection from program or patient abuse, effective and meaningful disclosure offers some protection against possible abuses of patient trust.[12]

Seventh, the financial incentives under the Proposed Arrangement are reasonably limited in duration and amount.

Eighth, because the Surgical Group's profits are distributed to its members on a per capita basis, any incentive for an individual surgeon to generate disproportionate cost savings is mitigated.

Our decision not to impose sanctions on the Requestors in connection with the Proposed Arrangement is an exercise of our discretion and is consistent with our Special Advisory Bulletin on "Gainsharing Arrangements and CMPs for Hospital Payments to Physicians to Reduce or Limit Services to Beneficiaries" (July 1999) (the "Special Advisory Bulletin"). We reiterate that the CMP applies to any payment by a hospital to a physician that is intended to induce the reduction or limitation of items or services to Medicare or Medicaid patients under the physician's direct clinical care. The Proposed Arrangement is markedly different from many "gainsharing" plans, particularly those that purport to pay physicians a percentage of generalized cost savings not tied to specific, identifiable cost-lowering activities. Importantly, the Proposed Arrangement sets out the specific actions to be taken and ties the remuneration to the actual, verifiable cost savings attributable to those actions. This transparency allows an assessment of the likely effect of the Proposed Arrangement on quality of care and ensures that the identified actions will be the cause of the savings.

By contrast, many gainsharing plans contain features that heighten the risk that payments will lead to inappropriate reductions or limitations of services. These features include, but are not limited to, the following:

- There is no demonstrable direct connection between individual actions and any reduction in the hospital's out-of-pocket costs (and any corresponding "gainsharing" payment).
- The individual actions that would give rise to the savings are not identified with specificity.
- There are insufficient safeguards against the risk that other, unidentified actions, such as premature hospital discharges, might actually account for any "savings."
- The quality of care indicators are of questionable validity and statistical significance.
- There is no independent verification of cost savings, quality of care indicators, or other essential aspects of the arrangement.

Simply put, many "gainsharing" plans present substantial risks for both patient and program abuse—risks that are not present in the Proposed Arrangement. Given the limited duration and scope of the Proposed Arrangement, the safeguards provide sufficient protections against patient and program abuse. Other arrangements, including those that are longer in duration or more expansive in scope than the Proposed Arrangement, are likely to require additional or different safeguards.

B. The Anti-Kickback Statute

The anti-kickback statute makes it a criminal offense knowingly and willfully to offer, pay, solicit, or receive any remuneration to induce or reward referrals of items or services reimbursable by a Federal health care program. See section 1128B(b) of the Act. Where remuneration is paid purposefully to induce or reward referrals of items or services payable by a Federal health care program, the anti-kickback statute is violated. By its terms, the statute ascribes criminal liability to parties on both sides of an impermissible "kickback" transaction. For purposes of the anti-kickback statute, "remuneration" includes the transfer of anything of value, directly or indirectly, overtly or covertly, in cash or in kind.

The statute has been interpreted to cover any arrangement where one purpose of the remuneration was to obtain money for the referral of services or to induce further referrals. United States v. Kats, 871 F.2d 105 (9th Cir. 1989); United States v. Greber, 760 F.2d 68 (3d Cir.), cert. denied, 474 U.S. 988 (1985). Violation of the statute constitutes a felony punishable by a maximum fine of $25,000, imprisonment up to five years, or both. Conviction will also lead to automatic exclusion from Federal health care programs, including Medicare and Medicaid. Where a party commits an act described in section 1128B(b) of the Act, the OIG may initiate administrative proceedings to impose civil monetary penalties on such party under section 1128A(a)(7) of the Act. The OIG may also initiate administrative proceedings to exclude such party from the Federal health care programs under section 1128(b)(7) of the Act.

The Department of Health and Human Services has promulgated safe harbor regulations that define practices that are not subject to the anti-kickback statute because such practices would be unlikely to result in fraud or abuse. See 42 C.F.R. § 1001.952. The safe harbors set forth specific conditions that, if met, assure entities involved of not being prosecuted or sanctioned for the arrangement qualifying for the safe harbor. However, safe harbor protection is afforded only to those arrangements that precisely meet all of the conditions set forth in the safe harbor.

The safe harbor for personal services and management contracts, 42 C.F.R. §1001.952(d), is potentially applicable to the Proposed Arrangement. In relevant part for purposes of this advisory opinion, the personal services safe harbor requires that the aggregate compensation paid for the services be set in advance and consistent with fair market value in arm's-length transactions. The Proposed Arrangement would not fit in the safe harbor because the Surgical Group will be paid on a percentage basis, and thus the compensation would not be set in advance. However, the absence of safe harbor protection is not fatal. Instead, the Proposed Arrangement must be subject to case-by-case evaluation.

Like any compensation arrangement between a hospital and a physician who admits or refers patients to such hospital, we are concerned that the Proposed Arrangement could be used to disguise remuneration from the Hospital to reward or induce referrals by the Surgical Group. Specifically, the Proposed Arrangement could encourage the surgeons to admit Federal health care program patients to the Hospital, since the surgeons would receive not only their Medicare Part B professional fee, but also, indirectly, a share of the Hospital's payment, depending on cost savings. In other words, the more procedures a surgeon performs at the Hospital, the more money he or she is likely to receive under the Proposed Arrangement.

While we believe the Proposed Arrangement could result in illegal remuneration if the requisite intent to induce referrals were present, we would not impose sanctions in the particular circumstances presented here and as qualified below.

First, the circumstances and safeguards of the Proposed Arrangement reduce the likelihood that the arrangement will be used to attract referring physicians or to increase referrals from existing physicians. Specifically, participation in the

Proposed Arrangement will be limited to surgeons already on the medical staff, thus limiting the likelihood that the Proposed Arrangement will attract other surgeons. In addition, the potential savings derived from procedures for Federal health care program beneficiaries will be capped based on the prior year's admissions of Federal health care program beneficiaries. Finally, the contract term will be limited to one year, reducing any incentive to switch facilities, and admissions will be monitored for changes in severity, age, or payor. Thus, while the incentive to refer will not necessarily be eliminated, it will be substantially reduced.

Second, the structure of the Proposed Arrangement eliminates the risk that the Proposed Arrangement will be used to reward cardiologists or other physicians who refer patients to the Surgical Group or its surgeons. The Surgical Group is the sole participant in the Proposed Arrangement and is composed entirely of cardiac surgeons; no cardiologists or other physicians are members of the Surgical Group or share in its profit distributions. Within the Surgical Group, profits are distributed to its members on a per capita basis, mitigating any incentive for an individual surgeon to generate disproportionate cost savings.

Third, the Proposed Arrangement sets out with specificity the particular actions that will generate the cost savings on which the payments are based. While many of the recommendations in the Practice Patterns Report are simple common sense, they do represent a change in operating room practice, for which the surgeon is responsible and will have liability exposure. While most of the recommendations would appear to present minimal risk, limitations on use of certain surgical supplies and product standardization each carry some increased liability risk for the physicians. It is not unreasonable for the surgeon to receive compensation for the increased risk from the proposed change in practice. Moreover, the payments will represent a portion of one year's worth of cost savings and will be limited in amount (i.e., the aggregate cap), duration (i.e., the limited contract term), and scope (i.e., the total savings that can be achieved from the implementation of any one recommendation are limited by appropriate utilization levels). The payments under the Proposed Arrangement do not appear unreasonable, given, among other things, the nature of the actions required of the physicians to implement the twenty-seven recommended actions, the specificity of the payment formula, and the cap on total remuneration to the Surgical Group.[13] We caution that payments of 50% of cost savings in other arrangements, including multi-year arrangements or arrangements with generalized cost savings formulae, could well lead to a different result.

In light of these circumstances and safeguards, the Proposed Arrangement poses a low risk of fraud or abuse under the anti-kickback statute.

III. Conclusion

Notwithstanding the foregoing, we reiterate our concerns regarding many arrangements between hospitals and physicians to share cost savings. Improperly designed or implemented arrangements risk adversely affecting patient care and could be vehicles to disguise payments for referrals. For example, an arrangement that cannot be adequately and accurately measured for quality of care would pose a high risk of fraud or abuse, as would one that rewards physicians based on overall cost savings without accountability for specific cost reduction measures. Moreover, arrangements structured so as to pose a heightened potential for patient steering and unfair competition would be considered suspect. In short, this opinion is predicated on the specific arrangement posed by the Requestors and is limited to that specific arrangement. Other apparently similar arrangements could raise different concerns and lead to a different result.

Based on the facts certified in your request for an advisory opinion and supplemental submissions, we conclude:

(i) the Proposed Arrangement would constitute an improper payment to induce reduction or limitation of services pursuant to sections 1128A(b)(1)-(2) of the Act, but that the OIG would not impose sanctions under sections 1128A(b)(1)-(2) on the Requestors in connection with the Proposed Arrangement; and (ii) the Proposed Arrangement would potentially generate prohibited remuneration under the anti-kickback statute, if the requisite intent to induce or reward referrals of Federal health care program business were present, but that the OIG would not impose administrative sanctions on the Requestors under sections 1128(b)(7) or 1128A(a)(7) of the Act (as those sections relate to the commission of acts described in section 1128B(b) of the Act) in connection with the Proposed Arrangement.

IV. Limitations

The limitations applicable to this opinion include the following:

- This advisory opinion is issued only to [names redacted], the Requestors of this opinion. This advisory opinion has no application to, and cannot be relied upon by, any other individual or entity.
- This advisory opinion may not be introduced into evidence in any matter involving an entity or individual that is not a requestor to this opinion.

- This advisory opinion is applicable only to the statutory provisions specifically noted above. No opinion is expressed or implied herein with respect to the application of any other Federal, state, or local statute, rule, regulation, ordinance, or other law that may be applicable to the Proposed Arrangement, including, without limitation, the physician self-referral law, section 1877 of the Act.
- This advisory opinion will not bind or obligate any agency other than the U.S. Department of Health and Human Services.
- This advisory opinion is limited in scope to the specific arrangement described in this letter and has no applicability to other arrangements, even those that appear similar in nature or scope.
- No opinion is expressed herein regarding the liability of any party under the False Claims Act or other legal authorities for any improper billing, claims submission, cost reporting, or related conduct.

This opinion is also subject to any additional limitations set forth at 42 C.F.R. Part 1008.

The OIG will not proceed against the Requestors with respect to any action that is part of the Proposed Arrangement taken in good faith reliance upon this advisory opinion, as long as all of the material facts have been fully, completely, and accurately presented, and the Proposed Arrangement in practice comports with the information provided. The OIG reserves the right to reconsider the questions and issues raised in this advisory opinion and, where the public interest requires, to rescind, modify, or terminate this opinion. In the event that this advisory opinion is modified or terminated, the OIG will not proceed against the Requestors with respect to any action taken in good faith reliance upon this advisory opinion, where all of the relevant facts were fully, completely, and accurately presented, and where such action was promptly discontinued upon notification of the modification or termination of this advisory opinion. An advisory opinion may be rescinded only if the relevant and material facts have not been fully, completely, and accurately disclosed to the OIG.

NOTES

Acknowledgments

1. Burns, L. R. *The Health Care Value Chain*. San Francisco: Jossey-Bass, 2002.
2. Kohn, L., Corrigan, J. M., and Donaldson, M. S. (eds.). *To Err Is Human: Building a Safer Health System*. Washington, D.C.: National Academy Press, 2000.

Introduction

1. Dranove, D., and Shanley, M. "Cost Reductions or Reputation Enhancement as Motives for Mergers: The Logic of Multihospital Systems." *Strategic Management Journal*, 1995, *16*(10), 55–74.
2. Efficient Healthcare Consumer Response. *Improving the Efficiency of the Healthcare Supply Chain*. Chicago: American Society for Healthcare Materials Management, 1996.
3. Hospitals spend approximately $125 billion on health care supplies each year. Marchula, D., and Shannon, E. G. *eHealth B2B Overview*. Minneapolis: Piper Jaffray Equity Research, 2000.
4. Lacy, R. G., and others. *The Value of eCommerce in the Healthcare Supply Chain*. New York: Andersen, 2001.
5. These data reflect a typical group of hospitals, in a very competitive environment, that we visited.
6. The idea of "useful knowledge" has been developed by Kilman, R., Slevin D. P., and Thomas, K. W. "The Problem of Producing Useful Knowledge." In R. H. Kilman and others (eds.), *Producing Useful Knowledge for Organizations*. New York: Praeger, 1983.

7. Chopra, S., and Meindl, P. *Supply Chain Management: Strategy, Planning, and Operations.* (2nd ed.) Upper Saddle River, N.J.: Prentice Hall, 2004, p. 4. This book provides a solid grounding in the general principles and ideas associated with this growing field.

8. In most instances, since patients only rarely demand specific products, a focus on the patient as client obscures the key issues involved in hospital supply chain management: strategically managing the supply chain to meet the needs of clinicians and others who bring value, through their activities, to accomplishing the goals of the hospital or system.

9. Chopra and Meindl, *Supply Chain Management.*

10. Fine, C. H. *Clockspeed: Winning Industry Control in the Age of Temporary Advantage.* New York: Basic Books, 1998.

11. Fine, *Clockspeed,* p. 144.

12. For a comprehensive description of reprocessing for single-use devices, see *Federal Register,* June 26, 2003, pp. 38071–38083. See the following at *Federal Register Online* via GPO Access [wais.access.gpo.gov][DOCID:fr26jn03–101]: "On October 26, 2002, MDUFMA (Public Law 107–250) amended the Federal Food, Drug, and Cosmetic Act (the act) by adding section 510(o) (21 U.S.C. 360(o)), which provided new regulatory requirements for reprocessed SUDs [single use devices]. According to this new provision, in order to ensure that reprocessed SUDs are substantially equivalent to predicate devices, 510(k)s for certain reprocessed SUDs identified by FDA must include validation data. These required validation data include cleaning and sterilization data, and functional performance data demonstrating that each SUD will remain substantially equivalent to its predicate device after the maximum number of times the device is reprocessed as intended by the person submitting the premarket notification."

13. U.S. Department of Health and Human Services, Centers for Medicare and Medicaid Services. *HHS/OIG Fiscal Year 2004 Work Plan.* Washington, D.C.: U.S. Government Printing Office. 2004. http://oig.hhs.gov/reading/workplan/2004/2-CMS%204.pdf.

14. Agency for Health Care Policy and Research. *Hospital Inpatient Statistics.* 1996. http://www.ahcpr.gov/data/hcup/his96/clinclas.htm.

15. Agency for Health Care Policy and Research, Hospital Inpatient Statistics.

16. For an excellent discussion on using frames for improved managerial analysis and decision making, see Bolman, L. G., and Deal, T. *Reframing Organizations: Artistry, Choice and Leadership.* San Francisco: Jossey-Bass, 1991.

17. Chopra and Meindl, *Supply Chain Management.*

18. Borys, B., and Jemison, D. "Hybrid Arrangements as Strategic Alliances: Theoretical Issues in Organizational Combinations." *Academy of Management Review,* 1989, *14*(2), 234–249.

19. Over the past five years, there has been a proliferation of GPOs and new GPO business models and strategies. This has led many hospitals and hospital systems to carefully rethink their relationships with their current GPO, carry out due diligence to assess the advisability of changing GPO partners, and even consider bringing the sourcing, contracting, and other services provided by the GPOs into the hospital.

20. Ragion, C. "Introduction: Cases of 'What Is a Case.'" In C. C. Ragion and H. S. Becker, *What Is a Case: Exploring the Foundations of Social Inquiry.* Cambridge: Cambridge University Press, 1992.

21. Kilman, R., Slevin, D. P., and Thomas, K. W. "The Problem of Producing Useful Knowledge." In R. H. Kilman and others (eds.), *Producing Useful Knowledge for Organizations.* New York: Praeger, 1983.

22. Burns, L. R. *The Health Care Value Chain.* San Francisco: Jossey-Bass, 2002.

23. Smeltzer, L., and Ramanathan, V. "Supply Chain Management: Can Progressive Manufacturing Practices Be Used by Health Care Providers?" "Health Sector Supply Chain Initiatives" working paper no. 1, W. P. Carey School of Business, Arizona State University, 2002.

24. Silverman, D. D. *Qualitative Research.* Thousand Oaks, Calif.: Sage, 1999.

25. Glaser, B., and Strauss, A. *The Discovery of Grounded Theory: Strategies for Qualitative Research.* Chicago: Aldine, 1967. Guba, E. *Toward a Methodology of Naturalistic Inquiry in Educational Evaluation.* Los Angeles: UCLA for the Study of Evaluation, 1978.

26. Ragion and Becker, *What Is a Case.*

27. See Glaser and Strauss, *The Discovery of Grounded Theory.*

Chapter One

1. Chapman, T. L., Gupta, A., and Mango, P. D. "Group Purchasing Is Not a Panacea for U.S. Hospitals." *McKinsey Quarterly,* 1998, no. 1, 160–165. Efficient Healthcare Consumer Response. *Improving the Efficiency of the Healthcare Supply Chain.* Chicago: American Society for Healthcare Materials Management, 1996. Muse & Associates. *Role of Group Purchasing Organizations in the U.S. Health Care System.* Washington, D.C.: Muse & Associates, Mar. 2000.

2. EHCR, *Efficient Healthcare Consumer Response.*

3. Hospitals spend approximately $125 billion on health care supplies each year. Marchula, D., and Shannon, E. G. "eHealth B2B Overview." Minneapolis: US Bancorp, Piper Jaffray Equity Research, 2000.

4. Lacy, R. G., and others. *The Value of eCommerce in the Healthcare Supply Chain.* New York: Andersen, 2001.

5. Romano, M. "A Good Education." *Modern Healthcare,* 2004, *34*(9), 6–14.

6. Bowersox, D. J., Closs, D. J., and Stank, T. P. "Ten Megatrends That Will Revolutionize Supply Chain Logistics." *Journal of Business Logistics,* 2000, *21*(2), 1–16.

7. Arndt, M., and Bigelow, B. "The Transfer of Business Practices into Hospitals: History and Implications." In J. D. Blair, M. D. Fottler, and G. T. Savage (eds.), *Advances in Health Care Management.* Greenwich, Conn.: JAI Press, 2000.

8. Luke, R. D., Walston, S. L., and Plummer, P. M. *Healthcare Strategy: In Pursuit of Competitive Advantage.* Chicago: Health Administration Press, 2004, p. 68.

9. Arndt and Bigelow, "The Transfer of Business Practices into Hospitals," p. 340.

10. A comprehensive discussion of group purchasing organization origins and development can be found in Burns, L. R. *The Health Care Value Chain.* San Francisco: Jossey-Bass, 2002. Chapter Two in this book addresses the role of GPOs in greater detail.

11. Schneller, E. S. *The Value of Group Purchasing.* Tempe: W. P. Carey School of Business, Arizona State University, 2000. This is Study 1, "The Value of Group Purchasing in the Health Care Supply Chain," in this book.

12. Chopra, S., and Meindl, P. *Supply Chain Management: Strategy, Planning, and Operations.* Upper Saddle River, N.J.: Prentice Hall, 2004, p. 4. This book provides a solid grounding in the general principles and ideas associated with the growing field of supply chain management.

13. Leenders, M. R., and Fearon, H. E. *Purchasing and Supply Management.* New York: McGraw-Hill, 1997, p. 6.

14. Byrnes, J. "Fixing the Healthcare Supply Chain." Apr. 2004. http://hbswk.hbs.edu/item.jhtml?id=4036&t=dispatch.

15. Smeltzer, L., and Ramanathan, V. "Supply Chain Management: Can Progressive Manufacturing Practices Be Used by Health Care Providers?" Health Sector Supply Chain Initiatives working paper no. 1, W. P. Carey School of Business, Arizona State University, 2002.

16. In an environment increasingly characterized by direct-to-patient marketing, this factor may well change. As discussed later in the book, there is increased activity by manufacturers of costly clinical items, including orthopedic implants and cardiac implants, to influence patient preference.

17. Dennis, M., and Wolf, A. "New Business Models in Service Management, Accenture Supply Chain Management Practice." Apr. 15, 2001. http://www.ascet.com/documents.asp?d_ID=526.

18. Leenders and Fearon, *Purchasing and Supply Management*, p. 7.

19. Luke, Walston, and Plummer, *Healthcare Strategy*.

20. Moncza, R., Trent, R., and Handfield, R. *Purchasing and Supply Chain Management*. Cincinnati, Ohio: South-Western Publishers, 2002, p. 15.

21. Moncza, Trent, and Handfield, *Purchasing and Supply Chain Management*, p. 15.

22. Moncza, Trent, and Handfield, *Purchasing and Supply Chain Management*, p. 15.

23. Moncza, Trent, and Handfield, *Purchasing and Supply Chain Management*, p. 11.

24. Harland, C., Lamming, M., Richard, C., and Cousins, P. D. "Developing the Concept of Supply Strategy." *International Journal of Operations and Production Management*, 1999, *19*(7), 663.

25. Harland, Lamming, and Cousins, "Developing the Concept of Supply Strategy," p. 663.

26. Drucker, P. F. *Managing the Non-Profit Organization*. New York: HarperBusiness, 1990.

27. Luke, Walston, and Plummer, *Healthcare Strategy*, p. 15.

28. Burns, *The Health Care Value Chain*.

29. Schneller, E. S., and Smeltzer, L. "Becoming Strategic/Being Ethical." Paper presented at the annual meeting of HCA, New Orleans, La., June 2004.

30. Leenders and Fearon, *Purchasing and Supply Management*, p. 68.

31. Leenders and Fearon, *Purchasing and Supply Management*, p. 68.

32. For an excellent discussion of the factors related to translating vision, values, and mission into strategy, see Luke, Walston, and Plummer, *Healthcare Strategy*.

33. See Study 1, "The Value of Group Purchasing in the Health Care Supply Chain."

34. Bolman, L. G., and Deal, T. *Reframing Organizations: Artistry, Choice and Leadership*. San Francisco: Jossey-Bass, 1997.

35. Smeltzer, L., and Manship, J. "How Good Are Your Cost Reduction Measures?" *Supply Chain Management Review*, May 2003, pp. 28–33.

36. Arndt and Bigelow, "The Transfer of Business Practices into Hospitals: History and Implications."

37. Harland, Lamming, Richard, and Cousins, "Developing the Concept of Supply Strategy."

38. Schneller, E. S., Harland, C., Knight, L., and Forrest, S. "Systems of Exchange and Health Sector Purchasing in the United Kingdom and the United States." Paper presented at the Eighth International Conference on System Science in Health Care (Health Care Systems: Public and Private Management), Geneva, Switzerland, Sept. 2004.

39. Saunders, C., quoted in Werner, C. "The Supply Chain Beast: Hospitals Slowly Coming to Grips with Importance of Supply Chain Strategies That Work." *FirstMoves*, July 2004.

40. Saunders, quoted in Werner, "The Supply Chain Beast."

41. Harland, Lamming, Richard, and Cousins, "Developing the Concept of Supply Strategy," p. 663.

42. Luthans, F., and Stewart, T. I. "A General Contingency Theory of Management." *Academy of Management Review*, 1977, *2*(2), 181–195.

43. Bolman, L. G., and Deal, T. E. *Reframing Organizations: Artistry, Choice, and Leadership.* San Francisco: Jossey-Bass, 1997.

44. For a better understanding of the concept of strategic fit, see Venkatraman, N. "The Concept of Fit in Strategy Research: Toward Verbal and Statistical Correspondence." *Academy of Management Review*, 1989, *14*(3), 423–444. Venkatraman, N., and Camillis, J. C. "Exploring the Concept of Fit in Strategic Management." *Academy of Management Review*, 1984, *9*(3), 513–525. Zajac, E. J., Kraatz, M. S., and Bressler, R.K.F. "Modeling the Dynamics of Strategic Fit: A Normative Approach to Strategic Change." *Strategic Management Journal*, 2000, *21*(4), 429–453.

45. Kohn, L., Corrigan, J. M., and Donaldson, M. S. (eds.). *To Err Is Human: Building a Safer Health System.* Washington, D.C.: National Academy Press, 2000.

46. Simchi-Levi, D., Kaminsky, P., and Simchi-Levi, E. *Designing and Managing the Supply Chain: Concepts, Strategies, and Case Studies.* New York: Irwin/McGraw-Hill, 2000.

47. Lee, H. L. "The Triple-A Supply Chain." Harvard Business School Case 8096, 2004.

48. Fine, C. *Clockspeed.* New York: HarperCollins, 1998, p. 12.

49. Miller, D., and Whitney, J. O. "Beyond Strategy: Configuration as a Pillar of Competitive Advantage." *Business Horizons*, 1999, *42*(3), 5–19.

50. Fine, *Clockspeed.*

51. Smeltzer and Ramanathan, "Supply Chain Management."

Chapter Two

1. Young, R. D. "Knowledge Management in Supply." Business briefing. Denver: Pharmatech, 2003, p. 4.

2. Coase, R. H. "The Nature of the Firm." *Economica*, 1937, *4*(16), 386–405, cited in A. T. Kronman and R. A. Posner (eds.), *The Economics of Contract Law.* New York: Little, Brown, 1979.

3. Williamson, O. E. "Transaction-Cost Economics: The Governance of Contractual Relations." *Journal of Law and Economics*, 1979, *22*(2), 233–261. Williamson, O. E. "Contract Analysis: The Transaction Cost Approach." In P. Burrows and C. G. Veljanovski (eds.), *The Economic Approach to Law.* Burlington, Mass.: Butterworth, 1981.

4. Tsang, E.W.K. "Transaction Cost and Resource-Based Explanations of Joint Ventures: A Comparison and Synthesis." *Organization Studies*, 2000, *21*(1), 215–242.

5. Buczynski, M. "Uncovering the Total Cost of Ownership of Storage Management." *Computer Technology Review*, 2002, *22*(1), 45–46.

6. Handfield, R., and Ernst, L. *Supply Chain Redesign: Transforming Supply Chains into Integrated Value Systems.* Upper Saddle River, N.J.: Prentice Hall, 2002.

7. "Cost of Ownership: New Ways to Calculate Costs." 2004. http://www.steelcase.com/na/knowledgedesign.aspx?f=10255&c=10903case.

8. Smeltzer, L. R., and Siferd, S. "Proactive Supply Management: The Management of Risk." *International Journal of Purchasing and Materials Management*, 1998, *34*, 38–45.

9. Yates, J. F., and Stone, E. R. "The Risk Construct." In J. Yates (ed.), *Risk Taking Behavior.* New York: Wiley, 1992.

10. Zsidisin, G. A., and Ellram, L. M. "An Agency Theory Investigation of Supply Risk Management." *Journal of Supply Chain Management,* 2003, *39*(3), 15–29.

11. Clouse, M., and Busch, J. "How to Identify and Manage Supply Risk." Oct. 2003. http://www.supplychainplanet.com/e_article000195015.cfm.

12. Barlow, R. D. "Team CS Captures 'Heart and Soul' of Virginia Mason." *Healthcare Purchasing News,* Dec. 2004, pp. 10–12.

13. Young, "Knowledge Management in Supply."

14. Schneller, E. S. *The Value of Group Purchasing.* Tempe: W. P. Carey School of Business, Arizona State University, 2000.

15. Ellram, L. M., and Carr, A. S. "Strategic Purchasing: A History and Review of the Literature." *International Journal of Purchasing and Materials Management,* 1994, *30*(2), 10–18.

16. Smeltzer, L. R., Manship, J., and Rosetti, C. L. "An Analysis of the Integration of Strategic Sourcing and Negotiation." *Journal of Supply Chain Management,* 2003, *39*(4), 16–25. Since the focus of this chapter is on strategic sourcing, issues pertaining to a final stage, supplier management, are not discussed.

17. The use of quadrants to scrutinize product categories and other aspects of supply chain can be traced to Kraljic, P. "Purchasing Must Become Supply Management." *Harvard Business Review,* 1983, *61*(5), 109–117. Cavinato, J. L. "The Quadrant Approach to Effective 1990s Procurement and Supply." *ARDC Spectrum,* 1993, *1*(1), 1–6.

18. Enthoven, A. "On the Ideal Market Structure for Third Party Purchasing of Health Care." *Social Science and Medicine,* 1994, *39*(10), 1413–1424.

19. Minahan, T., and Degnan, C. *Best Practices in Spending Analysis: Cure for a Corporate Epidemic.* Boston: Aberdeen Group, 2004.

20. Handfield, R., and Nichols, E. *Supply Chain Redesign: Transforming Supply Chains into Integrated Systems.* Upper Saddle River, N.J.: Prentice Hall, 2002, p. 213.

21. Sitt, W. "Patient Satisfaction and Clinical Excellence: A Materials Management Perspective." *Healthcare Purchasing News,* Dec. 2004, pp. 57–58.

22. A commodity is "a logical grouping of inventory based upon user-defined characteristics" (http://accuracybook.com/glossary.htm). Different industries define commodity classifications differently. For example, one industry may have a classification of building materials that encompasses anything that could be used to describe all construction materials, while another industry may have separate commodity classifications for framing lumber, decking materials, fasteners, and concrete products. In the health sector, *commodity* generally refers to items that are purchased at the discretion of the supply management staff. Broadlane, a group purchasing organization, distinguishes among health products as follows: low-volume commodities, such as soaps and slippers; high-volume commodities, such as IVs and custom packs; and clinical preference items, such as pacemakers and stents (http://www.broadlane.com/res/res_3.html).

23. Broadlane. "Frequently Asked Questions About Broadlane." http://www.broadlane.com/res/res_3.html. 2004.

24. Handfield, R. B., and Nichols E. Z. *Introduction to Supply Chain Management.* Upper Saddle River, N.J.: Prentice Hall, 1999.

25. Handfield and Nichols, *Introduction to Supply Chain Management,* pp. 126–127.

26. Handfield and Nichols, *Introduction to Supply Chain Management,* pp. 269–271.

27. Smeltzer, L. R., and Ogden, J. A. "Purchasing Professionals' Perceived Differences Between Purchasing Materials and Purchasing Services." *Journal of Supply Chain Management,* 2002, *38*(1), 54–70. Beall, S., and others. *The Role of Reverse Auctions in Strategic Sourcing.* Tempe,

Ariz.: CAPS Research, 2003; Smeltzer, L., and Carr, A. "Electronic Reverse Auctions: Promises, Risks and Conditions for Success." *Industrial Marketing Management*, 2000, *32*(4), 481–488. Smeltzer, L., and Carr, A. "Reverse Auctions in Industrial Marketing and Buying." *Business Horizons*, 2002, *45*(2), 470–520.

28. Porter, M. *Competitive Strategy: Techniques for Analyzing Industries and Competitors*. New York: Free Press, 1980.

29. Steele, P. T., and Court, B. H. *Profitable Purchasing Strategies: A Manager's Guide for Improving Organizational Competitiveness Through the Skills of Purchasing*. New York: McGraw-Hill, 1996.

30. These strategies are described in Handfield and Nichols, *Introduction to Supply Chain Management*, and Steele and Court, *Profitable Purchasing Strategies*.

31. Lambert, D., Adams, R., and Emmelhanz, M. "Supplier Selection Criteria in the Health-care Industry: A Comparison of Importance and Performance." *Journal of Supply Chain Management*, 1997, *33*(1), 16–22.

32. Ellram, L. M. *Total Cost Modeling in Purchasing*. Tempe, Ariz.: Center for Advanced Purchasing Studies, 1994.

33. Donohue, W. A., and Roberto, A. J. "An Empirical Investigation of Three Models of Integrative and Distributive Bargaining." *International Journal of Conflict Management*, 1996, *7*(3), 209–299.

34. Smeltzer, L. R., Manship, J., and Rosetti, C. L. "An Analysis of the Integration of Strategic Sourcing and Negotiation." *Journal of Supply Chain Management*, 2003, *39*(4),16–25.

35. Cyert, R., and March, J. *A Behavioral Theory of the Firm*. Upper Saddle River, N.J.: Prentice Hall, 1963.

36. Goldschmidt, H. J., Mann, M. H., and Weston, F. J. (eds.). *Industrial Concentration: The New Learning*. New York: Little, Brown, 1974.

Chapter Three

1. Iorio, R., and Healy, W. "Economic Concerns in Total Joint Arthroplasty: Problems and Solutions." *Medscape General Practice Medicine*, 1999, *1*(1). www.medscape/iewarticle/408479_pring?WebLogicSession=Py1k1tMTfMh.

2. Kowalski-Dickow Associates. *Managing Hospital Materials Management*. Chicago: American Hospital Publishers, 1994, p. 290.

3. Freidson, E. *Profession of Medicine: A Study of the Sociology of Applied Knowledge*. New York: HarperCollins, 1970.

4. Kohn, L. T., Corrigan, J. M., and Donaldson, M. S. (eds.). *To Err Is Human: Building a Safer Health System*. Washington, D.C.: National Academy Press, 2000.

5. Jones, J. "Medical Device Manufacturer Relationships." *Physician's News Digest*, Mar. 2005. http://www.physiciansnews.com/law/305jones.html.

6. Such involvement appears to be key for supply chain management in the United States as well as in national systems where physicians are employees of the system itself. NHS. *Working with Clinical Networks*. Version 3. 2002.

7. Murphy, J. "Value Analysis: An RX in Healthcare." *Purchasing Today*, Mar. 2000, p. 55.

8. Hesson, D. "Achieving Supply Chain Savings When You Least Expect It." *Healthcare Purchasing News*, Aug. 2004, p. 24.

9. Mintzberg, H. *The Structuring of Organizations*. Upper Saddle River, N.J.: Prentice Hall, 1979.

10. Pauley, M. V. *Doctors and Their Workshops: Economic Model of Physician Behavior.* Chicago: University of Chicago Press, 1980.

11. Omachonu, V. K. *Healthcare Performance Improvement.* Norcross, Ga.: Engineering and Management Press, 1988.

12. Schneller, E. S., and Epstein, K. R. *The Hospitalist Movement in the United States: Agency and Common Agency Issues.* Tempe: W. P. Carey School of Business, Arizona State University, 2004.

13. TheOrthoPeople. "Direct-to Consumer Education and Marketing in Orthopaedics: Perspectives from Surgeon and Consumer." 2000. http://www.orthoworld.com/knowledge/pubs/surveydtc0005h.htm.

14. Freidson, E. *Profession of Medicine: A Study in the Sociology of Applied Knowledge.* New York: Dodd, Mead, 1968.

15. Schön, D. *The Reflective Practitioner.* New York: Basic Books. 1983.

16. McGlynn, E. A., and others. "The Quality of Health Care Delivered to Adults in the United States." *New England Journal of Medicine,* 2003, *348*(26), 2635–2645.

17. Alford, J. M. "The People Mix." *Air University Review,* 1976, *27*(4), 2.

18. Gouldner, A. W. "Cosmopolitans and Locals: Toward an Analysis of Latent Social Roles." *Administrative Sciences Quarterly,* 1957, *2*(3), 281–306. Kornhauser, W. *Scientists in Industry: Conflict and Accommodation.* Berkeley: University of California Press, 1962.

19. Katz, R., and Allen, T. J. "Managing Dual Ladder Systems in RD&E Settings." In R. Katz (ed.), *The Human Side of Managing Technological Innovation.* New York: Oxford University Press, 2004.

20. Winkless, T., Pedler, M., and Mascie-Taylor, H. "Doctors and Dilemmas." In D. Sanderson and J. Brown (eds.), *Managing Medicine: A Survival Guide.* London: Financial Times Health Care, Maple House, 1997.

21. Winkless, Pedler, and Mascie-Taylor, "Doctors and Dilemmas."

22. Winkless, Pedler, and Mascie-Taylor, "Doctors and Dilemmas."

23. Winkless, Pedler, and Mascie-Taylor, "Doctors and Dilemmas."

24. Committee for Evaluating Medical Technologies in Clinical Use. *Assessing Medical Technologies.* Washington, D.C.: National Academy Press, 1985. Also see Rodgers, E. *Diffusion of Innovations.* New York: Free Press 1983.

25. Winkless, Pedler, and Mascie-Taylor, "Doctors and Dilemmas."

26. Schneller, E. S. "The Physician Executive: Role in the Adaptation of American Medicine." *Health Care Management Review,* 1997, *22*(2), 90–96.

27. Schneller, "The Physician Executive."

28. Neumann, L. "Streamlining the Supply Chain." *Healthcare Financial Management,* 2003, *57*(7), 56–62.

29. Gouldner, A. W. "Cosmopolitans and Locals." Kornhauser, *Scientists in Industry.*

30. Saner, R., and Yiu, L. "Challenges of the Twenty-First Century for Leadership Qualifications: Reflections and Responses." *Asian Journal of Public Administration,* 2000, *22*(1), 75–89.

31. Commodities in the hospital arena constitute undifferentiated items for which there may be several equivalencies in the marketplace. The training and deployment costs associated with conversion from one manufacturer to another are usually fairly low, with changes in products and vendors causing few disruptions.

32. Katzenbach, J. R., and Smith, D. K. "The Discipline of Teams." *Harvard Business Review,* 1993, *71*(2), 111–120.

33. Katzenbach and Smith, "The Discipline of Teams."

34. Lewin Group. "The Clinical Review Process Conducted by Group Purchasing Organizations and Health Systems." Arlington, Va.: Health Industry Group Purchasing Association, Apr. 2002.

35. Katz, R. "Managing Creative Performance in R&D Teams." In R. Katz (ed.), *The Human Side of Managing Technological Innovation*. New York: Oxford University Press, 2004, p. 168.

36. Cap Gemini Ernst and Young. *The New Road to System Profitability: Realizing the Opportunity in the Health Care Supply Chain*. New York: Cap Gemini Ernst and Young, Feb. 2001.

37. See Study 1, "The Value of Group Purchasing in the Health Care Supply Chain."

38. Alexander, J. A., and others. "The Ties That Bind: Interorganizational Linkages and Physician-System Alignment." *Medical Care*, 2001, *39*(7), I-30–I-45.

39. VHA. "Engaging Physicians in Supply Cost Reduction." 2002. www.vha.com.

40. Pettigrew, A. "On Studying Organizational Cultures." *Administrative Science Quarterly*, 1979, *24*, 570–581.

41. Deal, T., and Kennedy, A. *Corporate Cultures: The Rites and Rituals of Corporate Life*. Reading, Mass.: Addison-Wesley, 1982.

42. Deal and Kennedy, *Corporate Cultures*, p. 183.

43. Mohr, P. E., Newman, P. J., and Bausch, S. "Paying for New Medical Technology: Lessons for the Medicare Program from Other Large Health Care Purchasers." Washington, D.C.: Project Hope Center for Health Affairs, 2002, p. 16.

44. Healthcare Financial Management Association. *Resource Management: The Healthcare Supply Chain Survey Results*. Chicago: Health Care Financial Management Association, 2002.

45. Cap Gemini Ernst and Young. *The New Road to System Profitability*.

46. Cox, A., Lonsdale, C., Watson, G., and Sanderson, J. *Business Relationships for Competitive Advantage: Managing Alignment and Misalignment in Buyer and Supplier Transactions*. London: Palgrave Macmillan, 2004.

47. NHS. *Working with Clinical Networks*. Version 3. 2002.

48. Cox, A., Sanderson, J., and Watson, G. *Power Regimes: Mapping the DNA of Business and Supply Chain Relations*. Winteringham, UK: Earlsgate Press, 2000.

49. There is very little published literature on how physicians choose products. This section draws heavily on the OrthoPeople study: "Direct-to Consumer Education and Marketing in Orthopaedics."

50. TheOrthoPeople. "Direct-to Consumer Education and Marketing in Orthopaedics."

51. TheOrthoPeople. "Direct-to Consumer Education and Marketing in Orthopaedics."

52. VHA, *Engaging Physicians in Supply Cost Reduction*.

53. Akridge, J. "Orthopedic Strategies: Implanting Clinical Cooperation for Cost Savings." *Healthcare Purchasing News*, 2000, *28*(2), 28–29.

54. TheOrthoPeople, "Direct-to Consumer Education and Marketing in Orthopaedics."

55. The ASU/CHMR study participants secured a vast majority of these commodity items through GPOs, which, as described in the next chapter, act as the purchasing agents for many hospitals in the United States. In some instances, hospitals, believing that they can use their volume to influence prices, may engage the marketplace independently or in concert with the GPO. While there is evidence that hospitals engage in a substantial amount of comparative pricing on such items, progressive systems appear to reduce the time and effort associated with the purchase of such products.

56. VHA, *Engaging Physicians in Supply Cost Reduction*.

57. Singh, A., and Schneller, E. S. "The Role of the Physician Executive in Managing the Health Care Value Chain." *Hospital Quarterly*, Fall 2000, pp. 38–43.

58. Conrad, D. A., and Christianson, J. B. "Penetrating the 'Black Box': Financial Incentives for Enhancing the Quality of Physician Services." *Medical Care Research and Review*, 2004, *61*(3), 37S–68S.

59. Institute of Medicine. *Crossing the Quality Chasm: A New Health System for the Twenty-First Century.* Washington, D.C.: National Academy Press, 2001.

60. Harland, C., and Knight, L. A. "Supply Network Strategy: Role and Competence Requirements." *International Journal of Operations and Production Management,* 2001, *21*(4), 476–489.

61. Akridge, "Orthopedic Strategies."

62. Meltzer, L. R., and Ogden, J. A. "Purchasing Professionals' Perceived Differences Between Purchasing Materials and Purchasing Services." *Journal of Supply Chain Management,* 2002, *38*(1), 54–70. Beall, S., and others. *The Role of Reverse Auctions in Strategic Sourcing.* Tempe, Ariz.: Center for Advanced Purchasing Studies, 2003; Smeltzer, L., and Carr, A. "Electronic Reverse Auctions: Promises, Risks and Conditions for Success." *Industrial Marketing Management,* 2000, *32*(4), 481–488. Smeltzer, L., and Carr, A. "Reverse Auctions in Industrial Marketing and Buying." *Business Horizons,* 2002, *45*(2), 470–520.

Chapter Four

1. Zsidisin, G. "Managerial Perceptions of Supply Risk." *Journal of Supply Management,* 2003, *39*(1), 14–25.

2. At the time this book was written, the Medical Device Competition Act of 2004 (S. 2880) was introduced for consideration by Senators Mike DeWine (R-Ohio) and Herb Kohl (D-Wisconsin), chairman and ranking member, respectively, of the U.S. Senate Judiciary Subcommittee on Antitrust, Competition Policy and Consumer Rights. The bill was designed to increase GPO oversight and develop a set of rules and regulations to shape GPO marketplace behavior. This act was vigorously opposed by the Health Industry Group Purchasing Association of Arlington, Virginia, and many other key stakeholders, including hospitals. Although this bill did not gain traction, it is a signal of increased interest in regulating the GPO industry.

3. Nollet, J., and Beaulieu, M. "The Development of Group Purchasing: An Empirical Study in the Healthcare Sector." *Journal of Purchasing and Supply Management,* 2003, *9*(1), 3–10.

4. Anderson, M. G., and Katz, P. B. "Strategic Sourcing." *Internal Journal of Logistics Management,* 1998, *9*(1), 1–13.

5. Schneller, E. S., Harland, C., Knight, L., and Forrest, S. "Systems of Exchange and Health Sector Purchasing in the United Kingdom and the United States." Paper presented at the Eighth International Conference on System Science in Health Care (Health Care Systems: Public and Private Management), Geneva, Switzerland, Sept. 2004.

6. Schneller, Harland, Knight, and Forrest, "Systems of Exchange in the United Kingdom and the United States."

7. Williamson, O. E. "Transaction Cost Economics: How It Works and Where It Is Headed." *DE Economist,* 1998, *146*(1), 23–58.

8. Health Industry Group Purchasing Association. "GPOs Provide Measurable Savings to Health Care Providers," press release, May 21, 2003.

9. Muse & Associates. *The Role of Group Purchasing in the Health Care System and the Impact on Public Health Care Expenditures If Additional Restrictions Are Imposed on GPO Contracting Processes.* Arlington, Va.: Health Industry Group Purchasing Association, Mar. 2000.

10. Muse & Associates, *The Role of Group Purchasing.* Betz, R. Testimony before the U.S. Congress, Joint Hearings on Health Care and Competition Law and Policy on Group Purchasing Organizations, Sept. 26, 2003.

11. Hewitt, D. "The Consortium Option." *Purchasing and Supply Management,* Jan. 1995, p. 32, cited in Leenders, M. R., and Fearon, H. E. *Purchasing and Supply Management.* New York: Irwin/McGraw-Hill, 1998.

12. Group purchasing as an alliance strategy to bring together hospitals to aggregate volume is not limited to the investor-owned and nonprofit sector group purchasing organizations. The Veterans Administration, for example, has established a national formulary for pharmaceuticals, has engaged widely in standardization for the purpose of purchasing, and engages the marketplace in many ways that resemble large purchasing organizations. Although the VA is not formally a GPO, it behaves much like a GPO as it accrues the desires and commitments of its members to address the marketplace.

13. Hendrick, T. E. *Horizontal Alliances Among Firms Buying Common Goods and Services: What? Who? Why? How?* Tempe, Ariz.: Center for Advanced Purchasing Studies, 1997.

14. Plummer, M. "Collaborative GPO/IDN Relationships." Paper presented at the NCI, IDN Summit Expo, Scottsdale, Ariz., Oct. 2004.

15. Lewin Group. "The Clinical Review Process Conducted by Group Purchasing Organizations and Health Systems." Arlington, Va.: Health Industry Group Purchasing Association, Apr. 2002.

16. Burns, L. R. *The Health Care Value Chain.* San Francisco: Jossey-Bass, 2002.

17. Schneller, E. S. *The Value of Group Purchasing.* Tempe: W. P. Carey School of Business, Arizona State University, 2000.

18. Becker, C. "Hanging Tough." *Modern Healthcare,* Aug. 16, 2004, p. 22.

19. Ben Nur, A. "Task Force Report: Outsourcing for Nonprofit Organizations." N.d. http:.www.nationalcne.org/outsourcing.htm.

20. Handfield, R. B., and Nichols, E. L., Jr. *Supply Chain Redesign: Transforming Supply Chains into Integrated Value Systems.* Upper Saddle River, N.J.: Prentice Hall, 2002.

21. Ben Nur, "Task Force Report."

22. Williamson, "Transaction Cost Economics."

23. Williamson, "Transaction Cost Economics."

24. Schneller, E. S., and Williams, F. "Contract Management Requires Strategic Planning." *Healthcare Financial Management,* 1988, *43*(3), 56–61.

25. Harland, C., and Knight, L. "Supply Strategy: A Corporate Social Capital Perspective." *Research in the Sociology of Organizations,* 2001, *18,* 153.

26. Anderson and Katz, "Strategic Sourcing."

27. Figure adapted from Figure 2.6 in Chopra, S., and Meindl, P. *Supply Chain Management: Strategy, Planning and Operations.* Upper Saddle River, N.J.: Prentice Hall, 2004, p. 28.

28. Plummer, "Collaborative GPO/IDN Relationships."

29. The term *alliance* is used here to reflect the relationship between the GPO and this hospital or system. Some GPOs consider themselves to be "alliances" of multiple members that bring value by their affinity of interests and interaction. Others GPOs see those with whom they act as purchasing partners to be clients or customers rather than members of an alliance. The term *alliance* has not been employed in this manner in the chapter.

30. For a discussion of agency relationships, see Jensen, M. C., and Meckling, W. "Theory of the Firm: Managerial Behavior, Agency Costs, and Ownership Structure." *Journal of*

Financial Economics, 1983, *11,* 5–50, and Bergemann, D., and Valimaki, J. "Dynamic Common Agency." *Journal of Economic Theory,* 2003, *111*(1), 23–48.

31. Clouse, M., and Busch, J. "How to Identify and Manage Supply Risk Part 1." 2003. http://www.supplychainplanet.com/e_article000195015.cfm.

32. Handfield, R. B., and Nichols, E. L., Jr. *Supply Chain Redesign: Transforming Supply Chains into Integrated Value Systems.* Upper Saddle River, N.J.: Prentice Hall, 2002.

33. Handfield and Nichols, *Supply Chain Redesign.*

34. Luke, R. D., Walston, S. L., and Plummer, P. M. *Healthcare Strategy: In Pursuit of Competitive Advantage.* Chicago: Health Administration Press, 2004.

35. Mayer, R. C., Davis, J. H., and Schoorman, F. D. "An Integrative Model of Organizational Trust." *Academy of Management Review,* 1995, *20,* p. 715.

36. O'Hara, K. *Trust: From Socrates to Spin.* Cambridge: Icon Books, 2004. Hardin, R., Levi, M., Moe, M., and Buckley, T. "The Transaction Costs of Distrust: Labor and Management at the National Labor Relations Board." In K. Hardin (ed.), *Distrust.* New York: Russell Sage Foundation, 2004.

37. Handfield and Nichols, *Supply Chain Redesign,* pp. 164–169.

38. Handfield and Nichols, *Supply Chain Redesign,* p. 164.

39. Handfield and Nichols, *Supply Chain Redesign,* p. 164.

40. Handfield and Nichols, *Supply Chain Redesign.*

41. For more information on the GPO controversy, see Walsh, M. W. "When a Buyer for Hospitals Has a Stake in Drugs It Buys," *New York Times,* Mar. 26, 2002.

42. *Core competency* is defined as "the collective learning in the organization, especially how to coordinate diverse production skills and integrate multiple streams of technology." Monczka, R., Trent, R. J., and Handfield, R. B. *Purchasing and Supply Chain Management.* Cincinnati, Ohio: South-Western Publishers, 2002.

43. Nollet and Beaulieu, "The Development of Group Purchasing," p. 10.

44. Cox, A., and Thompson, I. "On the Appropriateness of Benchmarking." *Journal of General Management,* 1998, *23*(3), p. 2.

45. It is important to recognize that not all hospitals or systems are of sufficient size to assist GPOs in building volume commitments and, given the organization of the medical staff, not all are able to secure consensus on standardization. These systems report valuing the knowledge that GPO product analysis provides their physicians and report that they especially benefit from GPOs that carefully engage in product selection.

46. See Study 1, "The Value of Group Purchasing in the Health Care Supply Chain."

47. *Healthcare Purchasing News Online,* Sept. 30, 2003.

48. Handfield and Nichols, *Supply Chain Redesign,* p. 235.

49. Handfield and Nichols, *Supply Chain Redesign,* p. 236.

50. Scanlon, W. J. "Group Purchasing Organizations: Pilot Study Suggest Large Buying Groups Do Not Always Offer Hospitals Lower Prices." Testimony before the Subcommittee on Antitrust, Competition, and Business and Consumer Rights, Committee on the Judiciary, U.S. Senate, Apr. 30, 2002.

51. Scanlon, "Group Purchasing Organizations."

52. Schneller, *The Value of Group Purchasing.*

53. Muse and Associates, *The Role of Group Purchasing.*

54. Gorlin, R. A. (ed.). *Codes of Professional Responsibility: Ethics Standards in Business, Health and Law.* (4th ed.) Washington, D.C.: Bureau of National Affairs, 1999.

55. Mendes, E., and Mehmet, O. *Global Governance, Economy and Law: Waiting for Justice.* New York: Routledge, 2003. Also see Mendes, E. P., and Clark, J. A. "Five Generations of

Corporate Codes of Conduct and Their Impact on Corporate Social Responsibility." Human Rights Research and Education Center, Sept. 1996. http://www.uottawa.ca/hrrec/publicat/five.html.

56. Mendes and Clark, "Five Generations of Corporate Codes of Conduct and Their Impact on Corporate Social Responsibility."

57. Mendes and Clark, "Five Generations of Corporate Codes of Conduct and Their Impact on Corporate Social Responsibility."

58. Handfield and Nichols, *Supply Chain Redesign.*

59. Harland and Knight, "Supply Strategy."

Chapter Five

1. Simchi-Levi, D., Kaminsky, P., and Simchi-Levi, E. *Managing the Supply Chain: The Definitive Guide for the Business Professional.* New York: McGraw-Hill 2004, p. 4.

2. Efficient Healthcare Consumer Response. *Improving the Efficiency of the Healthcare Supply Chain.* Chicago: American Society for Healthcare Materials Management, 1996.

3. Burns, L. R., and DeGraaff, R. A. "Role of Wholesalers and Distributors." In L. R. Burns, *The Health Care Value Chain.* San Francisco: Jossey-Bass, 2000, p. 137.

4. Marchula, D., and Shannon, E. G. *eHealth B2B Overview.* Minneapolis: Piper Jaffray Equity Research, 2000.

5. Study 1 or Schneller, E. *The Value of Group Purchasing.* Tempe: Arizona State University, 2000.

6. McFadden, C. D., and Leahy, T. *U.S. Healthcare Distribution: Positioning the Health Care Supply Chain for the Twenty-First Century.* New York: Goldman Sachs, Jan. 20, 2000.

7. Fine, C. H. *Clockspeed: Winning Industry Control in the Age of Temporary Advantage.* New York: Basic Books, 1998, p. 89

8. Fine, *Clockspeed.*

9. Fine, *Clockspeed.*

10. Burns and Degraaff, "Role of Wholesalers and Distributors."

11. Burns and Degraaff, "Role of Wholesalers and Distributors."

12. Burns, L. R., and DeGraaff, R. A. "Threats of Disintermediation Facing Distributors." In L. R. Burns, *The Health Care Value Chain.* San Francisco: Jossey-Bass, 2000.

13. Burns and DeGraaff, "Threats of Disintermediation Facing Distributors."

14. Chopra, S., and Meindl, P. *Supply Chain Management: Strategy, Planning and Operations.* Upper Saddle River, N.J.: Prentice Hall, 2004.

15. Cardinal Corporate. One Partner. 2004. http://www.cardinal.com/ar2004/comp1b.asp.

16. Schneller, E. S. *Request for Proposals for the Health Sector Supply Chain Research Consortium.* Tempe: Arizona State University, 2005.

17. Leenders, M. R., and Fearon, H. E. *Purchasing and Supply Management.* New York: Irwin/McGraw-Hill, 1997, p. 206.

18. Schonberger, R. J. "Selecting the Right Manufacturing Inventory System: Western and Japanese Approaches." *Production and Inventory Management Journal,* 2nd quarter 1983, pp. 33–44.

19. Quinn, J. B. *Strategies for Change.* Homewood, Ill.: Irwin, 1980.

20. Frazelle, E. *Supply Chain Strategy.* New York: McGraw-Hill, 2002.

21. Frazelle, *Supply Chain Strategy.*

22. Leenders and Fearon, *Purchasing and Supply Management.*

23. Leenders and Fearon, *Purchasing and Supply Management,* p. 196.

24. Leenders and Fearon, *Purchasing and Supply Management.*

25. Hugos, M. *Essentials of Supply Chain Management.* New York: Wiley, 2003.

26. McFaddan and Lehay, *U.S. Healthcare Distribution,* p. 26.

27. Burns and DeGraaff, "Threats of Disintermediation Facing Distributors."

28. Burns and DeGraaff, "Threats of Disintermediation Facing Distributors."

29. Everard, L. J. "Defining Value in the Healthcare Supply Chain." *FirstMoves,* 2003, *3*(3), 9.

30. Hill, C.W.L., and Jones, G. R. *Strategic Management Theory.* (5th ed.) Boston: Houghton Mifflin, 2001.

31. Quinn, J. B., and Hilmer, F. G. "Strategic Outsourcing." *Sloan Management Review,* 1994, *35,* 43–55.

32. Stalk, E., and Shulman, L. E. "Competing on Capabilities: The New Rules of Corporate Strategy." *Harvard Business Review,* 1992, *70,* 57–69.

33. Ramsey, J., "Power Measurement." *European Journal of Purchasing and Supply Management,* 1996, *2*(2), 129–143.

34. Rem Associates. "Distributors: The Key Link in the Supply Chain." Presentation at the Council of Logistics Management Annual Conference, Oct. 2001.

35. Morgan, N. J., and Anderson, J. "Turn Your Industrial Distributors into Partners." *Harvard Business Review,* Mar.-Apr. 1986, pp. 66–71.

36. Burns, L., and Pauley, M. "Integrated Delivery Networks: A Detour on the Road to Integrated Healthcare?" *Health Affairs,* 2002, *21*(4), 128–143.

37. Lynk, W. "The Creation of Economic Efficiencies in Hospital Mergers." *Journal of Health Economics,* 1995, *14,* 507–530.

38. Chopra and Meindl, *Supply Chain Management.*

39. Burns and Pauley, "Integrated Delivery Networks."

40. Marino, A., and Edwards, D. J. "Give Logistics Its Own Place in the Price Equation." *Hospital Materials Management,* 1999, *24,* 10–11.

41. Simchi-Levi, Kaminsky, and Simchi-Levi, *Designing and Managing the Supply Chain.*

42. McFaddan and Leahy, *U.S. Healthcare Distribution.*

43. Lacy, R. G., and others. *The Value of eCommerce in the Healthcare Supply Chain.* New York: Andersen, 2001.

44. Barlow, R. D. "IT or Miss." *FirstMove,* 2003, *3*(1), 22–24. DeJohn, P. "Growing Pains: Glitches Mark New MMI Systems." *Hospital Materials Management,* 2001, *26,* 9.

45. Cooke, J. A. "Is XML the Next Big Thing?" *Logistics Management and Distribution Report,* 2002, *4*(5), 53.

46. Lacy and others, *The Value of eCommerce in the Healthcare Supply Chain.*

47. Besanko, D., Dranove, D., and Shanley, M. *Economics of Strategy.* New York: Wiley, 2000.

48. Burns, L. R. *The Health Care Value Chain.* San Francisco: Jossey-Bass, 2002. Marsh, L., Feinstein A., and Raskin, J. *HealthCare Information Technology and Outsourcing/Distribution Guidebook.* New York: Lehman Brothers, 2000. Hochstadt, B., and Lewis, D. *Bits of Paper to Bytes of Data: A White Paper on Healthcare Information and Internet.* San Francisco: Thomas Weisel Partners, 1999.

49. Leenders and Fearon, *Purchasing and Supply Management.*

50. Crawford, F., and Mathews, R. *The Myth of Excellence.* New York: Crown, 2001.

51. Crawford and Mathews, *The Myth of Excellence,* p. 258.

52. Simchi-Levi, Kaminsky, and Simchi-Levi, *Managing the Supply Chain.*

53. Crawford and Mathews, *The Myth of Excellence.*

54. Nonaka, I., and Takeuchi, H. *The Knowledge Creating Company.* New York: Oxford University Press, 1995. Also see Bahra, N. *Competitive Knowledge Management.* New York: Palgrave Press, 2001.

55. Schneller, *Request for Proposals for the Health Sector Supply Chain Research Consortium.*

Chapter Six

1. Chandler, A. *Strategy and Structure: Chapters in the History of the American Business Enterprise.* Cambridge, Mass.: MIT Press 1962.

2. Rogers, S. "Supply Management: Six Elements of Superior Design." *Supply Chain Management Review,* Apr. 1, 2004. http://www.manufacturing.net/scm/article/CA422114.html?stt+002&txt=steve+rogers.

3. Rogers, "Supply Management," p. 1.

4. Van de Ven, A., and Drazin, R. "The Concept of Fit in Contingency Theory." In L. Cummings and B. Staw (eds.), *Research in Organizational Behavior* (Greenwich, Conn.: JAI Press, 1985). Donaldson, L. (ed.) "Strategy and Structural Adjustment to Regain Fit and Performance: In Defense of Contingency Theory." *Journal of Management Studies,* 1987, *24,* 1–24.

5. Drucker, P. F. *Management: Tasks, Responsibilities, and Practices.* New York: HarperCollins, 1973, p. 517.

6. Herzlinger, R. *Market Driven Health Care.* Reading, Mass.: Addison-Wesley, 1997.

7. Porter, M. E. *Competitive Strategy: Techniques for Analyzing Industries and Competitors.* New York: Free Press, 1980.

8. Blackburn, R. S. "Dimensions of Structure: A Review and Reappraisal." *Academy of Management Review,* Jan. 1982, pp. 59–66.

9. Blackburn, "Dimensions of Structure."

10. Rogers, "Supply Management."

11. Rogers, "Supply Management."

12. Galbraith, J. R. *Organizational Design.* Reading, Mass.: Addison-Wesley, 1977. Huey, J. "Managing in the Midst of Chaos." *Fortune,* Apr. 5, 1993, pp. 38–48.

13. Dooley, K. "Organizational Complexity." In M. Warner (ed.), *International Encyclopedia of Business and Management.* London: Thompson Learning, 2002.

14. Fine, C. H. *Clockspeed: Winning Industry Control in the Age of Temporary Advantage.* New York: Basic Books, 1998.

15. Fine, *Clockspeed.*

16. Fine, *Clockspeed.*

17. Such observations for other industries have been made by Leenders, M., and Johnson, P. F. *Major Structural Changes in Supply Organizations.* Tempe, Ariz.: Center for Advanced Purchasing Studies, 2000. Johnson, P. F., Leenders, M., and Fearon, H. "Evolving Roles and Responsibilities of Purchasing Organizations." *International Journal of Purchasing and Materials Management,* Winter 1998, pp. 2–11.

18. Aldrich, H. *Organizations and Environments.* Upper Saddle River, N.J.: Prentice Hall, 1979.

19. Fine, *Clockspeed,* p. 103.

20. Fine, *Clockspeed,* p. 103.

21. Huey, "Managing in the Midst of Chaos."
22. Straub, C. "Chaos Theory." *Health Management Technology,* Sept. 1997. http://www. findarticles.com/p/articles/mi_m0DUD/is_n10_v18/ai_19802941.
23. Manuz, C. C., Keating, D., and Donnellon, A. "Preparing for an Organizational Change to Employee Self-Managed Teams: The Managerial Transition." *Organizational Dynamics,* Autumn 1990, pp. 15–26. Monczka, R., and Trent, R. *Cross-Functional Sourcing Team Effectiveness.* Tempe, Ariz.: Center for Advanced Purchasing Studies, 1993.
24. Adizes, I. *Corporate Lifecycles: How and Why Corporations Grow and Die and What to Do About It.* Upper Saddle River, N.J.: Prentice Hall, 1988.

Chapter Seven

1. Lummus, R., Alber, K., and Vokureka, R. J. "Self-Assessment: A Foundation for Supply Chain Success." *Supply Chain Management Review,* July-Aug. 2000, pp. 81–87.
2. Adizes, I. *Corporate Lifecycles: How and Why Corporations Grow and Die and What to Do About It.* Upper Saddle River, N.J.: Prentice Hall, 1988.
3. For a discussion of attributes of integrated delivery systems, see NCI: http://www. ncihome.com/idn_stage_list.aspt.
4. Burns, L., and Pauley, M. "Integrated Delivery Networks: A Detour on the Road to Integrated Healthcare?" *Health Affairs,* 2002, *21*(4), 128–143.
5. Burns and Pauley, "Integrated Delivery Networks," p. 131.
6. Zajac, E. J., Kraatz, M. S., and Bresser, R.F.K. "Modeling the Dynamics of Strategic Fit: A Normative Approach to Strategic Change." *Strategic Management Journal,* 2000, *21*(4), 429–455.
7. Venkatraman, N. "The Concept of Fit in Strategy Research: Toward Verbal and Statistical Correspondence." *Academy of Management Review,* 1989, *14*(3), 423–444. Venkatraman, N., and Camillus, J. C. "Exploring the Concept of Fit in Strategic Management." *Academy of Management Review,* 1984, *9*(3), 513–525. Miles, R. E., and Snow, C. C. *Fit, Failure and the Hall of Fame.* New York: Macmillan, 1994.
8. Zajac, Kraatz, and Bresser, "Modeling the Dynamics of Strategic Fit." Venkatraman and Camillus, "Exploring the Concept of Fit in Strategic Management."
9. Chopra, S., and Meindl, P. *Supply Chain Management: Strategy, Planning and Operations.* Upper Saddle River, N.J.: Prentice Hall, 2004.
10. Zajac, Kraatz, and Bresser, "Modeling the Dynamics of Strategic Fit."
11. Thallner, K. "OIG Approves Hospital-Physician Gainsharing." *Physician's News Digest,* 2001. http://www.physiciansnews.com/law/701.htm.
12. See Study 1, "The Value of Group Purchasing in the Health Care Supply Chain," and Schneller, E. S., Harland, C., Knight, L., and Forrest, S. "Systems of Exchange and Health Sector Purchasing in the United Kingdom and the United States." Paper presented at the Eighth International Conference on System Science in Health Care (Health Care Systems: Public and Private Management), Geneva, Switzerland, Sept. 2004.
13. Conrad, D. A., and Shortell, S. M. "Integrated Health Systems: Promises and Performance." *Frontiers of Health Services Management,* 1996, *13*(1), 3–42. Burda, D. "Study—Mergers Cut Costs, Services, Increase Profits." *Modern Healthcare,* 1993, *23*(60), 4. Zinn, J. S., Proenca, J., and Rosko, M. D. "Organizational and Environmental Factors in Hospital Alliance Membership and Contract Management: A Resource-Dependence Perspective." *Hospitals and Health Services Administration,* 1997, *42*(1), 67–86.

14. Zuckerman, H. S., and Kaluzny, A. D. "Strategic Alliances in Health Care: The Challenges of Cooperation." *Frontiers of Health Services Management,* 1991, *7*(3), 3–23.

15. Board on Manufacturing and Engineering Design. *Surviving Supply Chain Integration: Strategies for Small Manufacturers.* Washington, D.C.: National Academy Press, 2000.

16. Greene, J. "Mergers Monopolies." *Modern Healthcare,* 1994, *24*(49), 38–48.

17. Dranove, D., and Shanley, M. "Cost Reductions or Reputations Enhancement as Motives for Mergers: The Logic of Multi-Hospital Systems." *Strategic Management Journal,* 1995, *16*(1), 55–74.

18. Spang, H. R., Bazzoli, G., and Arnould, R. "Hospital Mergers and Savings for Consumers: Exploring New Evidence." *Health Affairs,* 2001, *20*(4), 150–158.

19. Cuellar, A. E., and Gertler, P. J. "Trends in Hospital Consolidation: The Formation of Local Systems." *Health Affairs,* 2003, *22*(6), 77–78.

20. Williamson, O. "Comparative Economic Organizations: The Analysis of Discrete Structural Alternatives." *Administrative Science Quarterly,* 1991, *36*(20), 269–296.

21. Conrad and Shortell, "Integrated Health Systems: Promises and Performance."

22. NCI. "Levels of Integration." 2004. ncihome.com/idn_stage_list.asp.

23. For a discussion of the idea of functional prerequisites, see Parsons, T. *The Social System.* New York: Free Press, 1951.

24. Schneller, E. S., Harland, C., Knight, L., and Forrest, S. "Systems of Exchange and Health Sector Purchasing in the United Kingdom and the United States." Paper presented at the Eighth International Conference on System Science in Health Care (Health Care Systems: Public and Private Management), Geneva, Switzerland, Sept. 2004.

25. Burns, L. R., Bazzoli, G. J., Dynam, L., and Douglas, R. "Managed Care, Market Stages and Integrated Delivery Systems: Is There a Relationship?" *Health Affairs,* 1998, *16,* 204–218.

26. Quinn, R. E., and Cameron, K. "Organizational Life Cycles and Shifting Criteria of Effectiveness: Some Preliminary Evidence." *Management Science,* 1983, *29,* 33–51.

27. Greiner, L. E. "Evolution and Revolution as Organizations Grow." *Harvard Business Review,* 1972, *50,* 37–46.

28. See Study 1, "The Value of Group Purchasing in the Health Care Supply Chain."

29. Ellram, L. *Total Cost of Ownership.* Tempe, Ariz.: Center for Advanced Purchasing Studies, 1993.

30. Ellram, L. M. *Total Cost Modeling in Purchasing.* Tempe, Ariz.: Center for Advanced Purchasing Studies, 1994.

31. Monczka, R., Trent, R., and Handfield, R. *Purchasing and Supply Chain Management.* (2nd ed.) Cincinnati: South-Western, 2002.

32. Speckman, R. E. "Strategic Supplier Selection: Understanding Long-Term Buyer Relationships." *Business Horizons,* 1988, *31*(4), 75–81.

33. Oliver, A. L., and Montgomery, K. "A System Cybernetic Approach to the Dynamics of Individual- and Organizational-Level Trust." *Human Relations,* 2001, *54,* 1045–1063.

34. Schein, E. H. "Organizational Culture." *American Psychologist,* 1990, *45,* 109–119.

35. Longest, B. B. Jr., Rakich, J. S., and Darr, K. *Managing Health Services Organizations and Systems.* (4th ed.) Baltimore: Health Professions Press, 2000.

36. Deal, T. E. "Healthcare Executives as Symbolic Leaders." *Healthcare Executives,* 1990, pp. 24–27.

37. Zuckerman, H. S. "Redefining the Role of the CEO: Challenges and Conflicts." *Hospital and Health Services Administration,* 1989, *34,* 35–36.

38. Kavaler, F., and Spiegel, A. D. *Risk Management in Health Care Institutions: A Strategic Approach.* Sudbury, Mass.: Jones & Bartlett, 1997.

Chapter Eight

1. Clouse, M., and Busch, J. "How to Identify and Manage Supply Risk." Oct. 2003. http://www.supplychainplanet.com/e_article000195015.cfm.

2. Zsidisin, G. "Managerial Perceptions of Supply Risk." *Journal of Supply Chain Management*, Winter 2003, pp. 14–25.

3. Chopra, S., and Meindl, P. *Supply Chain Management: Strategy, Planning, and Operations.* (2nd ed.) Upper Saddle River, N.J.: Prentice Hall, 2004.

4. Montgomery, K., and Schneller, E. Working paper on value analysis teams, May 2005.

5. PricewaterhouseCoopers. *Financial and Cost Management Team, CFO: Architect of the Corporation's Future.* New York: Wiley, 1997.

6. Deloitte and Touche. *CIO 2.0: The Changing Role of the Chief Information Officer.* New York: Deloitte Development, 2004. http://www.deloitte.com/dtt/article/0,1002,sid%253D26551%2526cid%253D65595,00.html.

7. Deloitte and Touche, *CIO 2.0.*

8. PricewaterhouseCoopers. *Financial and Cost Management Team, CFO.* Deloitte and Touche. *CIO 2.0.*

9. Johnsen, T., and others. "Networking Activities in Supply Networks." *Journal of Strategic Marketing*, 2000, *8*, 161–181.

10. Johnsen and others, "Networking Activities in Supply Networks."

11. Harland, C., and Knight, L. "Supply Network Strategy, Roles and Competence Requirements." *International Journal of Operations and Production Management*, 2001, *21*(4), 476–489.

12. Neumann, L. "Streamlining the Supply Chain." *Healthcare Financial Management*, July 2003, pp. 22–30.

13. NHS Purchasing and Supply Agency. "Developing a Research Agenda for Supply in the NHS." Reading, England: NHS Purchasing and Supply Agency, Oct. 2002.

14. "Small IDN Manages Speedy Integration, Starting with Materials Management." *Hospital Materials Management*, Dec. 3, 2002. p. 22.

15. Whitman, M. "Pyramid Power: A Plan for Continuous Materials Management Improvement." *Healthcare Purchasing News*, Jan. 2004, pp. 27–30.

16. Glassberg, T. "Integrated Supply Chains." *Delta News*, Spring 2001, p. 2.

17. HCI. "PDCA Cycle." N.d. http://www.hci.com.au/hcisite2/toolkit/pdcacycl.htm. See also Kaisen, M. I. *The Key to Japan's Competitive Success.* New York: McGraw-Hill, 1986.

18. Chopra and Meindl, *Supply Chain Management.*

19. Harland and Knight, "Supply Network Strategy, Roles and Competence Requirements."

20. Harland and Knight, "Supply Network Strategy, Roles and Competence Requirements."

21. Deloitte and Touche, *CIO 2.0.*

22. Deloitte and Touche, *CIO 2.0.*

23. Werner, C. "Thoughtful Supply Chain Management Plans Can Make a Big Difference." *Healthcare Purchasing News*, Apr. 2002. http://www.hpnonline.com/inside/apr02.html.

24. Simchi-Levi, D., Kaminsky, P., and Simchi-Levi, E. *Managing the Supply Chain: The Definitive Guide for the Business Professional.* New York: McGraw-Hill, 2004.

25. PricewaterhouseCoopers, *Financial and Cost Management Team, CFO.*

26. Temkin, B. "Preparing for the Coming Shake-Out in Online Markets." Apr. 15, 2001. http://temkin.ascet.com.

27. Burns, L. R. *The Health Care Value Chain*. San Francisco: Jossey-Bass, 2002.
28. Burns, L. R., and DeGraff, R. A. "E-Commerce in Health Care: Manufacturers, Distributors and GPOs." In L. Burns, *The Health Care Value Chain*. San Francisco: Jossey-Bass, 2002.
29. Florian, E. "IT Takes On the ER." *Fortune Magazine*, Nov. 24, 2003, p. 193.
30. Ernst & Young. "The Health Care Supply Chain Solution (SCS): The Supply Chain Advantage Driving Vision to Value." Mimeo., 1999, cited in Burns and DeGraff, "E-Commerce in Health Care," p. 367.
31. Jaklevic, M. C. "Making It Click." *Modern Healthcare*, Oct. 27, 2003, p. 24.
32. Patterson, P. "Get with the Program." *Materials Management in Health Care*, May 1998, p. 16.
33. Rauber, C. "Information, Please." *Modern Healthcare*, Mar. 29, 1999, p. 22.
34. Kowalski-Dickow Associates. *Managing Hospital Materials Management*. Chicago: American Hospital Publishers, 1994.
35. National Coordinator for Health Information Technology. *Health IT Strategic Framework Attachment 4*. Washington, D.C.: Federal Health Information Technology Programs, U.S. Department of Health and Human Services, Apr. 27, 2004. http://www.os.dhhs.gov/healthit/attachment_4.html.
36. Florian, "IT Takes On the ER."
37. Burns and DeGraff, "E-Commerce in Health Care: Manufacturers, Distributors and GPOs," p. 301. Skinner, R. "The Value of Information Technology in Healthcare." *Frontiers of Health Services Management*, 2001, *19*(3), 3–15.
38. Lieber, H. S. "Can IT Transform Healthcare?" *Frontiers of Health Services Management*, 2003, *19*(3), 31.
39. Ovretveit, J. "The Convergence of Evidence-Based Health Care and Quality Assessment." *Healthcare Review—Online*, 1998, *2*(9). http://www.enigma.co.nz/hcro/website/index.cfm?fuseaction=articledisplay&featureid=42. Kovner, A. R., Elton, J. J., and Billings, J. "Evidence Based Management." *Frontiers of Health Services Management*, 2000, *16*(4), 3–24.
40. Grol, R. "Research and Development in Quality of Care: Establishing the Research Agenda." *Quality in Health Care*, 1996, *5*, 235–242.
41. Whitman, "Pyramid Power."
42. Kaczmarek, D. "Supply Chain Managers Must Close Credibility Gap with Bosses." *FirstMoves*, July-Aug. 2002, p. 1.

Study 1

1. A GPO is an organization whose primary product or service is the development of purchasing contracts for its membership to access. GPOs derive a significant portion, if not all, of their revenue from supplier administrative fees. Their membership may be composed of affiliate subgroups and health care delivery facilities that are charged annual or monthly fees or that simply sign a membership form (in these cases, the GPO covers all of its expenses and derives all of its income from administrative fees). Their membership is typically a mixture of for-profit and nonprofit facilities, and the GPO may be national or regional in scope. HIGPA has pointed out that GPOs cover virtually everything hospitals, nursing homes, and other health care providers require, offering discounted prices on supplies and equipment related to almost every aspect of a health care facility.

2. Muse & Associates. *The Role of Group Purchasing in the Health Care System and the Impact on Public Health Care Expenditures If Additional Restrictions Are Imposed on GPO Contracting Processes.* Arlington, Va.: Health Industry Group Purchasing Association, Mar. 2000.

3. Hewitt, D. "The Consortium Option." *Purchasing and Supply Management,* Jan. 1995, p. 32, cited in Leenders, M. R., and Fearon, H. E. *Purchasing and Supply Management.* New York: McGraw-Hill, 1997, p. 69.

4. Molina, S. L. "A Cure for Contract Compliance." *Health Industry Today,* 1998, *61*(7).

5. Betz, R. "Vendor Perspectives on Compliance." *Repertoire Magazine,* 1996, *6.*

6. Hendrick, T. W. *Purchasing Consortiums: Horizontal Alliances Among Firms Buying Common Goods and Services: What? Who? Why? How?* Tempe, Ariz.: Center for Advanced Purchasing Studies, 1997.

7. Stodgill, R. II, "Attack of the Health-Care Colossus." *Business Week,* May 20, 1996, p. 40. Muse & Associates, *The Role of Group Purchasing in the Health Care System and the Impact on Public Health Care Expenditures If Additional Restrictions Are Imposed on GPO Contracting Processes.*

8. The projected increments in hospital and nursing home group purchasing will be fueled by growth in the elderly population, new technologies, the emergence of entirely new lines of pharmaceuticals, and a focus on managing the care of patients throughout episodes of care. These estimates of savings, however, are grounded in very macro measurements of the total cost of goods purchased by health care organizations and gross estimates by purchasing executives regarding savings.

9. Novation. *Marketing Supply Costs Market Research Report.* Irving, Tex.: Novation, Sept. 1999.

10. Appel, G. "The IDN/GPO Relationship: Its Evolution in an Era of Direct Contracting Advantages." *Health Strategist,* 1999, *6*(6), 2.

11. Appel, "The IDN/GPO Relationship."

12. Muse & Associates, *The Role of Group Purchasing in the Health Care System and the Impact on Public Health Care Expenditures If Additional Restrictions Are Imposed on GPO Contracting Processes,* p. 2.

13. Novation, *Marketing Supply Costs Market Research Report.*

14. G. Firestone quoted in Betz, "Vendor Perspectives on Compliance."

15. Carr, A. S., and Smeltzer, L. R. "The Relationship Among Purchasing Benchmarking, Strategic Purchasing, Firm Performance and Size." *Journal of Supply Chain Management,* Fall 1999, pp. 51–59.

16. Bogan, C., and English, M. J. *Benchmarking for Best Practices: Winning Through Innovative Adaptation.* New York: McGraw-Hill, 1994. Carr, A. S., and Smeltzer, L. R. "The Relationship of Strategic Purchasing to Supply Chain Management." *European Journal of Purchasing and Supply Management,* 1999, *5,* 43–51.

17. VHA. "West Coast Materials Management Report Card." Summer 1999.

18. Hurwich, M. R., and Lanigan, E. P. *In Vivo,* Sept.-Oct. 1999. A. T. Kearney. "Leveraging the Strategic Nature of Procurement." A. T. Kearney, 1998.

19. A. T. Kearney, "Leveraging the Strategic Nature of Procurement."

20. A. T. Kearney, "Leveraging the Strategic Nature of Procurement."

21. Schneller, E. "Healthcare System Change and the Twenty-First Century: Observations from South of the Border." *Hospital Quarterly,* Fall 1999, p. 26.

22. Schneller, "Healthcare System Change and the Twenty-First Century."

23. "E-Commerce Coming to Health Care Industry." *Wall Street Journal,* Feb. 28, 2000, p. B4.

24. Muse & Associates. *The Role of Group Purchasing in the Health Care System and the Impact on Public Health Care Expenditures If Additional Restrictions Are Imposed on GPO Contracting Processes.*

25. Sarpong, D. F. "Application of Pharmacoeconomics and Outcomes Research in Formulary Decision Making." *Drug Benefit Trends,* 1999, *11*(8), 53–57.

26. Maltz, A., and Ellram, L. "Outsourcing Supply Management." *Journal of Supply Chain Management,* Spring 1999, p. 12.
27. Maltz and Ellram, "Outsourcing Supply Management," p. 12.

Study 3

1. Metropolitan Hospital is a fictitious name for one of the large hospital systems visited during the ASU/CHMR study.
2. Zelman, W. A. *The Changing Healthcare Marketplace.* San Francisco: Jossey-Bass, 1996.
3. Dranove, D., and Shanley, M. "Cost Reductions or Reputation Enhancement as Motives for Mergers: The Logic of Multihospital Systems." *Strategic Management Journal,* 1995, *16*(10), 55–74.
4. Hill, R., Wang, J., and Nahrstedt, K. "Quantifying Non-Functional Requirements: A Process Oriented Approach." Paper presented at the Requirements Engineering Conference, Twelfth IEEE International Conference, Kyoto, Japan, Sept. 6–10, 2004.

Study 4

1. The Surgical Group performs the majority of cardiac surgery cases at the Hospital. The surgeons in the Surgical Group also practice at one other hospital in the region.
2. The Program Administrator has developed software products that measure cost, quality, and utilization on a national basis. The products are certified by both the American College of Cardiology and the Society of Thoracic Surgery.
3. The Practice Patterns Report for the Surgical Group, dated October 2004, is attached to this advisory opinion as Appendix A [redacted]. The Requestors' original submission included additional cost savings recommendations that posed an unacceptable risk of fraud and abuse. The Requestors withdrew those recommendations from the Proposed Arrangement.
4. We note that the Practice Patterns Report identifies with specificity the vendors and products at issue.
5. The Practice Patterns Report clearly identifies with specificity each substitution recommendation under this category.
6. We note that for product substitution recommendations that are of clinical significance, we would require additional safeguards, such as the establishment of quality thresholds beyond which no cost savings would be credited.
7. The current year will be the twelve-month term of the contract for which the Surgical Group will be compensated under the Proposed Arrangement.
8. The "base year" will be the twelve months preceding the effective date of the contract. For purposes of this opinion, the Proposed Arrangement is limited to the one-year term of the contract; accordingly, this opinion is without force and effect with respect to any future renewal or extension of the Proposed Arrangement. Notwithstanding, we note that any renewal or extension of the Proposed Arrangement should incorporate updated base year costs.
9. In addition, nonprofit hospital arrangements raise issues of private inurement and private benefit under the Internal Revenue Service's income tax regulations in connection with section 501(c)(3) of the Internal Revenue Code. See Rev. Rul. 69–383, 1969–2 C.B. 113.

We express no opinion on the application of the Internal Revenue Code to the Proposed Arrangement.

10. Physician incentive arrangements related to Medicare risk-based managed care contracts, similar Medicaid contracts, and Medicare Advantage plans (formerly Medicare + Choice) are subject to regulation by the Secretary pursuant to sections 1876(i)(8),1903(m)(2)(A)(x), and 1852(j)(4) of the Act (respectively), in lieu of being subject to sections 1128A(b)(1)-(2). See OIG letter regarding hospital-physician incentive plans for Medicare and Medicaid beneficiaries enrolled in managed care plans (dated August 19, 1999), available at http://oig.hhs.gov/fraud/docs/alertsandbulletins/gsletter.htm. See also 42 C.F.R. § 417.479 (Medicare HMOs or competitive medical plans); 42 C.F.R. § 422.208 (Medicare Advantage plans); 42 C.F.R. § 438.6 (Medicaid risk plans).

11. We have had the Proposed Arrangement reviewed by a government medical expert who concluded that the proposed cost savings measures, as described in the advisory opinion request and supplemental submissions, should not adversely affect patient care. For purposes of this opinion, however, we rely solely on the Requestors' certifications, and nothing in this advisory opinion should be construed as an endorsement or conclusion as to the medical propriety of the specific activities being undertaken as part of the Proposed Arrangement.

12. Ordinarily, we would expect patient disclosures to be coupled with patient satisfaction surveys that closely monitor patient perceptions of their care. However, in the context of the Proposed Arrangement, which focuses on items and medications used in operating rooms, we believe that patient satisfaction surveys would not be effective.

13. We are precluded by statute from opining on whether fair market value shall be or was paid for goods, services, or property. See 42 U.S.C. § 1320a–7d(b)(3)(A). While the Requestors have certified that the payments under the Proposed Arrangement are consistent with fair market value, we do not rely on that certification in this opinion, nor have we have made an independent fair market value assessment.

INDEX

CPSIA information can be obtained at www.ICGtesting.com
Printed in the USA
BVOW09s0851120614

356171BV00005B/61/P

9 781118 193426